Nephrology: An Evidence-Based Approach

Nephrology: An Evidence-Based Approach

Edited by Valentina Houston

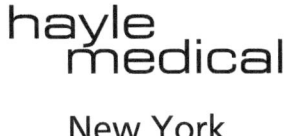

New York

Hayle Medical,
750 Third Avenue, 9th Floor,
New York, NY 10017, USA

Visit us on the World Wide Web at:
www.haylemedical.com

© Hayle Medical, 2019

This book contains information obtained from authentic and highly regarded sources. Copyright for all individual chapters remain with the respective authors as indicated. All chapters are published with permission under the Creative Commons Attribution License or equivalent. A wide variety of references are listed. Permission and sources are indicated; for detailed attributions, please refer to the permissions page and list of contributors. Reasonable efforts have been made to publish reliable data and information, but the authors, editors and publisher cannot assume any responsibility for the validity of all materials or the consequences of their use.

ISBN: 978-1-63241-660-5

Trademark Notice: Registered trademark of products or corporate names are used only for explanation and identification without intent to infringe.

Cataloging-in-Publication Data

Nephrology : an evidence-based approach / edited by Valentina Houston.
    p. cm.
Includes bibliographical references and index.
ISBN 978-1-63241-660-5
1. Nephrology. 2. Kidneys--Diseases. I. Houston, Valentina.
RC902 .N47 2019
616.61--dc23

Table of Contents

Preface XI

Chapter 1 **A Case of Proliferative Glomerulonephritis with Monoclonal IgG Deposits that showed Predominantly Membranous Features** 1
Homare Shimohata, Kentaro Ohgi, Hiroshi Maruyama, Yasunori Miyamoto, Mamiko Takayashu, Kouichi Hirayama and Masaki Kobayashi

Chapter 2 **Delayed Manifestation of Shunt Nephritis: A Case Report** 6
Michael Babigumira, Benjamin Huang, Sherry Werner and Wajeh Qunibi

Chapter 3 **Kinetics of Rituximab Excretion into Urine and Peritoneal Fluid in Two Patients with Nephrotic Syndrome** 15
Klaus Stahl, Michelle Duong, Anke Schwarz, A. D. Wagner, Hermann Haller, Mario Schiffer and Roland Jacobs

Chapter 4 **New Thrombolytic Infusion Application of Dissolving Renal Artery Embolic Thrombosis: Low-Dose Slow-Infusion Thrombolytic Therapy** 23
Ahmet Karakurt

Chapter 5 **De Novo Atypical Haemolytic Uremic Syndrome after Kidney Transplantation** 26
Arnaud Devresse, Martine de Meyer, Selda Aydin, Karin Dahan and Nada Kanaan

Chapter 6 **In Acute IgA Nephropathy, Proteinuria and Creatinine are in the Spot, but Podocyturia Operates in Silence: Any Place for Amiloride?** 30
H. Trimarchi, M. Paulero, R. Canzonieri, A. Schiel, A. Iotti, C. Costales-Collaguazo, A. Stern, M. Forrester, F. Lombi, V. Pomeranz, R. Iriarte, T. Rengel, I. Gonzalez-Hoyos, A. Muryan and E. Zotta

Chapter 7 **Rhabdomyolysis Induced by Coadministration of Fusidic Acid and Atorvastatin** 34
Dimitrios Patoulias, Theodoros Michailidis, Thomas Papatolios, Rafael Papadopoulos and Petros Keryttopoulos

Chapter 8 **A Report of Two Cases of Hazards Associated with High Flow Arteriovenous Fistula in ESRD Patients** 38
Vipuj Shah, Rakesh Navuluri, Yolanda Becker and Mary Hammes

Chapter 9 **Clinical Relapses of Atypical HUS on Eculizumab: Clinical Gap for Monitoring and Individualised Therapy** 43
Chia Wei Teoh, Kathleen Mary Gorman, Bryan Lynch, Timothy H. J. Goodship, Niamh Marie Dolan, Mary Waldron, Michael Riordan and Atif Awan

Chapter 10	**Fatal Pneumococcus Sepsis after Treatment of Late Antibody Mediated Kidney Graft Rejection** 47
	Gunilla Einecke, Jan Hinrich Bräsen, Nils Hanke, Hermann Haller and Anke Schwarz

Chapter 11	**Antiglomerular Basement Membrane Disease in a Pediatric Patient** 53
	Vimal Master Sankar Raj, Diana Warnecke, Julia Roberts and Sarah Elhadi

Chapter 12	**Sticky Platelet Syndrome: An Unrecognized Cause of Acute Thrombosis and Graft Loss** 60
	Fabio Solis-Jimenez, Hector Hinojosa-Heredia, Luis García-Covarrubias, Virgilia Soto Abraham and Rafael Valdez-Ortiz

Chapter 13	**A Rare Benign Tumor in a 14-Year-Old Girl** 66
	Meral Hassan Abualjadayel, Osama Y. Safdar, Maysaa Adnan Banjari, Sherif El Desoky, Ghadeer A. Mokhtar and Raed A. Azhar

Chapter 14	**A Rare Case of Transient Proximal Renal Tubular Acidosis in Pregnancy** 70
	Dennis Narcisse, Manyoo Agarwal and Aneel Kumar

Chapter 15	**Atypical Haemolytic Uraemic Syndrome Associated with *Clostridium difficile* Infection Successfully Treated with Eculizumab** 73
	Joshua M. Inglis, Jeffrey A. Barbara, Rajiv Juneja, Caroline Milton, George Passaris and Jordan Y. Z. Li

Chapter 16	**Therapeutic Approach to the Management of Severe Asymptomatic Hyponatremia** 76
	Thaofiq Ijaiya, Sandhya Manohar and Kameswari Lakshmi

Chapter 17	**Severe Symptomatic Hyponatremia Secondary to Escitalopram-Induced SIADH** 80
	Rishi Raj, Aasems Jacob, Ajay Venkatanarayan, Mohankumar Doraiswamy and Manjula Ashok

Chapter 18	**Cisplatin-Induced Renal Salt Wasting Requiring over 12 Liters of 3% Saline Replacement** 87
	Phuong-Chi Pham, Pavani Reddy, Shaker Qaqish, Ashvin Kamath, Johana Rodriguez, David Bolos, Martina Zalom and Phuong-Thu Pham

Chapter 19	**Scleroderma Renal Crisis Debute with Thrombotic Microangiopathy: A Successful Case Treated with Eculizumab** 91
	Maite Hurtado Uriarte, Carolina Larrarte and Laura Bravo Rey

Chapter 20	**Acute Hypocalcemia and Metabolic Alkalosis in Children on Cation-Exchange Resin Therapy** 95
	Aadil Kakajiwala, Kevin T. Barton, Elisha Rampolla, Christine Breen and Madhura Pradhan

Chapter 21 **Denosumab-Induced Severe Hypocalcaemia in Chronic Kidney Disease** 100
Ryan Jalleh, Gopal Basu, Richard Le Leu and Shilpanjali Jesudason

Chapter 22 **Porphyria Cutanea Tarda in a Patient with End-Stage Renal Disease: A Case of Successful Treatment with Deferoxamine and Ferric Carboxymaltose** 107
Natacha Rodrigues, Fernando Caeiro, Alice Santana, Teresa Mendes and Leonor Lopes

Chapter 23 **Extended Peritoneal Dialysis and Renal Recovery in HIV-Infected Patients with Prolonged AKI** 111
Donlawat Saengpanit, Pongpratch Puapatanakul, Piyaporn Towannang and Talerngsak Kanjanabuch

Chapter 24 **Discontinuation of Hemodialysis in a Patient with Anti-GBM Disease by the Treatment with Corticosteroids and Plasmapheresis despite Several Predictors for Dialysis-Dependence** 115
Yoshihide Fujigaki, Chikayuki Morimoto, Risa Iino, Kei Taniguchi, Yosuke Kawamorita, Shinichiro Asakawa, Daigo Toyoki, Shinako Miyano, Wataru Fujii, Tatsuru Ota, Shigeru Shibata and Shunya Uchida

Chapter 25 **Rifampicin in Nontuberculous Mycobacterial Infections: Acute Kidney Injury with Hemoglobin Casts** 120
Rishi Kora, Sergey V. Brodsky, Tibor Nadasdy, Dean Agra and Anjali A. Satoskar

Chapter 26 **Cisplatin-Induced Nephrotoxicity and HIV Associated Nephropathy: Mimickers of Myeloma-Like Cast Nephropathy** 125
Muhammad Siddique Khurram, Ahmed Alrajjal, Warda Ibrar, Jacob Edens, Umer Sheikh, Ameer Hamza and Hong Qu

Chapter 27 **Multiple Electrolyte and Metabolic Emergencies in a Single Patient** 130
Caprice Cadacio, Phuong-Thu Pham, Ruchika Bhasin, Anita Kamarzarian and Phuong-Chi Pham

Chapter 28 **Bilateral Testicular Infarction from IgA Vasculitis of the Spermatic Cords** 136
Mazen Toushan, Ashka Atodaria, Stephen D. Lynch, Hassan D. Kanaan, Limin Yu, Mitual B. Amin, Mamon Tahhan, Ping L. Zhang, Paul S. Kellerman and Abhishek Swami

Chapter 29 **Acute Renal Failure due to a Tobramycin and Vancomycin Spacer in Revision Two-Staged Knee Arthroplasty** 141
Ronak A. Patel, Hayden P. Baker and Sara B. Smith

Chapter 30 **A Case of Hepatic Glomerulosclerosis with Monoclonal IgA1-κ Deposits** 145
Yusuke Okabayashi, Nobuo Tsuboi, Naoko Nakaosa, Kotaro Haruhara, Go Kanzaki, Kentaro Koike, Akihiro Shimizu, Akira Fukui, Hideo Okonogi, YoichiMiyazaki, Tetsuya Kawamura, Makoto Ogura, Akira Shimizu and Takashi Yokoo

Chapter 31 **Cetuximab-Associated Crescentic Diffuse Proliferative Glomerulonephritis............................150**
Sukesh Manthri, Sindhura Bandaru, Anthony Chang and Tamer Hudali

Chapter 32 **Nontraumatic Exertional Rhabdomyolysis Leading to Acute Kidney Injury in a Sickle Trait Positive Individual on Renal Biopsy 154**
Kalyana C. Janga, Sheldon Greenberg, Phone Oo, Kavita Sharma and Umair Ahmed

Chapter 33 *Achromobacter xylosoxidans* **Relapsing Peritonitis and** *Streptococcus suis* **Peritonitis in Peritoneal Dialysis Patients...159**
Rafal Donderski, Magdalena Grajewska, Agnieszka Mikucka, Beata Sulikowska, Eugenia Gospodarek-Komkowska and Jacek Manitius

Chapter 34 **Posttransplant Lymphoproliferative Disorder Presenting as Testicular Lymphoma in a Kidney Transplant Recipient 163**
Steve Omoruyi Obanor, Michelle Gruttadauria, Kayla Applebaum, Mohammad Eskandari, Michelle Lieberman Lubetzky and Stuart Greenstein

Chapter 35 **Mucin-1 Gene Mutation and the Kidney: The Link between Autosomal Dominant Tubulointerstitial Kidney Disease and Focal and Segmental Glomerulosclerosis...169**
H. Trimarchi, M. Paulero, T. Rengel, I. González-Hoyos, M. Forrester, F. Lombi, V. Pomeranz, R. Iriarte and A. Iotti

Chapter 36 **Successful Resuscitation of a Patient with Life-Threatening Metabolic Acidosis by Hemodialysis: A Case of Ethylene Glycol Intoxication..............................173**
Ikuyo Narita, Michiko Shimada, Norio Nakamura, Reiichi Murakami, Takeshi Fujita, Wakako Fukuda and Hirofumi Tomita

Chapter 37 *Bartonella* **Endocarditis Mimicking Crescentic Glomerulonephritis with PR3-ANCA Positivity..177**
Joseph Vercellone, Lisa Cohen, Saima Mansuri, Ping L. Zhang and Paul S. Kellerman

Chapter 38 **Nephrologists Hate the Dialysis Catheters: A Systemic Review of Dialysis Catheter Associated Infective Endocarditis..181**
Kalyana C. Janga, Ankur Sinha, Sheldon Greenberg and Kavita Sharma

Chapter 39 **Renal Tubular Acidosis and Hypokalemic Paralysis as a First Presentation of Primary Sjögren's Syndrome...188**
Arun Sedhain, Kiran Acharya, Alok Sharma, Amir Khan and Shital Adhikari

Chapter 40 **Early Renal Involvement in a Girl with Classic Fabry Disease 192**
Fernando Perretta, Norberto Antongiovanni and Sebastián Jaurretche

Chapter 41 **Ureteropelvic Junction Obstruction and Parathyroid Adenoma: Coincidence or Link?** 196
Salah Termos, Majd AlKabbani, Tim Ulinski, Sami Sanjad, Henri Kotobi,
Francois Chalard and Bilal Aoun

Permissions

List of Contributors

Index

Preface

The in-depth study of kidneys along with their diseases is known as nephrology. Nanonephrology and onconephrology are two significant and upcoming branches of nephrology. Nanopherology deals with the study of kidney cells and the nanoparticles which are useful in treating several kidney diseases. Onconephrology deals with the study of kidney diseases in cancer patients. Kidney diseases cause a loss of kidney function which can potentially result in renal failure and the complete loss of kidney function. The most common and the most effective treatments for treating kidney diseases include renal replacement therapy, proper diet and medications. Renal replacement therapy involves dialysis and kidney transplantation. This book unfolds the innovative aspects of nephrology which will be crucial for the progress of this field in the future. The topics included herein are of utmost significance and bound to provide incredible insights to readers. This book, with its detailed analyses and data, will prove immensely beneficial to professionals and students involved in this field at various levels.

The information shared in this book is based on empirical researches made by veterans in this field of study. The elaborative information provided in this book will help the readers further their scope of knowledge leading to advancements in this field.

Finally, I would like to thank my fellow researchers who gave constructive feedback and my family members who supported me at every step of my research.

Editor

A Case of Proliferative Glomerulonephritis with Monoclonal IgG Deposits That Showed Predominantly Membranous Features

Homare Shimohata, Kentaro Ohgi, Hiroshi Maruyama, Yasunori Miyamoto, Mamiko Takayashu, Kouichi Hirayama, and Masaki Kobayashi

Department of Nephrology, Tokyo Medical University Ibaraki Medical Center, Ibaraki, Japan

Correspondence should be addressed to Homare Shimohata; h-shimo@tokyo-med.ac.jp

Academic Editor: Ichiei Narita

In 2004, the novel category of monoclonal IgG deposition disease has been proposed and termed "proliferative glomerulonephritis with monoclonal IgG deposits" (PGNMID). This disease is characterized by membranoproliferative glomerulonephritis and staining for a single light-chain isotype and gamma heavy-chain subclass. A 76-year-old male who had monoclonal gammopathy was referred to our hospital because of proteinuria. The renal biopsy showed diffuse thickening of the glomerular capillary walls with focal mesangial proliferation. On immunofluorescence study, only IgG1 among the four subclasses and lambda light chains were detected mainly in the glomerular capillary walls. From these results, we diagnosed our case as PGNMID showing predominantly membranous features. Almost all pathological findings on light microscopy of PGNMID are membranoproliferative GN or endocapillary proliferative GN, while membranous GN cases are rare. Here, we present the case of PGNMID that showed predominantly membranous features on light microscopy.

1. Introduction

Although AL amyloidosis and monoclonal immunoglobulin deposition disease (light-chain deposition disease and heavy-chain deposition disease, resp.) are both characterized by monoclonal immunoglobulin deposits in tissues, these diseases are distinguishable strictly by Congo red staining and characteristic appearance on electron microscopy. Furthermore, almost all fragments of light-chain deposition in AL amyloidosis are of the lambda type, whereas LCDD depositions are of the kappa type. In 2004, Nasr et al. reported the novel category of monoclonal IgG deposition disease characterized by membranoproliferative glomerulonephritis or endocapillary glomerulonephritis on light microscopic findings, staining for a single light-chain isotype and a single gamma heavy-chain subclass on immunofluorescence findings, and granular electron-dense deposits on electron microscopic findings [1]. Thereafter, they gathered 37 similar cases and termed this novel category of glomerular involvement "proliferative glomerulonephritis with monoclonal IgG deposits" (PGNMID) [2]. After their disease concept proposal, further cases were reported by other groups [3, 4].

According to Nasr et al.'s report, almost all pathological findings on light microscopy of PGNMID are membranoproliferative GN or endocapillary proliferative GN, while membranous GN cases are rare. Here, we present the case of PGNMID that showed predominantly membranous features on light microscopy.

2. Case Presentation

A 76-year-old Japanese male was referred to our hospital because of pretibial edema and proteinuria. On examination, his blood pressure was 124/90 mmHg and the pulse rate was 74 beats/min (regular sinus rhythm). Laboratory data showed serum creatinine and blood urea nitrogen of 3.6 and 46.7 mg/dL, respectively. Hemoglobin and serum albumin were 9.7 and 2.7 g/dL, respectively. C-reactive protein, alanine aminotransferase, aspartate aminotransferase, lactate dehydrogenase, blood glucose, hemoglobin A1c, and electrolytes

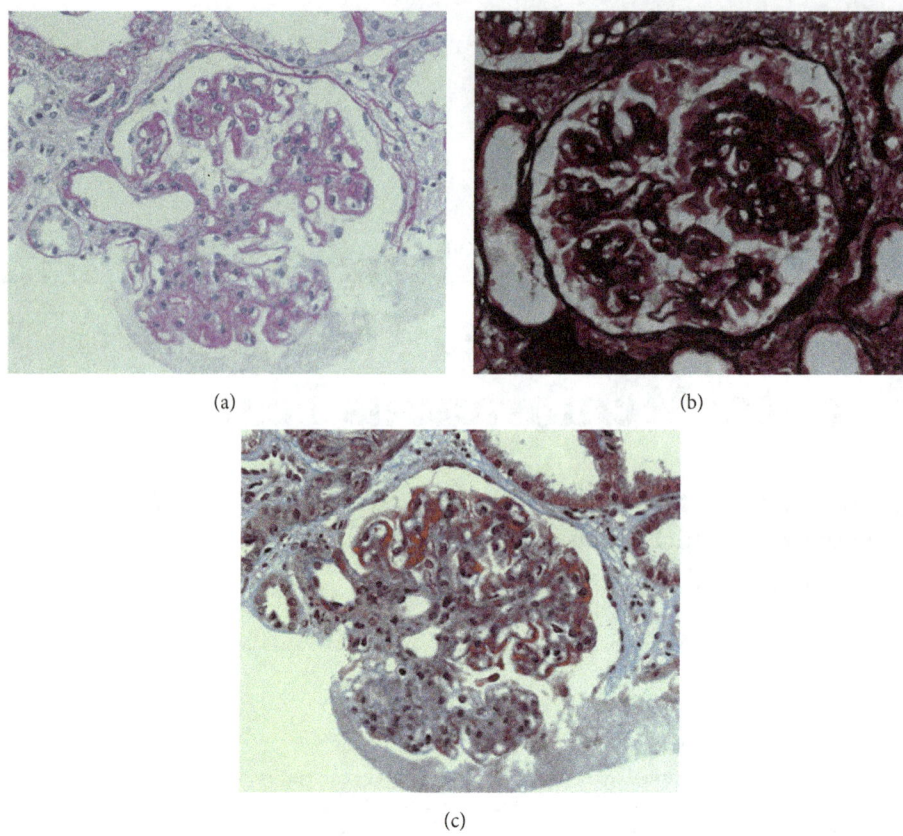

Figure 1: Light microscopy findings. (a) Periodic acid-Schiff stain (PAS) staining showed focal mesangial proliferation (original magnification ×400). (b) Periodic acid-methenamine silver (PAM) staining showed thickening of glomerular capillary walls (original magnification ×400). (c) Masson trichrome (MT) staining showed red staining in the subepithelial area (original magnification ×400).

were all normal. Serum cryoglobulin, hepatitis B virus surface antigen, and hepatitis C virus antibodies were negative. Urinalysis showed proteinuria (4.9 g/day) and hematuria (5–9 erythrocytes per high-power field) with granular casts (5–9 per high-power field) and lipid casts (5–9 per whole field). Proteinuria was in the nephrotic range. Immunoglobulin and complement levels were all within normal limits. We detected monoclonal IgG-kappa protein, not Bence-Jones protein, by serum and urine immunoelectrophoretic study. Because the bone marrow examination showed 3.3% plasma cells and the patient had no features of hematologic malignancy, he was diagnosed with monoclonal gammopathy of renal significance [5]. Renal biopsy was performed to investigate the reason for the proteinuria and elevated serum creatinine levels. Light microscopy showed diffuse thickening of the glomerular capillary walls with focal mesangial proliferation (Figures 1(a) and 1(b)), and red staining was observed in the subepithelial area by Masson's trichrome stain (Figure 1(c)). Severe tubular atrophy, interstitial fibrosis, and monocyte infiltration were observed in the tubulointerstitium. On immunofluorescence study, IgG and C3 granular deposits were detected in the peripheral capillary walls. Moreover, only IgG1 among the four subclasses (Binding-Site, Birmingham, UK) and only lambda light chains were detected in the glomerular capillary walls (Figures 2 and 3).

Granular electron-dense deposits were observed in subepithelial, intramembranous, and mesangial area by electron microscopy (Figure 4). From the above pathological findings, we considered that our case was consistent with the conception of PGNMID. Thereafter, in spite of conservative therapy such as angiotensin-converting enzyme inhibitors, calcium blocker, and erythropoietin-stimulating agents, hemodialysis therapy was started because of the progression to end-stage renal disease two years after the renal biopsy.

3. Discussion

Glomerular disease with monoclonal immunoglobulin deposition is divided into two categories by electron microscopy, those with organized deposits and those with disorganized deposits [6]. Amyloidosis, type 1 cryoglobulinemic glomerulonephritis, and immunotactoid glomerulonephritis are included in the first group and monoclonal immunoglobulin deposition disease is included in the second group. In 2004, Nasr et al. reported a novel form of glomerular injury related to monoclonal IgG deposition and termed the disease "proliferative glomerulonephritis with monoclonal IgG deposits" [4]. Although they described typical features of light microscopy as membranoproliferative glomerulonephritis or endocapillary proliferative glomerulonephritis,

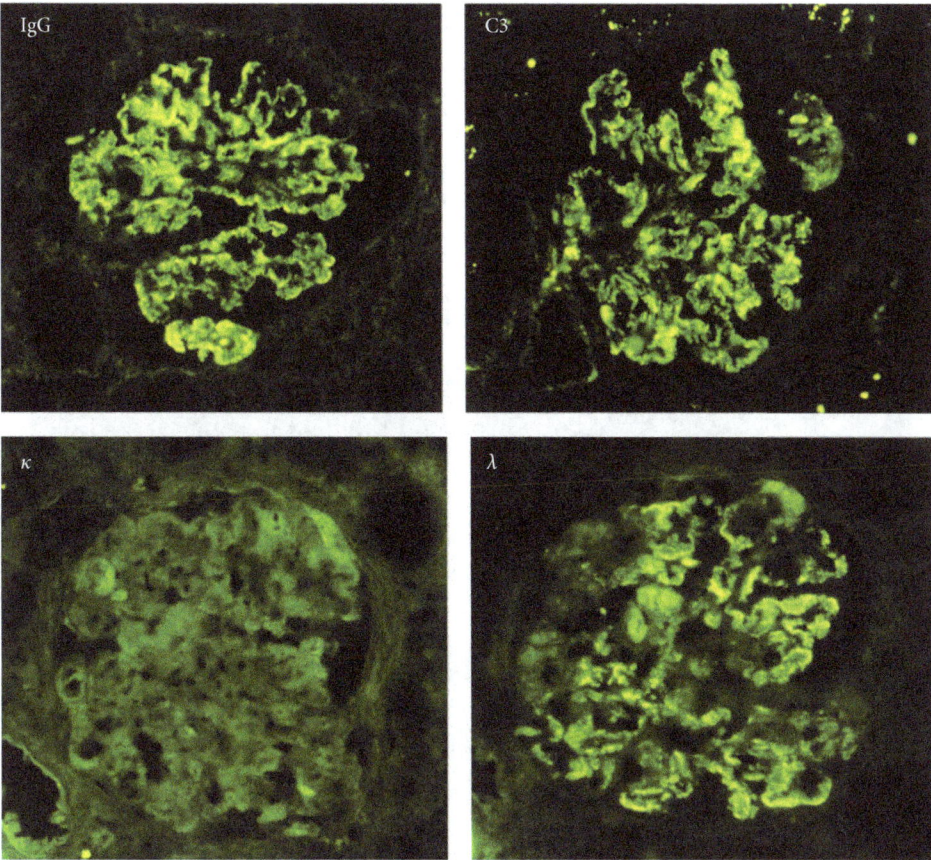

Figure 2: Immunofluorescence findings. IgG was strongly positive mainly in the peripheral capillary walls. C3 was also positive in peripheral pattern. In light-chain staining, kappa chain was entirely negative, but lambda chain was positive in the peripheral capillaries (original magnification ×400).

various histologic patterns have been reported. However, according to their report, membranous glomerulonephritis is a rare pathological finding in PGNMID, like mesangial proliferative glomerulonephritis. In the present report, we report a case of membranous glomerulonephritis associated with focal mesangial proliferation with monoclonal IgG deposits.

Komatsuda et al. reported a case of immunoglobulin deposition disease with a membranous pattern. Their case showed IgG lambda bands in serum electrophoresis and IgG1-lambda immunofluorescence staining in glomeruli. Although the pathological features and underling disease were similar to our case, their case had no mesangial hypercellularity whereas our case showed a serum light-chain isotype that differed from the glomerular immune deposits. The reason for this discrepancy is not obvious, but there have been some previous reports of glomerulonephritis with monoclonal IgG deposits without detection of monoclonal proteins in serum or LCDD without the deposition of light chains in the glomerulus [7, 8]. Furthermore, Nasr et al. demonstrated that thirty percent of PGNMID patients had a detectable circulating monoclonal protein with the same light-chain isotype as the glomerular deposits [9]. Therefore, discordance between the light-chain isotypes of serum and glomerular deposits is not a rare situation.

Komatsuda et al. also reported monoclonal immunoglobulin deposition disease associated with membranous features [10]. They described the light microscopic findings of their cases as thickening of the glomerular capillary walls and spike formation without proliferative lesions and immunofluorescence staining of glomerular deposits that were all of IgG-kappa type. Furthermore, steroid therapy was very effective in their cases and renal function was preserved in all patients. On the other hand, Nasr et al. summarized clinical outcomes of 32 patients who had PGNMID, of whom 21.9% progressed to end-stage renal disease [4]. At the time of renal biopsy, our patient showed the elevation of serum creatinine, and he progressed to end-stage renal disease within two years after renal biopsy. This poor clinical outcome was similar to those of Nasr et al.'s report. Light microscopy of our case revealed membranous glomerulonephritis with focal mesangial proliferation and lambda-type light-chain deposits. These findings are more similar to the pathological features of PGNMID. From these above considerations, we diagnosed our case as PGNMID with a predominantly membranous glomerulonephritis character. It

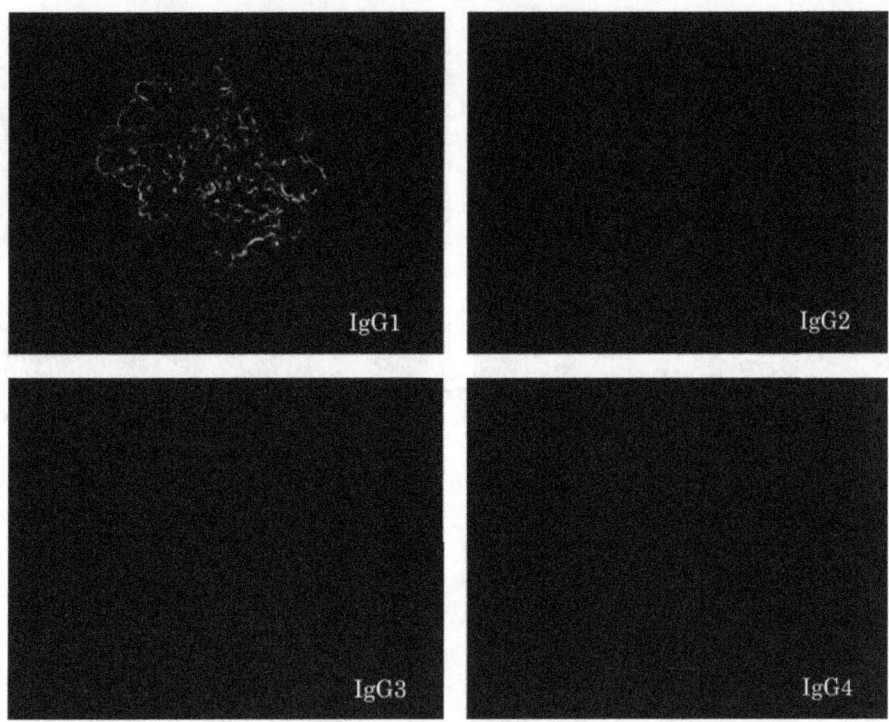

FIGURE 3: Findings of IgG subclass staining. IgG1 was positive in peripheral granular pattern. On the other hand, IgG2, IgG3, and IgG4 were all negative (original magnification ×400).

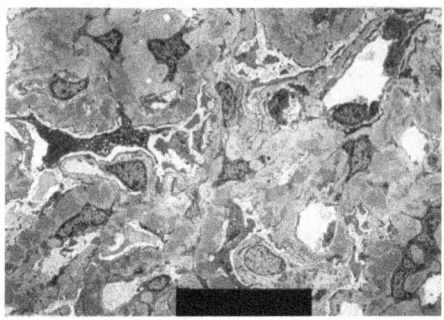

FIGURE 4: Electron microscopic finding. Electron microscopy showed huge electron-dense deposits in subepithelial, intramembranous, and mesangial lesions (original magnification ×3,000).

is unclear whether monoclonal immunoglobulin deposition disease associated with membranous features reported by de Seigneux et al. and Komatsuda et al. is a distinct disease concept from PGNMID. Further accumulation of cases of monoclonal immunoglobulin deposition disease associated with membranous features is needed to confirm whether these pathological features belong to PGNMID.

Here, we present the case of PGNMID that showed predominantly membranous features on light microscopy. Whenever membranous glomerulonephritis with monoclonal gammopathy is diagnosed, immunoglobulin staining for IgG subclass and immunoglobulin light chains should be conducted to clarify the immunoglobulin deposit disease.

Acknowledgments

The authors would like to thank Professor Yoshihiko Ueda of Department of Diagnostic Pathology, Dokkyo Medical University Koshigaya Hospital, Saitama, Japan, for staining IgG subclasses.

References

[1] S. H. Nasr, G. S. Markowitz, M. B. Stokes et al., "Proliferative glomerulonephritis with monoclonal IgG deposits: a distinct entity mimicking immune-complex glomerulonephritis," *Kidney International*, vol. 65, no. 1, pp. 85–96, 2004.

[2] S. H. Nasr, A. Satoskar, G. S. Markowitz et al., "Proliferative glomerulonephritis with monoclonal IgG deposits," *Journal of the American Society of Nephrology*, vol. 20, no. 9, pp. 2055–2064, 2009.

[3] R. Masai, H. Wakui, A. Komatsuda et al., "Characteristics of proliferative glomerulonephritis with monoclonal IgG deposits associated with membranoproliferative features," *Clinical Nephrology*, vol. 72, no. 1, pp. 46–54, 2009.

[4] S. de Seigneux, P. Bindi, H. Debiec et al., "Immunoglobulin Deposition Disease With a Membranous Pattern and a Circulating Monoclonal Immunoglobulin G With Charge-Dependent Aggregation Properties," *American Journal of Kidney Diseases*, vol. 56, no. 1, pp. 117–121, 2010.

[5] N. Leung, F. Bridoux, C. A. Hutchison et al., "Monoclonal gammopathy of renal significance: when MGUS is no longer undetermined or insignificant," *Blood*, vol. 120, no. 22, pp. 4292–4295, 2012.

[6] P. M. Ronco, M.-A. Alyanakian, B. Mougenot, and P. Aucouturier, "Light chain deposition disease: A model of glomerulosclerosis defined at the molecular level," *Journal of the American Society of Nephrology*, vol. 12, no. 7, pp. 1558–1565, 2001.

[7] A. Komatsuda, H. Ohtani, K. Sawada, K. Joh, and H. Wakui, "Proliferative glomerulonephritis with discrete deposition of monoclonal immunoglobulin γ1 CH2 heavy chain and κ light chain: A new variant of monoclonal immunoglobulin deposition disease," *Pathology International*, vol. 63, no. 1, pp. 63–67, 2013.

[8] S. Darouich, R. Goucha, M. H. Jaafoura, S. Zekri, A. Kheder, and H. B. Maiz, "Light-chain deposition disease of the kidney: A case report," *Ultrastructural Pathology*, vol. 36, no. 2, pp. 134–138, 2012.

[9] S. H. Nasr, S. Sethi, L. D. Cornell et al., "Proliferative glomerulonephritis with monoclonal IgG deposits recurs in the allograft," *Clinical Journal of the American Society of Nephrology*, vol. 6, no. 1, pp. 122–132, 2011.

[10] A. Komatsuda, R. Masai, H. Ohtani et al., "Monoclonal immunoglobulin deposition disease associated with membranous features," *Nephrology Dialysis Transplantation*, vol. 23, no. 12, pp. 3888–3894, 2008.

Delayed Manifestation of Shunt Nephritis: A Case Report and Review of the Literature

Michael Babigumira,[1] Benjamin Huang,[2] Sherry Werner,[1] and Wajeh Qunibi[1]

[1]Division of Nephrology, University of Texas Health Science Center at San Antonio, 7703 Floyd Curl Drive, MSC 7882, San Antonio, TX 78229, USA
[2]San Antonio Uniformed Services Health Education Consortium, San Antonio, TX, USA

Correspondence should be addressed to Michael Babigumira; babigumira@uthscsa.edu

Academic Editor: Kouichi Hirayama

We present an unusual case of shunt nephritis in a 39-year-old male who presented 21 years after placement of a ventriculoperitoneal (VP) shunt. He complained of fevers, headaches, dizziness, and urticarial plaques on arms, trunks, and legs and was found to have anemia, low complement levels, elevated serum creatinine, proteinuria, and new onset microhematuria. Blood and urine cultures were negative. Renal biopsy showed features of acute tubulointerstitial nephritis attributed to vancomycin use. Glomeruli showed increased mesangial hypercellularity and segmental endocapillary proliferation. Immunofluorescence showed focal IgM and C3 staining. Electron microscopy revealed small subendothelial electron-dense deposits. Symptoms and renal insufficiency appeared to improve with antibiotic therapy. He was discharged and readmitted 2 months later with similar presentation. CSF grew *Propionibacterium acnes* and shunt hardware grew coagulase-negative *Staphylococcus*. He completed an intravenous antibiotic course and was discharged. On 1-month follow-up, skin lesions persisted but he was otherwise asymptomatic. Follow-up labs showed significant improvement. We did a brief systematic review of the literature on shunt nephritis and report our findings on 79 individual cases. In this review, we comment on the presentation, lab findings, pathological features, and management of this rare, potentially fatal, but curable disease entity.

1. Introduction

Hydrocephalus is a pathophysiologic condition due to the accumulation of cerebrospinal fluid (CSF) in the cerebral ventricles [1]. The usual surgical treatment of hydrocephalus is drainage of excess CSF from the brain to another body cavity [shunting]. Historically, the shunts employed were ventriculoatrial (VA), ventriculoperitoneal (VP), and ventriculojugular (VJ) [2, 3], although nonshunt surgical techniques such as endoscopic third ventriculostomy (ETV) are increasingly being accepted [4]. These shunts are associated with a myriad of complications [5, 6] and unique among these is an immunologic phenomenon termed shunt nephritis. This refers to a glomerulonephritis characterized by proteinuria and hematuria which is associated with chronically infected shunts and usually resolves after treatment of the infection, removal of the shunt, or both. Since the description of the first case by Black et al. in 1965 [7], several patients in the literature have been reported to have shunt nephritis. While the overall incidence of shunt infections can range from 7% to 27% [6, 8], the rate of shunt nephritis is considerably much lower with some estimates suggesting its occurrence as low as 0.8% [6].

2. Case Report

A 39-year-old male was admitted for work-up of occult infection due to recurrent fevers, nausea, nonbilious emesis, and occipital headache for three weeks. Prior history was notable for traumatic brain injury in 1995 complicated by subarachnoid hemorrhage with subsequent placement of a ventriculoperitoneal (VP) shunt.

At presentation, the patient was tachycardic (HR: 130 per minute) and febrile (103 F) with urticarial plaques involving trunk, arms, and legs. Initial laboratory studies were notable

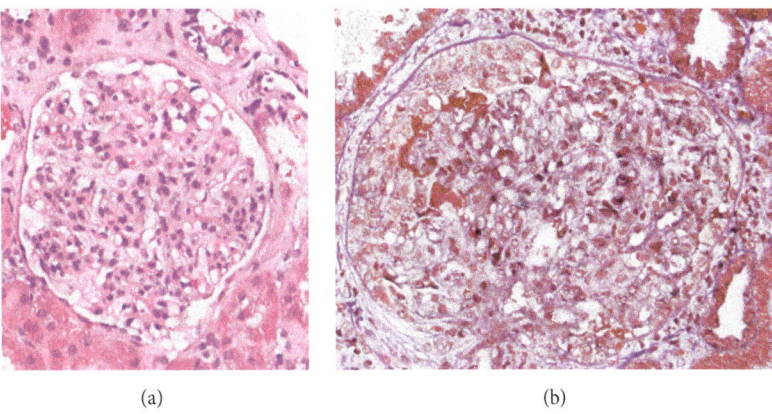

FIGURE 1: Light microscopy H&E (a) and PAS (b) showing mesangial hypercellularity.

for serum creatinine of 2.0 mg/dL, hemoglobin of 9.7 g/dL, C3 of 45 mg/dL (normal: 98–162), C4 of 9 mg/dL (normal: 16–43), and rheumatoid factor > 100 international units/mL (normal: <15). Urine microscopy did not reveal dysmorphic red cells or cellular casts. Cerebrospinal fluid showed elevated protein, decreased glucose, and gram stain with moderate leukocytosis but no organisms. Brain computed tomography indicated stable findings of his prior surgeries. The patient was given intravenous vancomycin. During the admission, a 24-hour urine collection revealed 1.4 grams of protein. Blood and cerebrospinal cultures remained negative for growth. However, serum creatinine only improved to 1.6 mg/dL (baseline: 0.98–1.1 mg/dL), so a renal biopsy was performed. Following the biopsy, the patient's renal insufficiency began improving, and this recovery was thought to be secondary to successful treatment of the infection. Vancomycin was discontinued at this time in light of negative blood cultures and the consultant neurosurgeon did not feel shunt removal was necessary at that time.

With regard to the renal biopsy, the glomeruli showed mesangial hypercellularity and segmental endocapillary proliferation with a single glomerular crescent containing hyaline droplets. Another glomerulus showed a sclerotic segment. There was no evidence of tubular cell vacuoles. The glomerular basement membranes were not thickened. Immunofluorescence was done with fluorochrome conjugated antibodies against human IgG, IgA, IgM, C3, C1q, fibrin, kappa light chain, and lambda light chain, using appropriate controls. A total of four glomeruli were identified. The glomeruli showed focal segmental 2+ IgM and 3+ C3 mesangial staining in three of the glomeruli. The glomeruli were negative for the other stains. The tubular basement membranes were negative for all of the aforementioned stains.

Electron microscopy showed that the foot processes of the podocytes were subtotally effaced. Rare, small, subendothelial osmiophilic electron-dense deposits were identified. Subepithelial deposits were not present. Spikes or duplicated basement membranes were not identified. Segmentally, there were increased numbers of endothelial and mononuclear cells. The mesangial matrix was mildly expanded and there was slightly increased mesangial cellularity with a few osmiophilic electron-dense deposits identified in the mesangium. These electron-dense deposits were not identified in the tubular basement membranes (see Figures 1–3). The final biopsy report's diagnosis was acute interstitial nephritis with tubular epithelial necrosis and segmental endocapillary proliferation with increased mesangial hypercellularity.

Two months after the renal biopsy, the patient was readmitted for recurrent symptoms similar to his initial presentation. Vital signs and exam were unremarkable. Laboratory data on readmission were notable for serum creatinine of 1.7 mg/dL, hemoglobin of 8.8 g/dL, C3 of 63 mg/dL, C4 of 15 mg/dL, and rheumatoid factor > 100 international units/mL. Cranial imaging did not show acute findings. On subsequent hospital day, the patient had repeat cerebrospinal fluid studies which showed the presence of Gram-positive organisms. He was restarted on antibiotics and the VP shunt was removed emergently. Cerebrospinal fluid culture resulted in the growth of *Propionibacterium acnes* and shunt hardware culture grew coagulase-negative *Staphylococcus*. As per infectious disease consultant's recommendations, the patient was treated with two weeks of intravenous vancomycin and ampicillin. Repeat blood cultures were negative and no further antimicrobial treatment was required.

At 1-month follow-up in the clinic, the patient had persistent skin lesions; he was otherwise asymptomatic with no headaches, dizziness, nausea, vomiting, fevers, or chills. Microscopic hematuria had completely resolved, C3 had increased to near normal levels, and serum creatinine had improved but not to baseline. Mild proteinuria persisted. Rheumatoid factor was normal. Serum creatinine was 1.2 and hemoglobin was 11.2 g/dL.

3. Discussion

3.1. Methodology. We ran the MeSH terms "shunt" and "nephritis" through 3 medical databases, PUBMED, SCOPUS, and Web of Science, yielding a combined total of 243 search results. After eliminating duplicates, articles not relevant to our search, and those written in a language other than English, we were left with 76 relevant articles that

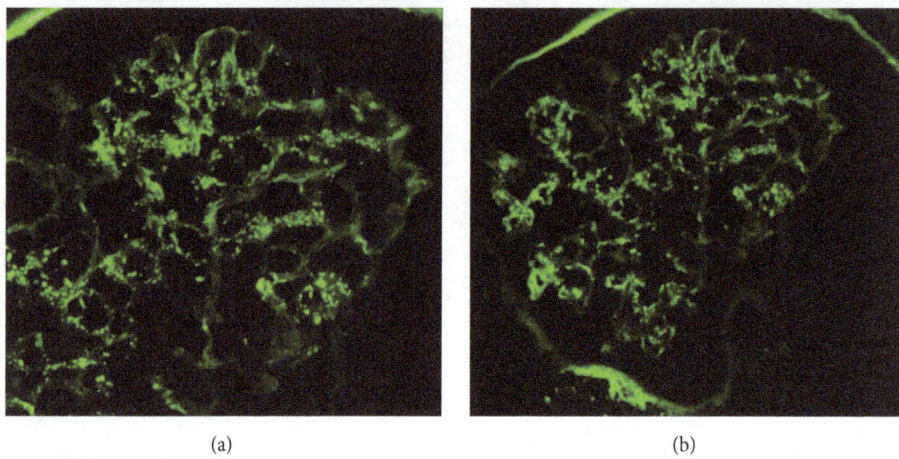

Figure 2: Immunofluorescence positive for C3 (a) and IgM (b) deposition in the mesangium.

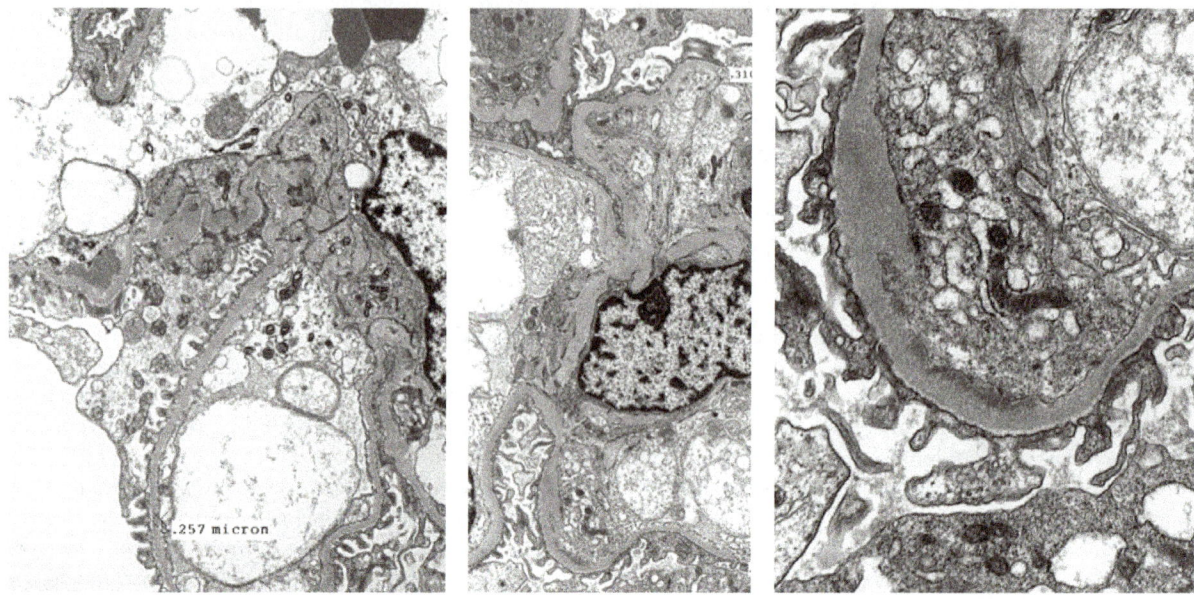

Figure 3: Electron microscopy images showing subendothelial electron-dense deposits.

included editorials, case reports, case series, and discussions. We identified 79 individual cases of shunt nephritis from 58 articles in this literature, which we further reviewed [7, 9–65].

3.2. Pathogenesis. The pathogenetic mechanism of shunt nephritis is not clear. It is hypothesized that the hydrophobic shunt material, acting as a nidus of infection, coupled with biofilm produced by bacteria promotes bacterial growth and bacteremia [10]. The released bacterial antigen results in formation of circulating immune complexes [66, 67], which are deposited in the glomeruli and activate the complement system [29, 32]. In this regard, Dobrin et al. demonstrated low total hemolytic complement, C1–C7, and elevated C9 in 3 patients with shunt nephritis, suggesting classical pathway activation [68]. While Strife et al. noted similar findings in a series of 4 patients with shunt nephritis, they also observed an association of elevated mixed serum cryoglobulins with the hypocomplementemia [69]. These mixed cryoglobulins decreased with treatment of the nephritis along with resolution of hypocomplementemia, suggesting a role in the pathogenesis of the disease. Although the composition of the serum cryoglobulins was different from that of the glomerular deposits, they posited that deposition of these immune complexes in the glomeruli and inability to penetrate the basement membrane result in subendothelial immune complex accumulation, mesangial proliferation, and mesangial interposition, all frequently encountered on renal pathology [70]. Several authors have also demonstrated bacterial antigens in the glomeruli, further bolstering this hypothesis [13, 14, 25, 45]. On the contrary, Vella et al. propose

Table 1: Microbiologic characteristics of shunt nephritis.

Microorganism	Blood cultures (%)	CSF cultures (%)	Shunt cultures (%)
Negative*	27	56	53
C. bovis	3	1	0
M. bovis	1	1	0
Diphtheroids	3	3	1
Micrococcus	3	1	4
G. morbillorum	1	1	1
P. aeruginosa	1	0	4
S. viridans	1	0	0
P. acnes	10	6	10
Staphylococcus epidermidis	19	11	9
Staphylococcus albus	15	9	11
Coagulase-negative Staphylococcus	13	8	5
Proteus	1	0	0
Staphylococcus aureus	3	1	1
Mixed infection	0	1	0
Total	100	100	100

*Culture results reported as negative or not reported at all.

Table 2: Characteristics of shunts in shunt nephritis.

Type of Shunt	%
Ventriculoatrial (VA)	76
Ventriculojugular (VJ)	9
Ventriculoperitoneal (VP)	5
Revisions, VP/VA	10
Total	100

Table 3: Presenting signs and symptoms of shunt nephritis.

Clinical finding	%
Hematuria	87
Fever	67
Hypertension	35
Hepatosplenomegaly	23
Edema	15
Skin rash	8
Splenomegaly	6
Arthralgia	4
Altered mental status	4
Seizure	4
Failure to thrive	4

that the source of antigen is the bioprosthetic shunt material which independently triggers a humoral immune response that results in shunt nephritis [71].

3.3. Microbiology. Analysis of microbiology from the 79 patients we reviewed is shown in Table 1. Approximately half of the CSF and shunt cultures were negative, while close to one-third of the blood cultures were negative. Four patients had negative blood, CSF, and shunt cultures, so-called culture-negative shunt nephritis [9, 43, 60, 61]. When cultures were positive, the *coagulase-negative Staphylococcal* (CNS) species (including *Staphylococcus epidermidis* and *Staphylococcus albus*) were predominant, irrespective of the type of culture specimen. These were closely followed by *Propionibacterium acnes (P. acnes)*. One patient had a CSF culture positive for more than one bacterium [72], while another grew different bacteria in blood and CSF [9]. Our patient grew *P. acnes* in CSF and shunt cultures grew *Staphylococcus epidermidis* (mixed infection) which is unusual. It is important to note that, in the past, *P. acnes* and CNS were considered contaminants. But the demonstration of the respective bacterial antigens in the blood and glomeruli of patients with shunt nephritis suggests a pathogenic role in the disease process [11, 32]. Of note also is the fact that it may take up to 14 days to grow *Propionibacterium* in cultures [73] and the diagnosis may be missed by terminating cultures prematurely.

3.4. Epidemiology. From the 79 patients with shunt nephritis that we reviewed, there is a slight male predominance, that is, 43 males versus 36 females. Patients' ages at presentation range from 1 year to 74 years, with an average age of 21 years. More than 75% of patients had a VA shunt, with a minority having either a VP or VJ shunt. 10% of patients had their shunt modality revised before onset of nephritis. Shunt characteristics are outlined in Table 2. We defined shunt duration as time from index insertion of shunt to onset of first nephritic symptoms irrespective of shunt revision surgery. We recognize that revision surgeries may influence shunt infections, but this information was not easily obtainable from the literature we reviewed. Our shunt duration definition is a departure from the definition used in a recent review, that is, time from last shunt surgery to onset of clinical signs and symptoms [74]. In our series, average shunt duration was 5.8 years. The range of shunt duration was 1 month to 20 years. Our patient presented 21 years after VP shunt placement, making his case rather unusual.

3.5. Clinical Presentation. Shunt nephritis may present with variable nonspecific signs and symptoms, most commonly hematuria, fever, hypertension, and hepatosplenomegaly (see Table 3). Less commonly, shunt nephritis may manifest with skin rashes and arthralgia. One case report noted very unusual and unexplained symptoms of fevers and myalgia only when the patient was taking showers [16]. Anemia is thought to be due to decreased erythropoietin production and/or iron deficiency [50] and hepatosplenomegaly secondary to removal of formed immune complexes by the reticuloendothelial system [75]. Arthritis and arthralgia have been attributed to the formation of circulating immune complexes in the synovium [56]. The pathophysiology of urticaria and skin rashes is less well understood but is thought

Table 4: Lab findings in shunt nephritis.

Lab finding		Number
Proteinuria	Median, 19.4 g (range: 0.5–38)	68
Anemia	Avg., 7.8 g/dL (range: 4–11.5)	58
Serum complements	Low	57
Serum creatinine	Greater than 1/abnormal	43
Acute renal failure	Significant rise in serum creatinine above baseline or decline in estimated GFR	46
Serum cryoglobulins	Positive	7
Serum ANCA	Positive	4
Serum RF	Positive	4

to be immune-mediated [34]. Common lab abnormalities include proteinuria, anemia, hypocomplementemia, and elevated serum creatinine. Positive serum cryoglobulins and rheumatoid factor are seen infrequently.

Nephrotic range proteinuria can be as massive as 38 g per day [63] and the anemia can be severe with hemoglobin as low as 4 g/dL [55]. Acute renal failure (ARF), defined as significant rise in serum creatinine above baseline or significant decline in estimated glomerular filtration rate (GFR), was reported in 46 patients. However, unlike serum creatinine, ARF was not consistently or uniformly reported in all the literatures reviewed. We therefore opted to use serum creatinine of greater than or equal to 1 (arbitrary value) as an alternative marker of renal dysfunction, even though it is inherently less accurate than the ARF definition cited above. Using this measure, over half of the patients reviewed had abnormal renal function (see Table 4). We do recognize the limitations of using serum creatinine as a gauge of renal function since it does not account for ARF in patients with baseline chronic kidney disease. But since no other measure of renal function was consistently reported in all of the reviewed cases, we settled for serum creatinine as a compromise. Some patients do present with positive anti-neutrophil cytoplasmic antibody (ANCA) titers, all antiproteinase 3 positive, with decrease in titers after treatment of the shunt nephritis [15, 31, 36, 42]. The exact mechanism of ANCA production is unclear [31]. The low complements, as discussed previously, may represent activation of the classical pathway as the disease unfolds [69]. For disease screening and diagnostic purposes, Bayston et al. have proposed the use of Anti Staphylococcus Epidermidis Titer (ASET) after they demonstrated that ASET rises predictably in patients with VA shunts colonized by *Staphylococcus epidermidis* [61, 76, 77]. While the ASET is a welcome addition to the diagnostic armamentarium, no single symptom, sign, or lab finding should be considered in isolation when shunt nephritis is suspected. Wyatt et al. suggest that complement levels be monitored until normalization and only be repeated when a relapse of nephritis is suspected [62]. Our patient presented with fever, anemia, microscopic hematuria, proteinuria, hypocomplementemia, renal insufficiency, positive rheumatoid factor, and urticarial plaques, all consistent with features of shunt nephritis described above.

3.6. Pathology. Of the 79 shunt nephritis patients reviewed, 62 had renal biopsies with 8 of these patients having repeat

Table 5: Light microscopy renal biopsy findings.

Biopsy findings	%
Mesangial proliferative GN	52
MPGN	45
Amyloidosis	2
End-stage kidney	2
Total	100

biopsies after treatment of the nephritis. The majority of these biopsies reveal a mesangial proliferative and membranoproliferative (MPGN) pattern of glomerulonephritis on light microscopy (see Table 5).

Immunofluorescence was done in approximately two-thirds of the renal biopsies with mesangial IgM, C1q, and C3 deposition being the most common finding. Relative intensities of immunoglobulin deposition were inconsistently reported, so we excluded them from our analysis (see Table 6). Out of the 62 biopsies reported in this literature review, electron microscopy was performed in only 28 instances, of which 18 (64%) had subendothelial deposits and 11 (39%) had mesangial deposits. Only 1 biopsy reported subepithelial deposits [53]. This further confirms the immune complex nature of the disease. Six biopsies had crescents [9, 19, 21, 53, 59, 64]. All the patients that had repeat biopsies after treatment of shunt nephritis demonstrated improvement in histologic findings [24, 28, 59, 60, 62, 63, 65]. One renal biopsy was initially read as amyloidosis but later retrospectively changed to "shunt nephritis" after signs and symptoms resolved with therapy [78].

Our patient's biopsy report showed features of tubulointerstitial nephritis that was attributed to vancomycin use. The glomeruli showed increased mesangial hypercellularity and segmental endocapillary proliferation, while immunofluorescence was positive for IgM and C3. Electron microscopy showed subendothelial deposits (see Figure 3).

3.7. Treatment. Therapy for this unique form of glomerulonephritis is multifaceted, including medical (antibiotics) and surgical approaches (shunt removal). Even though some cases of shunt nephritis show improvement with antibiotics alone [13, 14, 37, 40, 44, 54], best results are achieved with removal of the infected shunt, along with a course of IV antibiotics to clear the infection. If hydrocephalus remains

TABLE 6: Renal biopsy immunofluorescence findings.

Immunofluorescence	% (out of 42)
IgM	83
C3	71
IgG	57
C1q	83
IGA	26
C4	24
Lambda	5
Positive complement	5

TABLE 7: Renal outcomes after shunt nephritis treatment.

	Full renal recovery	Partial renal recovery	Progressed to ESRD	Death
Shunt removed	16	19	3	2
Shunt replaced	5	6	1	1
Converted to VP shunt	7	9	0	0
Antibiotics alone	0	6	0	3
Total*	29	40	4	6

Full renal recovery: complete resolution of hematuria, proteinuria, and renal dysfunction. Partial renal recovery: resolution of 1 or more of hematuria, proteinuria, and renal dysfunction but not all.
*Case of deceased kidney donor with shunt nephritis is excluded.

TABLE 8: Time to renal recovery after shunt nephritis treatment versus average shunt duration.

	%	Time to renal recovery in months (range)	Average shunt duration in years (range)
Death	8	—	4.79 (3.5–15)
Progressed to ESRD	5	—	8.75 (4–14)
Full renal recovery	37	10.8 (1–48)	4.94 (0.25–19)
Partial renal recovery	51	8.4 (0.25–72)	6.28. (0.1–20)
Total	100	9.5 (0.25–72)	5.8 (0.1–20)

Full renal recovery: complete resolution of hematuria, proteinuria, and renal dysfunction. Partial renal recovery: resolution of 1 or more of hematuria, proteinuria, and renal dysfunction but not all.

TABLE 9: Proportion of patients that received concurrent antibiotic therapy.

	Full renal recovery	Partial renal recovery	Progressed to ESRD	Death
Shunt removed	81%	84%	100%	100%
Shunt replaced	80%	100%	100%	100%
Converted to VP shunt	71%	100%	—	—

a clinical concern, a temporary external ventricular drain may be placed. Some authors advocate administration of intraventricular antibiotics during this period [74]. Once the infection is resolved, it may be prudent to consider nonshunt surgical techniques such as ventriculocisternostomy for persistent hydrocephalus [16]. If a shunt is still necessary, VP shunts appear to be more preferable to VA or VJ shunts (see Table 7). The use of antibiotic-coated shunts and perioperative antibiotic prophylaxis may play a role in the prevention of shunt infection [79, 80].

For the purposes of this review, we defined full renal recovery as complete resolution of hematuria, proteinuria, and renal dysfunction, while partial renal recovery was defined as resolution of one or more of hematuria, proteinuria, or renal dysfunction but not all. As described earlier, renal dysfunction was arbitrarily defined as serum creatinine greater than or equal to 1. The average time to achieve renal recovery (complete or partial resolution of hematuria, proteinuria, and renal dysfunction) is 9.5 months. As illustrated in Table 8, the majority of patients with renal recovery had the shunt removed. From our analysis, it appears that patients with full renal recovery had shorter average duration of shunt placement as compared to the ones with partial renal recovery and those that progressed to ESRD. This may suggest that longer residence of an infected shunt correlates with worse renal outcomes. While concurrent antibiotic therapy may play an additional role in renal recovery, only a small minority of patients in this review did not receive any antibiotics (see Table 9). Our brief analysis did not account for other factors, such as age or significant comorbidities, which may influence renal recovery in shunt nephritis.

Of the 6 deaths that were reported, only 1 was conclusively attributed to renal failure [40], with the rest being unknown or secondary to surgical complications of hydrocephalus [7, 32, 49, 64]. It appears that immune suppression therapy does not attenuate this disease process and may even contribute to negative outcomes [31, 32, 34, 64]. Indeed, one patient got steroids for 2 years followed by cyclophosphamide for presumed ANCA disease, but nephritis resolved only after removal of the shunt [15]. An unusual case of kidney donation by a deceased patient with shunt nephritis described remarkable resolution of renal disease in the recipient [26]; this observation further supports the notion that removal of the injurious immunologic environment is a means of cure. Our patient had the shunt in place for 21 years; the infection was initially treated with antibiotics, but meaningful symptomatic and renal recovery was not achieved until the shunt was removed. In hindsight, our patient's initial presumed diagnosis of acute interstitial nephritis attributed to vancomycin therapy was flawed and should have been revised to "shunt nephritis."

4. Conclusion

Shunt nephritis may manifest with many nonspecific symptoms, signs, and lab findings. If not quickly recognized, diagnostic delay may lead to irreversible chronic renal disease and possibly death. So nephrologists should maintain a high degree of suspicion in patients who present with indwelling CSF shunts and renal disease suggestive of nephritis.

Acknowledgments

Dr. Balakuntalam Kasinath and Dr. Brent Wagner helped with the editing of this manuscript.

References

[1] K. T. Kahle, A. V. Kulkarni, D. D. Limbrick Jr., and B. C. Warf, "Hydrocephalus in children," *The Lancet*, vol. 387, no. 10020, pp. 788–799, 2016.

[2] A. Aschoff, P. Kremer, B. Hashemi, and S. Kunze, "The scientific history of hydrocephalus and its treatment," *Neurosurgical Review*, vol. 22, no. 2-3, pp. 67–93, 1999.

[3] R. S. Tubbs, P. Vahedi, M. Loukas, and A. A. Cohen-Gadol, "Harvey Cushing's experience with treating childhood hydrocephalus: in his own words," *Child's Nervous System*, vol. 27, no. 6, pp. 995–999, 2011.

[4] M. G. Hamilton, "Treatment of hydrocephalus in adults," *Seminars in Pediatric Neurology*, vol. 16, no. 1, pp. 34–41, 2009.

[5] S. Iglesias, B. Ros, Á. Martín et al., "Surgical outcome of the shunt: 15-year experience in a single institution," *Child's Nervous System*, vol. 32, no. 12, pp. 2377–2385, 2016.

[6] A. R. Al-Schameri, J. Hamed, G. Baltsavias et al., "Ventriculoatrial shunts in adults, incidence of infection, and significant risk factors: a single-center experience," *World Neurosurgery*, vol. 94, pp. 345–351, 2016.

[7] J. A. Black, D. N. Challacombe, and B. G. Ockenden, "Nephrotic syndrome associated with bacteræmia after shunt operations for hydrocephalus," *The Lancet*, vol. 286, no. 7419, pp. 921–924, 1965.

[8] S. C. Schoenbaum, P. Gardner, and J. Shillito, "Infections of cerebrospinal fluid shunts: epidemiology, clinical manifestations, and therapy," *Journal of Infectious Diseases*, vol. 131, no. 5, pp. 543–552, 1975.

[9] R. S. Arze, H. Rashid, R. Morley, M. K. Ward, and D. N. Kerr, "Shunt nephritis: report of two cases and review of the literature," *Clinical Nephrology*, vol. 19, no. 1, pp. 48–53, 1983.

[10] R. A. Balogun, J. Palmisano, A. A. Kaplan, H. Khurshid, H. Yamase, and N. D. Adams, "Shunt nephritis from Propionibacterium acnes in a solitary kidney," *American Journal of Kidney Diseases*, vol. 38, no. 4, article E18, 2001.

[11] B. A. Beeler, J. G. Crowder, J. W. Smith, and A. White, "Propionibacterium acnes: pathogen in central nervous system shunt infection. Report of three cases including immune complex glomerulonephritis," *The American Journal of Medicine*, vol. 61, no. 6, pp. 935–938, 1976.

[12] R. Bogdanović, B. Marjanović, V. Nikolić et al., "Shunt nephritis associated with *Moraxella bovis*," *Acta Paediatrica*, vol. 85, no. 7, pp. 882–883, 1996.

[13] W. K. Bolton, M. A. Sande, and D. E. Normansell, "Shunt nephritis with Corynebacterium bovis (C.b.): successful therapy (Rx) with antibiotics," *Kidney International*, vol. 6, no. 6, article 26, 1974.

[14] W. K. Bolton, M. A. Sande, D. E. Normansell, B. C. Sturgill, and F. B. Westervelt Jr., "Ventriculojugular shunt nephritis with Corynebacterium bovis. Successful therapy with antibiotics," *The American Journal of Medicine*, vol. 59, no. 3, pp. 417–423, 1975.

[15] H. Bonarek, F. Bonnet, C. Delclaux, C. Deminière, V. De Précigout, and M. Aparicio, "Reversal of c-ANCA positive mesangiocapillary glomerulonephritis after removal of an infected cysto-atrial shunt," *Nephrology Dialysis Transplantation*, vol. 14, no. 7, pp. 1771–1773, 1999.

[16] G. Burström, M. Andresen, J. Bartek, and A. Fytagoridis, "Subacute bacterial endocarditis and subsequent shunt nephritis from ventriculoatrial shunting 14 years after shunt implantation," *BMJ Case Reports*, vol. 2014, 2014.

[17] P. Byrne, P. McArdle, G. K. Hayes, M. Archer, A. R. Pate, and S. Dundon, "Shunt nephritis," *Irish Medical Journal*, vol. 75, no. 9, p. 326, 1982.

[18] A. Cornér, K. Kaartinen, S. Aaltonen, A. Räisänen-Sokolowski, H. Helin, and E. Honkanen, "Membranoproliferative glomerulonephritis complicating Propionibacterium acnes infection," *Clinical Kidney Journal*, vol. 6, no. 1, pp. 35–39, 2013.

[19] R. S. Dobrin, N. K. Day, P. G. Quie et al., "The role of complement, immunoglobulin and bacterial antigen in coagulase-negative staphylococcal shunt nephritis," *The American Journal of Medicine*, vol. 59, no. 5, pp. 660–673, 1975.

[20] H. J. Dodd, H. J. Goldsmith, and J. L. Verbov, "Necrotizing cutaneous vasculitis occurring as an early feature of 'shunt nephritis'," *Clinical and Experimental Dermatology*, vol. 10, no. 3, pp. 284–287, 1985.

[21] K. P. Dawson, H. Lees, W. M. I. Smeeton, and P. B. Herdson, "Glomerulonephritis associated with an infected ventriculoatrial shunt," *New Zealand Medical Journal*, vol. 91, no. 659, pp. 342–344, 1980.

[22] J. A. Frank Jr., H. S. Friedman, D. M. Davidson, J. M. Falletta, and T. R. Kinney, "Propionibacterium shunt nephritis in two adolescents with medulloblastoma," *Cancer*, vol. 52, no. 2, pp. 330–333, 1983.

[23] H. L. Finney and T. S. Roberts, "Nephritis secondary to chronic cerebrospinal fluid—vascular shunt infection: 'shunt nephritis'," *Child's Brain*, vol. 6, no. 4, pp. 189–193, 1980.

[24] Y. Fukuda, Y. Ohtomo, K. Kaneko, and K. Yabuta, "Pathologic and laboratory dynamics following the removal of the shunt in shunt nephritis," *American Journal of Nephrology*, vol. 13, no. 1, pp. 78–82, 1993.

[25] A. B. J. Groeneveld, F. E. Nommensen, H. Mullink, E. C. Ooms, and W. A. Bode, "Shunt nephritis associated with Propionibacterium acnes with demonstration of the antigen in the glomeruli," *Nephron*, vol. 32, no. 4, pp. 365–369, 1982.

[26] F. Guerville, S. Lepreux, D. Morel et al., "Transplantation with pathologic kidneys to improve the pool of donors: an example of shunt nephritis," *Transplantation*, vol. 93, no. 8, pp. e34–e35, 2012.

[27] M. Guner, K. Yucesoy, and H. Ozer, "Shunt nephritis," *Turkish Neurosurgery*, vol. 8, no. 1-2, pp. 47–49, 1998.

[28] G. M. Halmagyi and J. S. Horvath, "Acute glomerulonephritis in an adult with infected ventriculoatrial shunt," *Medical Journal of Australia*, vol. 1, no. 4, pp. 136–137, 1979.

[29] G. D. Harkiss, D. L. Brown, and D. B. Evans, "Longitudinal study of circulating immune complexes in a patient with Staphylococcus albus-induced shunt nephritis," *Clinical and Experimental Immunology*, vol. 37, no. 2, pp. 228–238, 1979.

[30] D. Hettiarachchi, R. Gajanayaka, and M. Gilbert, "A case of shunt nephritis induced by propionibacterium acnes," *American Journal of Kidney Diseases*, vol. 67, no. 5, p. A53, 2016.

[31] Y. Iwata, S. Ohta, K. Kawai et al., "Shunt nephritis with positive titers for ANCA specific for proteinase 3," *American Journal of Kidney Diseases*, vol. 43, no. 5, pp. e11–e16, 2004.

[32] D. B. Kaufman and R. McIntosh, "The pathogenesis of the renal lesion in a patient with Streptococcal disease, infected ventriculoatrial shunt, cryoglobulinemia and nephritis," *The American Journal of Medicine*, vol. 50, no. 2, pp. 262–268, 1971.

[33] K. Kiryluk, D. Preddie, V. D. D'Agati, and R. Isom, "A young man with Propionibacterium acnes-induced shunt nephritis," *Kidney International*, vol. 73, no. 12, pp. 1434–1440, 2008.

[34] P. Kravitz and N. I. Stahl, "Urticarial vasculitis, immune complex disease, and an infected ventriculoatrial shunt," *Cutis*, vol. 36, no. 2, pp. 135–141, 1985.

[35] M. Kubota, Y. Sakata, N. Saeki, A. Yamaura, and M. Ogawa, "A case of shunt nephritis diagnosed 17 years after ventriculoatrial shunt implantation," *Clinical Neurology and Neurosurgery*, vol. 103, no. 4, pp. 245–246, 2001.

[36] B. Kumar and N. Munshi, "Antineutrophil cytoplasmic autoantibody specific for proteinase 3 in a patient with shunt nephritis induced by Staphylococcus epidermidis," *American Journal of Kidney Diseases*, vol. 53, no. 4, p. A48, 2009.

[37] H. S. Lee, S. H. Cha, B. S. Cho, and M. H. Yang, "A case of shunt nephritis," *Journal of Korean Medical Science*, vol. 10, no. 1, pp. 62–65, 1995.

[38] N. Legoupil, P. Ronco, and F. Berenbaum, "Arthritis-related shunt nephritis in an adult," *Rheumatology*, vol. 42, no. 5, pp. 698–699, 2003.

[39] G. Marini, P. W. Gabriele, B. Tanghetti, A. Castellani, G. Olivetti, and E. Zunin, "Membranoproliferative glomerulonephritis associated with infected ventriculoatrial shunt. Report of two cases recovered after removal of the shunt," *Modern Problems in Paediatrics*, vol. 18, pp. 207–210, 1976.

[40] S. A. McKenzie and K. Hayden, "Two cases of 'shunt nephritis,'" *Pediatrics*, vol. 54, no. 6, pp. 806–808, 1974.

[41] S. W. Moss, N. E. Gary, and R. P. Eisinger, "Nephritis associated with a diphtheroid-infected cerebrospinal fluid shunt," *The American Journal of Medicine*, vol. 63, no. 2, pp. 318–319, 1977.

[42] T. Nagashima, D. Hirata, H. Yamamoto, H. Okazaki, and S. Minota, "Antineutrophil cytoplasmic autoantibody specific for proteinase 3 in a patient with shunt nephritis induced by Gemella morbillorum," *American Journal of Kidney Diseases*, vol. 37, no. 5, article E38, 2001.

[43] H. N. Noe and S. Roy III, "Shunt nephritis," *The Journal of Urology*, vol. 125, no. 5, pp. 731–733, 1981.

[44] E. Noiri, S. Kuwata, K. Nosaka et al., "Shunt nephritis: efficacy of an antibiotic trial for clinical diagnosis," *Internal Medicine*, vol. 32, no. 4, pp. 291–294, 1993.

[45] S. O'Regan and S. P. Makker, "Shunt nephritis: demonstration of diphtheroid antigen in glomeruli," *American Journal of the Medical Sciences*, vol. 278, no. 2, pp. 161–172, 1979.

[46] C. Paliouras, F. Lamprianou, G. Ntetskas et al., "Membranoproliferative glomerulonephritis type 1 secondary to an infected ventriculoperitoneal shunt: a case report," *BANTAO Journal*, vol. 12, no. 2, pp. 117–119, 2014.

[47] W. Peeters, M. Mussche, I. Becaus, and S. Ringoir, "Shunt nephritis," *Clinical Nephrology*, vol. 9, no. 3, pp. 122–125, 1978.

[48] B. J. Pereira, S. Kumari, K. L. Gupta et al., "Shunt nephritis associated with Staphylococcus aureus septicaemia," *The Journal of the Association of Physicians of India*, vol. 35, no. 11, pp. 796–798, 1987.

[49] C. Ravindranath and F. J. Takacs, "Shunt nephritis glomerulonephritis associated with ventriculoatrial shunts," *Lahey Clinic Foundation Bulletin*, vol. 23, no. 2, pp. 48–52, 1974.

[50] S. Rifkinson-Mann, N. Rifkinson, and T. Leong, "Shunt nephritis. Case report," *Journal of Neurosurgery*, vol. 74, no. 4, pp. 656–659, 1991.

[51] M. Rodriguez Girones and A. Genoves, "Bacteraemia by P. aeruginosa associated with nephrotic syndrome after shunt operation for hydrocephalus," *Chemotherapy*, vol. 23, supplement 1, pp. 423–427, 1977.

[52] M. Schoeneman, B. Bennett, and I. Greifer, "Shunt nephritis progressing to chronic renal failure," *American Journal of Kidney Diseases*, vol. 2, no. 3, pp. 375–377, 1982.

[53] M. Searle and H. A. Lee, "Ventriculo-atrial shunt nephritis," *Postgraduate Medical Journal*, vol. 58, no. 683, pp. 566–569, 1982.

[54] U. Setz, U. Frank, K. Anding, F. D. Daschner, and A. Garbe, "Shunt nephritis associated with *Propionibacterium acnes*," *Infection*, vol. 22, no. 2, pp. 99–101, 1994.

[55] U. G. Stauffer, "'Shunt nephritis': diffuse glomerulonephritis complicating ventriculo-atrial shunts," *Developmental Medicine and Child Neurology. Supplement*, vol. 22, supplement 22, p. 161, 1970.

[56] E. J. ter Borg, M. H. Van Rijswijk, and C. G. Kallenberg, "Transient arthritis with positive tests for rheumatoid factor as presenting sign of shunt nephritis," *Annals of the Rheumatic Diseases*, vol. 50, no. 3, pp. 182–183, 1991.

[57] M. Thomas, M. Ralston, J. Harkness, and J. Hayes, "Resolution of shunt nephritis," *Australian and New Zealand Journal of Medicine*, vol. 7, no. 4, p. 452, 1977.

[58] R. Topaloglu, A. Bakkloglu, U. Saatci, N. Basbas, and T. Ozgen, "Consequences of delayed treatment on shunt nephrities. A case report," *Turkish Neurosurgery*, vol. 1, no. 4, pp. 174–175, 1990.

[59] Y. Wakabayashi, Y. Kobayashi, and H. Shigematsu, "Shunt nephritis: histological dynamics following removal of the shunt. Case report and review of the literature," *Nephron*, vol. 40, no. 1, pp. 111–117, 1985.

[60] W. Wegmann and E. P. Leumann, "Glomerulonephritis associated with (infected) ventriculo-atrial shunt," *Virchows Archiv. A, Pathological Anatomy and Histology*, vol. 359, no. 3, pp. 185–200, 1973.

[61] H. Wood, G. McCarthy, R. Fluck, and R. Bayston, "Shunt nephritis: fortuitous diagnosis and confirmation by serology (ASET)," *European Journal of Pediatric Surgery, Supplement*, vol. 8, supplement 1, pp. 66–67, 1998.

[62] R. J. Wyatt, J. W. Walsh, and N. H. Holland, "Shunt nephritis. Role of the complement system in its pathogenesis and management," *Journal of Neurosurgery*, vol. 55, no. 1, pp. 99–107, 1981.

[63] B. P. Yeh, H. F. Young, P. F. Schatzki, and E. S. Bear, "Immune complex disease associated with an infected ventriculo-jugular shunt: a curable form of glomerulonephritis," *Southern Medical Journal*, vol. 70, no. 9, pp. 1141–1146, 1977.

[64] I. Zamora, A. Lurbe, and A. Alvarez-Garijo, "Shunt nephritis: a report on five children," *Child's Brain*, vol. 11, no. 3, pp. 183–187, 1984.

[65] C. Zunin, A. Castellani, G. Olivetti, G. Marini, and P. W. Gabriele, "Membranoproliferative glomerulonephritis associated with infected ventriculoatrial shunt: report of two cases recovered after removal of the shunt," *Pathologica*, vol. 69, no. 991-992, pp. 297–305, 1977.

[66] W. Samtleben, G. Bauriedel, T. Bosch, C. Goetz, B. Klare, and H. J. Gurland, "Renal complications of infected ventriculoatrial shunts," *Artificial Organs*, vol. 17, no. 8, pp. 695–701, 1993.

[67] F. P. Schena, G. Pertosa, A. Pastore, A. De Tommasi, M. T. Montagna, and L. Bonomo, "Circulating immune complexes in infected ventriculoatrial and ventriculoperitoneal shunts," *Journal of Clinical Immunology*, vol. 3, no. 2, pp. 173–177, 1983.

[68] R. Dobrin, N. Day, P. Quie et al., "The role of complement, immunoglobulin and bacterial antigen in coagulase-negative staphylococcal shunt nephritis," *The American Journal of Medicine*, vol. 59, no. 5, pp. 660–673, 1975.

[69] C. F. Strife, B. M. McDonald, E. J. Ruley, A. J. McAdams, and C. D. West, "Shunt nephritis: the nature of the serum cryoglobulins and their relation to the complement profile," *Journal of Pediatrics*, vol. 88, no. 3, pp. 403–413, 1976.

[70] C. Strife, B. McDonald, E. Ruley, A. McAdams, and C. West, "Shunt nephritis: the nature of the serum cryoglobulins and their relation to the complement profile," *The Journal of Pediatrics*, vol. 88, no. 3, pp. 403–413, 1976.

[71] J. Vella, M. Carmody, E. Campbell, O. Browne, G. Doyle, and J. Donohoe, "Glomerulonephritis after ventriculo-atrial shunt," *QJM*, vol. 88, no. 12, pp. 911–918, 1995.

[72] P. Futrakul, L. O. Surapathana, and R. A. Campbell, "Review of shunt nephritis," *Journal of the Medical Association of Thailand*, vol. 53, no. 4, pp. 265–274, 1970.

[73] E. D. Everett, T. C. Eickhoff, and R. H. Simon, "Cerebrospinal fluid shunt infections with anaerobic diphtheroids (Propionibacterium species)," *Journal of Neurosurgery*, vol. 44, no. 5, pp. 580–584, 1976.

[74] D. Haffner, F. Schindera, A. Aschoff, S. Matthias, R. Waldherr, and K. Schärer, "The clinical spectrum of shunt nephritis," *Nephrology Dialysis Transplantation*, vol. 12, no. 6, pp. 1143–1148, 1997.

[75] S. L. Wald and R. L. McLaurin, "Shunt-associated glomerulonephritis," *Neurosurgery*, vol. 3, no. 2, pp. 146–150, 1978.

[76] R. Bayston and J. Rodgers, "Role of serological tests in the diagnosis of immune complex disease in infection of ventriculoatrial shunts for hydrocephalus," *European Journal of Clinical Microbiology & Infectious Diseases*, vol. 13, no. 5, pp. 417–420, 1994.

[77] R. Bayston, J. Rodgers, and Z. B. Tabara, "Ventriculoatrial shunt colonisation and immune complex nephritis," *European Journal of Pediatric Surgery*, vol. 1, supplement 1, pp. 46–47, 1991.

[78] H. Lee Finney and T. S. Roberts, "Nephritis secondary to chronic cerebrospinal fluid—vascular shunt infection: "Shunt nephritis"," *Pediatric Neurosurgery*, vol. 6, no. 4, pp. 189–193, 1980.

[79] A. A. Konstantelias, K. Z. Vardakas, K. A. Polyzos, G. S. Tansarli, and M. E. Falagas, "Antimicrobial-impregnated and -coated shunt catheters for prevention of infections in patients with hydrocephalus: a systematic review and meta-analysis," *Journal of Neurosurgery*, vol. 122, no. 5, pp. 1096–1112, 2015.

[80] X. Wu, Q. Liu, X. Jiang, and T. Zhang, "Prevention options for ventriculoperitoneal shunt infections: a retrospective analysis during a five-year period," *International Journal of Clinical and Experimental Medicine*, vol. 8, no. 10, pp. 19775–19780, 2015.

Kinetics of Rituximab Excretion into Urine and Peritoneal Fluid in Two Patients with Nephrotic Syndrome

Klaus Stahl,[1] Michelle Duong,[2] Anke Schwarz,[1] A. D. Wagner,[1] Hermann Haller,[1] Mario Schiffer,[1] and Roland Jacobs[3]

[1]Department of Nephrology, Hannover Medical School, Carl-Neuberg-Strasse 1, 30625 Hannover, Germany
[2]Department of Hospital Pharmacy, Hannover Medical School, Carl-Neuberg-Strasse 1, 30625 Hannover, Germany
[3]Department of Clinical Immunology and Rheumatology, Hannover Medical School, Hannover, Germany

Correspondence should be addressed to Klaus Stahl; stahl.klaus@mh-hannover.de and Michelle Duong; duong.michelle@mh-hannover.de

Academic Editor: Kandai Nozu

Clinical observations suggest that treatment of Rituximab might be less effective in patients with nephrotic range proteinuria when compared to nonnephrotic patients. It is conceivable that the reason for this is that significant amounts of Rituximab might be lost in the urine in a nephrotic patient and that these patients require a repeated or higher dosage. However, this has not been systematically studied. In this case report we describe two different patients with nephrotic range proteinuria receiving Rituximab. The first patient received Rituximab for therapy resistant cryoglobulinemic membranoproliferative glomerulonephritis and the other for second line treatment of Felty's syndrome. We employed flow cytometry to determine the amount of Rituximab excretion in both urine and peritoneal fluid specimens in these patients following administration of Rituximab. We found that a significant amount of Rituximab is lost from the circulation by excretion into the urine. Furthermore we saw a close correlation of the excretion of Rituximab to the excretion of IgG molecules suggesting selectivity of proteinuria as the determining factor of Rituximab excretion. Further larger scale clinical studies could have the potential to evaluate an optimal cut-off value of IgG urinary loss before a possible administration of Rituximab therefore contributing to a more individualized treatment approach in patients with nonselective and nephrotic range proteinuria.

1. Introduction

Rituximab is a chimeric monoclonal antibody targeting CD20+ expressing B-cells and is clinically used for a wide range of neoplastic diseases, including indolent and aggressive forms of B-cell non-Hodgkin's lymphoma and B-cell chronic lymphocytic leukaemia, and autoimmune-mediated diseases, such as systemic lupus erythematosus, anti-neutrophil cytoplasmic antibody associated vasculitis, and multiple sclerosis [1–3]. More recently, Rituximab has been also recognized more and more as a second line treatment option in therapy of patients in a wide range of nephrotic diseases, refractory to standard treatment, including steroid dependant and steroid resistant [4–6] or frequent relapsing nephrotic syndrome in children and adults [7, 8], refractory focal and segmental glomerular sclerosis (FSGS) [9], and recurrence of FSGS after renal transplantation [10] as well as membranous nephropathy (MN) [11].

Several clinical observations suggest that treatment with Rituximab in nephrotic patients might be less effective compared to nonnephrotic patients [4, 12]. It is intuitive to speculate that the excretion of 145 kDa Rituximab into the urine due to nonselective large molecular size proteinuria might contribute to this clinical important issue.

Here, we report on two patients with nephrotic range proteinuria receiving Rituximab. We measured Rituximab excretion into the urine and in one case where continuous ambulatory peritoneal dialysis (CAPD) was already initiated in the peritoneal fluid as well, using a flow cytometry based approach. We could demonstrate a significant loss of Rituximab both into the urine and in the peritoneal dialysis fluid.

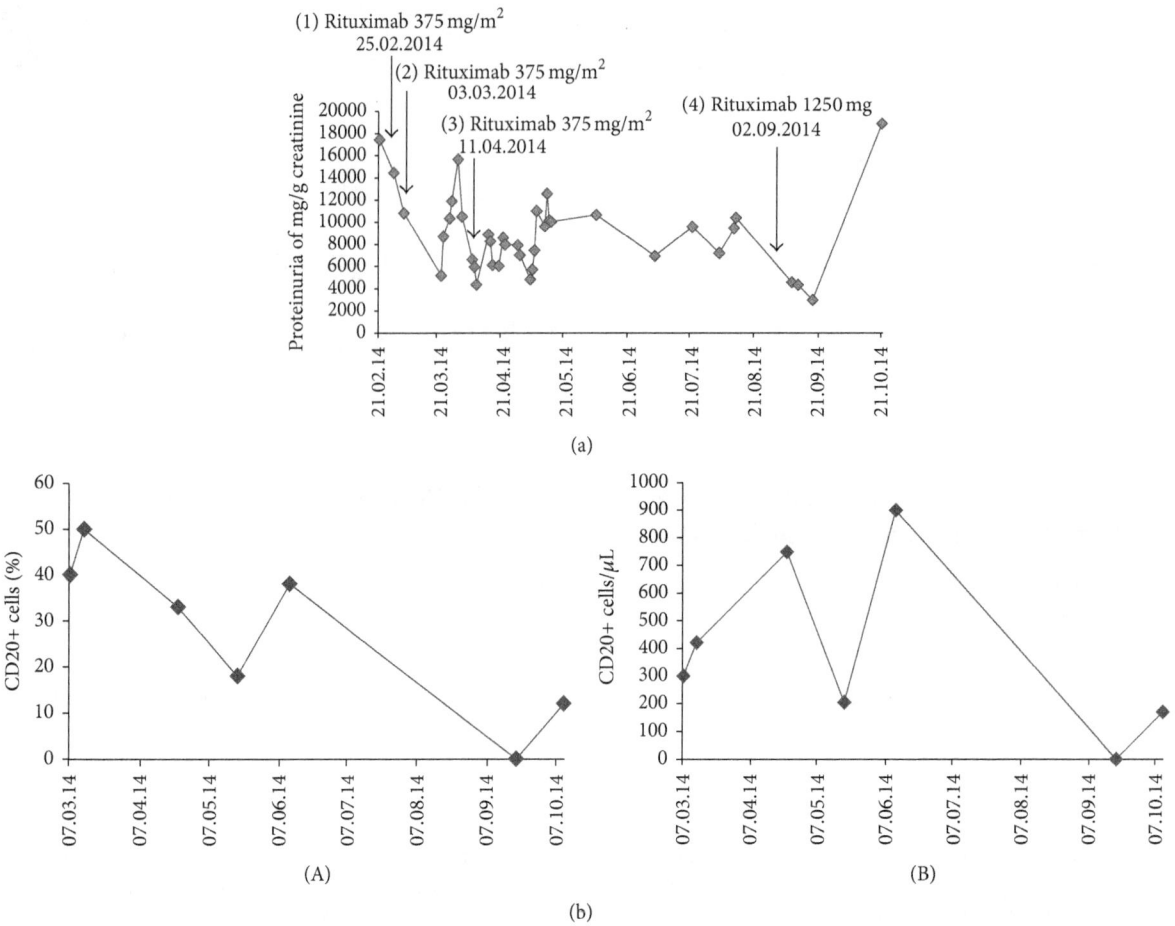

FIGURE 1: Kinetic of proteinuria (a) and CD20 cell count (b) in the first case. CD20 cell count is both displayed as absolute values (A) as well as percentage (B). Time points of Rituximab administrations are marked accordingly.

2. Case Presentation

2.1. Case One: Rituximab Excretion into the Urine in MPGN Associated Nephrotic Syndrome

2.1.1. History. A 62-year-old male patient was transferred to our renal care unit with a severe case of nephrotic membranoproliferative-glomerulonephritis (MPGN) with mixed cryoglobulinemia. At admission he displayed signs of heavy volume overload, including generalized severe body edema as well as pericardial and pleural effusions. Breathing appeared to be very difficult for the patient and walking or even standing supine was not possible anymore. Severe proteinuria and hypogammaglobulinemia despite regular parenteral immunoglobulin supplementation had caused diverse infectious complications like recurrent pneumonia, erysipelas of both legs, and urinary tract infections. Since we excluded all other possible infectious, autoimmune, and neoplastic differential diagnoses for MPGN and the existing cryoglobulinemia, we attributed his disease to an active but low replicative hepatitis B infection acquired years earlier. The patient had an initial proteinuria of 17450 mg/g creatinine and a serum creatinine of 126 μmol/L corresponding to an estimated glomerular filtration rate (eGFR) of 51 mL/min. eGFR in both patients was calculated using the Chronic Kidney Disease Epidemiology Collaboration (CKD-EPI) equation. The patient showed no signs of peripheral vasculitis or panarteritis nodosa type lesions.

The patient was refractory to high doses of steroids. Supportive therapy such as introduction of maximum therapeutic doses of an angiotensin-converting-enzyme inhibitor, aldosterone antagonist, and a high dose diuretic therapy was started and pleural drainage was performed several times. However, the clinical state did not improve nor could the volume overload significantly be reduced by this measures. We therefore decided to administer Rituximab twice in a dose of 375 mg/m² each and seven days apart from each other. The patient additionally received a permanent prophylactic medication of entecavir, which successfully inhibited increased viral replication or a flare of hepatitis under treatment with Rituximab. Proteinuria initially decreased to a minimal of 5206 mg/g creatinine but quickly increased again to the previous treatment value range. The time course of proteinuria is shown in Figure 1(b). Surprisingly, we did not see a substantial suppression of CD20+ B-cells following the first two Rituximab applications, as seen in

Figure 1(b). Given the fact that neither proteinuria could be decreased nor did we see a suppression of the target immune cells, we proceeded, about 6 weeks after the first Rituximab administration, to give another dose of 375 mg/m^2 Rituximab. Again, we only saw a temporal decrease of proteinuria and no substantial suppression of CD20+ B-cell count. Already a few days later, proteinuria rose up again in the high nephrotic range. Unfortunately, the patient developed a severe episode of *Clostridium difficile* associated diarrhea, which leads to sigma colon perforation and required emergency surgery. Postoperative catecholamine dependent sepsis could be managed by broad-spectrum antibiotics and a week of continuous-venovenous-hemodialysis. Although following discharge from intensive care the patient was not dependent on dialysis any more, a cimino fistula was created in prophylactic intention. He made an incomplete recovery, was completely dependent on nursing care, and again severely decompensated with a massive fluid overload and edema. We suspected that a high urinary excretion of Rituximab in this highly nephrotic patient could account for the missing effect of the three preceding Rituximab administrations. Due to the unfavorable prognosis of his disease course we decided following very close informed consent of the patient to administer Rituximab in a higher dose of 1250 mg in total. This time proteinuria indeed decreased to a minimum of 2977 mg/g creatinine and 14 days later CD20+ B-cell count eventually was completely depressed. Unfortunately, he suffered a relapse of peritonitis due to occult perforation. Infection progressed to severe sepsis and because the patient was assessed to be in no adequate condition for repeated surgery, interventional drainage of a paravesical abscess was performed. The patient survived this second severe infectious complication but remained this time dependent on dialysis. Proteinuria and CD20+ B-cell count could not steadily be suppressed and increased again soon after the fourth administration of Rituximab. He refused further treatment and all therapeutic measures including hemodialysis were terminated. The patient was discharged to a palliative care nursery facility and passed away a few weeks later.

2.1.2. Rituximab Kinetics. The amount of Rituximab excretion into the urine was measured from spot urine samples collected about 24 hours after each of the four Rituximab administrations using flow cytometry. Daudi cells as a CD20 expressing B-cell line were used to determine the Rituximab concentration and Octagam® instead of Rituximab as a negative control. Total IgG levels were determined by nephelometry using a BN ProSpec analyzer (Siemens, Erlangen, Germany). The principle of Rituximab detection by flow cytometry and representative FACS plots are shown in Figure 2. 10000 events of each sample were acquired after gating on Daudi cells according to their FCS/SSC properties. Offline data analyses were performed by using FCS Express V5 and determining mean fluorescence intensity (MFI) of each sample. Values of standard samples with known Rituximab concentration were subjected to statistical analysis in order to calculate nonlinear regression by using Graphpad Prism V6. Based on this calculation MFIs of urine samples were transformed into corresponding Rituximab concentrations.

Results of Rituximab and IgG measurement in the first case are shown in Figure 3. Since the amount of urinary output and the urine concentration ability of the patient varied significantly between the different probes, we additionally determined urine creatinine and calculated Rituximab/creatinine ratios for all samples. Figure 3(a) shows Rituximab urine concentrations and Figure 3(b) the corresponding Rituximab/creatinine urine ratios. A significant excretion of Rituximab into the urine is found in all four urine samples. Rituximab urine concentration steadily increases from only 144.67 µg/L after the first Rituximab application up to 3513.57 µg/L after the fourth Rituximab application. The same kinetics are seen when the corresponding Rituximab/creatinine ratios are studied. After the first Rituximab administration the Rituximab/creatinine ratio was only 0.018 µg/µmoL, while the ratio increased after the fourth application to 1.57 µg/µmoL. This conforms to a 25-fold increase of Rituximab concentration and an 84-fold increase of the Rituximab/creatinine ratio.

We measured Rituximab urinary loss in three patients without proteinuria receiving Rituximab for different indications (two for induction treatment of cANCA associated vasculitis, one for rescue treatment of stiff persons syndrome). In all three control patients no Rituximab could be detected in the patient urine.

Furthermore, to correlate excretion of Rituximab to excretion of IgG molecules, we determined IgG concentration and IgG/creatinine ratios in all samples. Significant amounts of IgG could be detected in all four urine samples. IgG showed varying urine concentrations ranging from 308 mg/L after the fourth up to 788 mg/L after the second Rituximab administration with no clear increasing kinetics. However, when IgG urine excretion was standardized to urine creatinine, an increase of IgG excretion could again be observed ranging from 0.078 mg/µmoL after the first up to 0.138 mg/µmoL following the last Rituximab administration, which marks an about 2-fold increase. Increasing loss of glomerular selectivity indicated by increased urinary IgG/Creatinine ratio therefore appeared to correlate with increment of Rituximab urinary loss.

2.2. Case Two: Rituximab Excretion into the Urine and Peritoneal Dialysate Fluid in IgA-GN Associated Nephrotic Syndrome

2.2.1. History. A 56-year-old male patient presented to our outpatient clinic with chronic symmetric arthralgias of multiple joints, pancytopenia, and a C-reactive protein of 340 U/mL. The patient's blood count was measured as a leukocytopenia of 1.9 Tsd./µL with a neutropenia of 0.7 Tsd./µL, a hemoglobin concentration of 9.2 g/dL, and a thrombocytopenia of 110 Tsd./µL. Rheumatic factor was measured in the normal range but the cyclic citrullinated peptide (CCP) antibody appeared to be very high with 340 U/mL. After infectious, neoplastic, and other rheumatologic differential diagnoses could be ruled out, he was diagnosed with Felty syndrome taking into account the combination of chronic polyarthritis, leukocytopenia, and splenomegaly. Since a combination of colchicum with a course of high dose

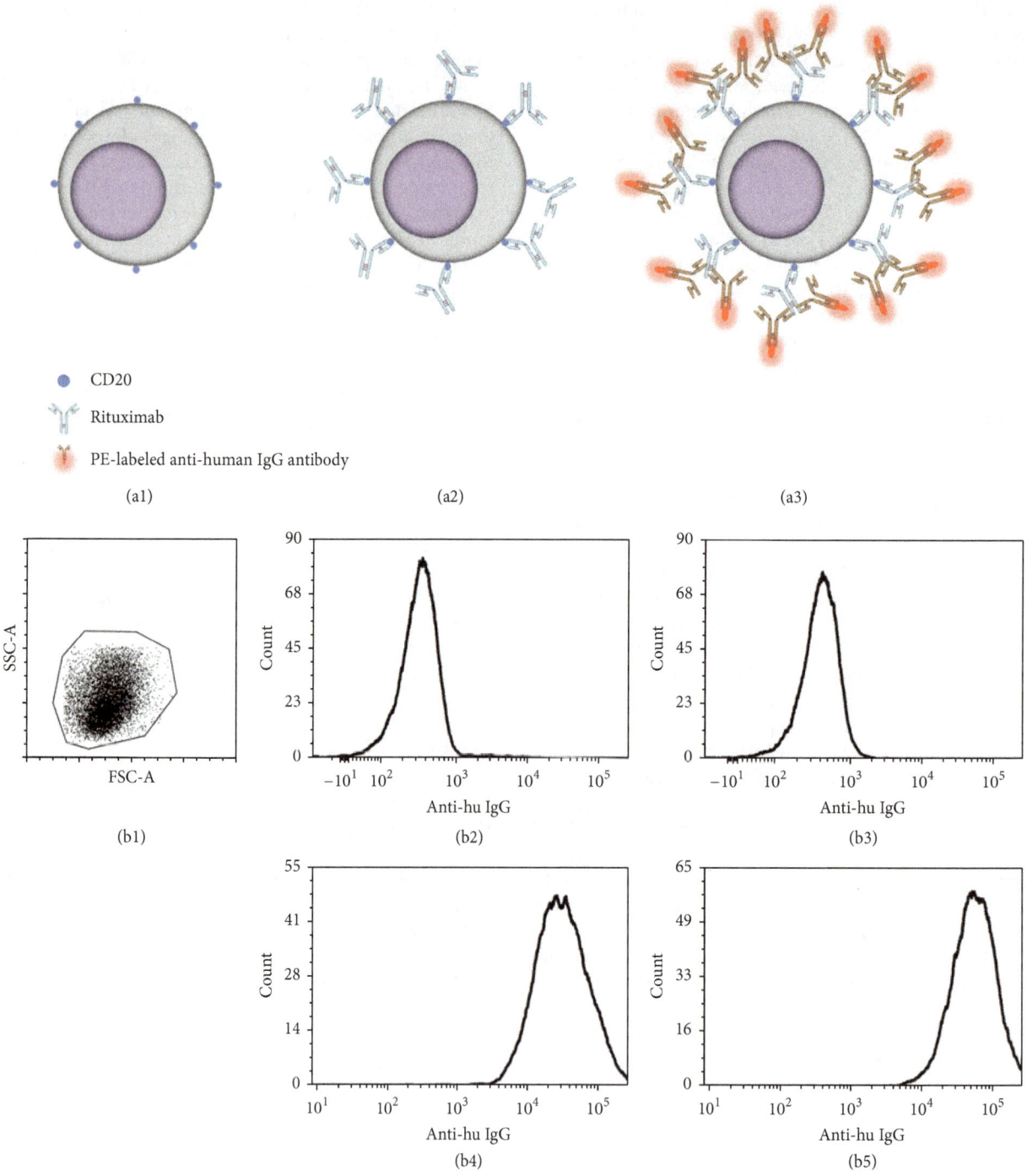

FIGURE 2: CD20 expressing Daudi cells (a1) were incubated with urine for 20 min to enable suspected Rituximab to bind the CD20 antigen (a2). After three washes in PBS/BSA, cells were incubated with a PE-labeled anti-human IgG antibody and incubated for 20 min (a3). After three washes in PBS/BSA, cells were subjected to flow cytometry analysis. Controls were identically performed but by using Octagam solution instead of urine. Flow cytometric analysis of Daudi cells. Daudi cells were gated according to their FSC/SSC properties (b1). Histograms of Daudi after incubation with PBS (b2), Octagam (b3), urine of the first patient (b4), and peritoneal dialysate fluid of the second patient (b5) are shown. Cell numbers are shown on y-axis and relative fluorescence intensity of the secondary (anti-human IgG) antibody on x-axis.

steroid medication (1 mg/kg equivalent of decortin) did not lead to a clinical remission, it was decided to treat this patient in second line with Rituximab and he was therefore admitted to our renal unit. Additionally, the patient was diagnosed about nine years earlier with IgA-nephropathy with proteinuria in the high nephrotic range. Despite treatment with steroids and cyclophosphamide he eventually progressed to end stage renal disease and started dialysis two years earlier.

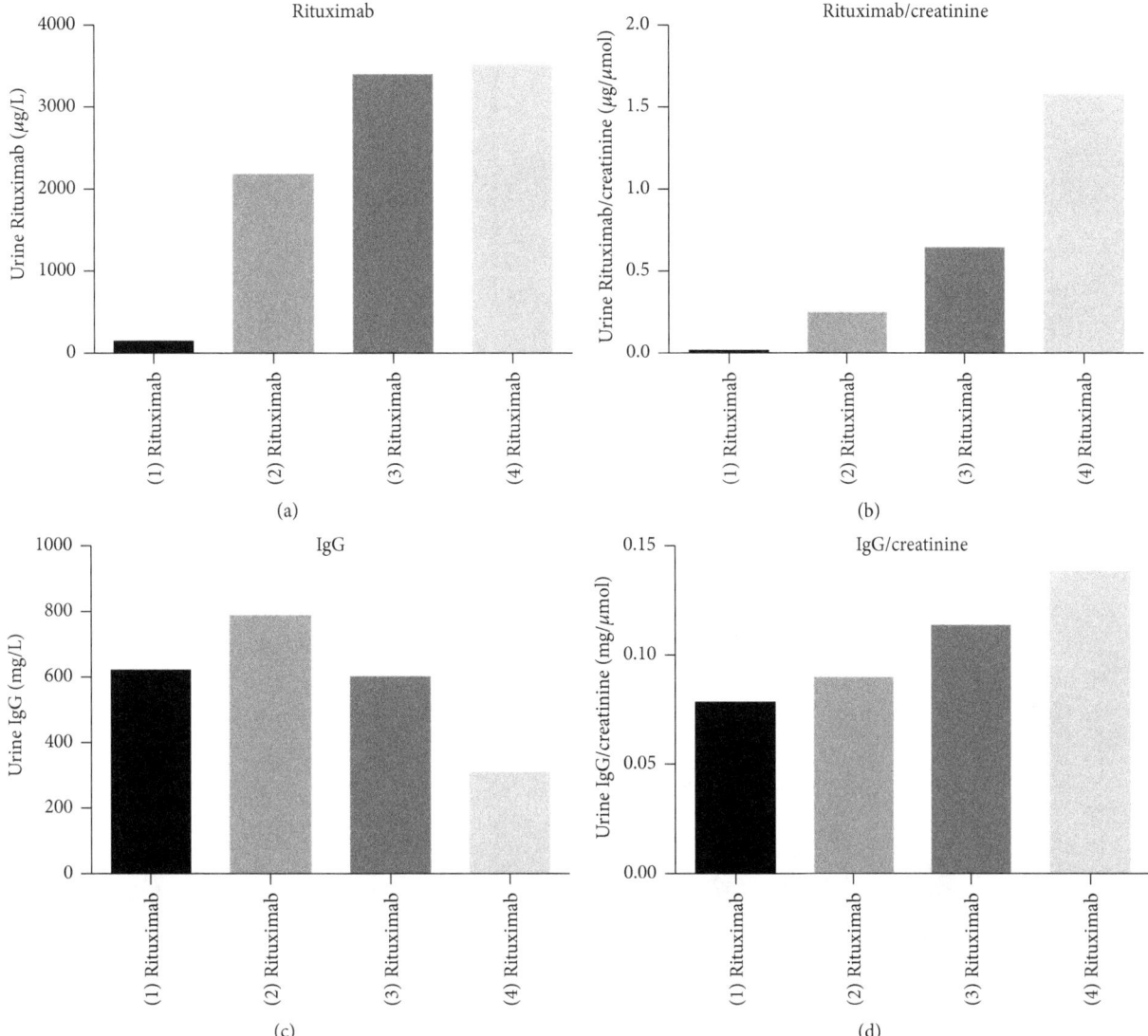

FIGURE 3: Rituximab urine concentrations (a), urine Rituximab/creatinine ratios as well as IgG urine concentrations (c), and IgG/creatinine ratios in the first case.

Because the patient still had a preserved urine output of about 2 l/d it was decided to treat him with continuous ambulatory peritoneal dialysis, which he tolerated well. The patient continued to show proteinuria with 1.95 g/L and a proteinuria to creatinine ratio of 3138 mg/g. He received 500 mg of Rituximab intravenously twice two days apart from each other and tolerated both administrations without experiencing any side effects. CD19/20+ cell count measured about three weeks after Rituximab administration was completely suppressed at 0%. Indeed, arthralgia in all previously affected joint regions subjectively improved significantly about 4 weeks after administration of Rituximab. However, leukocytopenia, anemia, and thrombocytopenia showed no significant signs of recovery until the present time point, which is about 12 weeks after Rituximab administration. Leukocytes were 1.8 Tsd./μL with a neutropenia of 1.0 Tsd./μL, hemoglobin concentration was 9.4 g/dL, and thrombocytes were of 149 Tsd./μL. Proteinuria was unchanged in the nephrotic range with 2.19 g/L and a proteinuria/creatinine ratio of 3800 mg/g.

2.2.2. Rituximab Kinetics. The amount of Rituximab excretion into the urine was measured from 24-hour urine collections, which were started to be collected instantly after each of the two Rituximab administrations. Furthermore, Rituximab concentration was determined from the different bags of effluent of the peritoneal dialysis solution collected after each Rituximab administration. Rituximab was measured in all probes applying FACS technology as described previously.

Results are shown in Figure 4. Rituximab was found in high concentrations in both urine and all peritoneal fluid samples that were analyzed. The highest Rituximab excretion into the urine was measured with 2314 μg/L after the first Rituximab administration. The highest excretion into the peritoneal fluid was 3518 μg/L in the third bag after the second Rituximab administration. When Rituximab concentration was standardized to creatinine concentration, Rituximab excretion into the urine and the peritoneal dialysate did increase by time and it showed a slightly additive effect after the second administration.

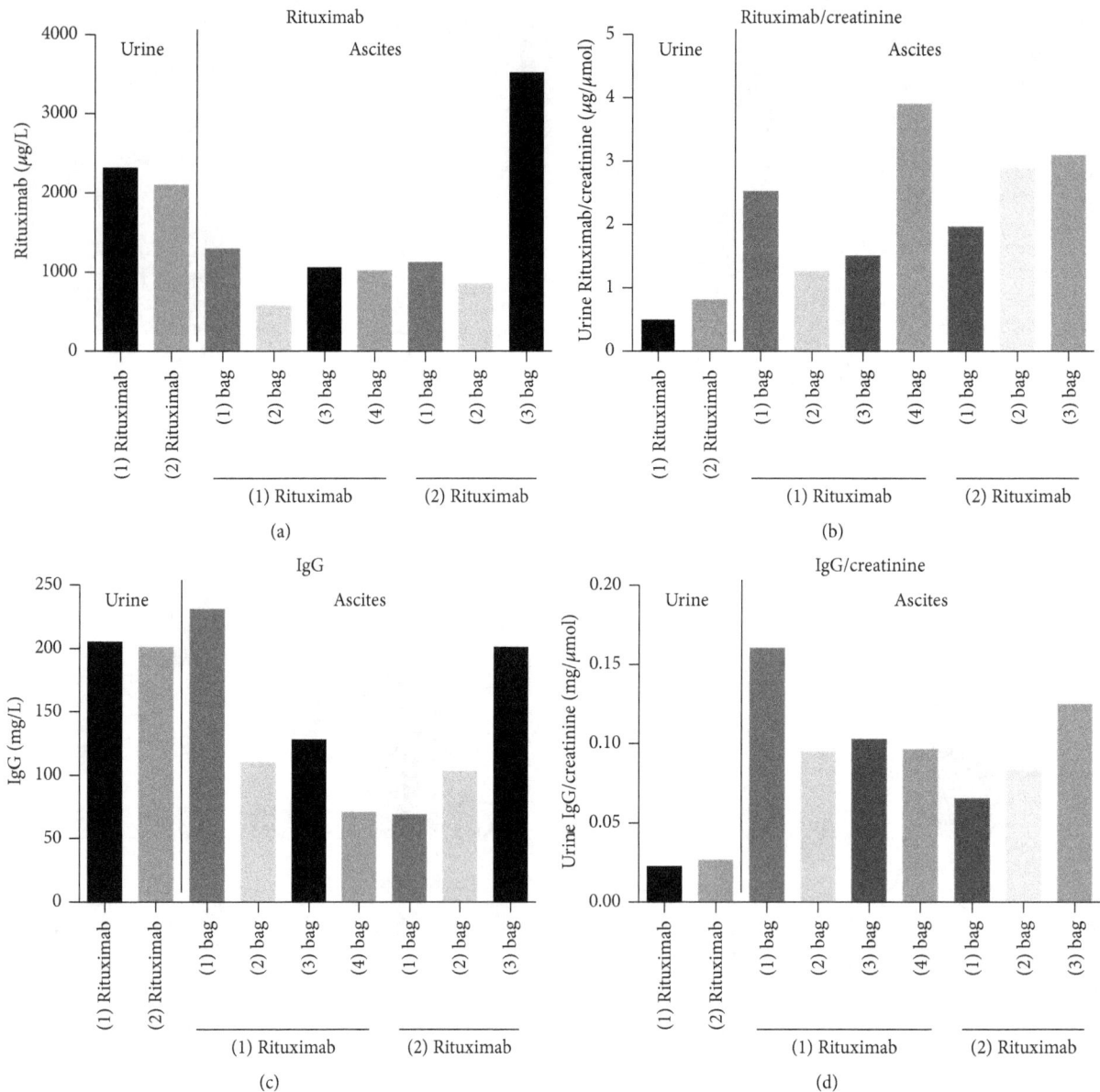

FIGURE 4: Rituximab urine and peritoneal fluid Rituximab concentrations (a) and Rituximab/creatinine ratios (b), as well as IgG urine and peritoneal fluid concentrations (c), and IgG/creatinine ratios (d) of the second case. Since the second patient performed CAPD with three to four peritoneal fluid bag changes per day, the corresponding effluent bags are numbered in chronological order.

A significant amount of IgG was found in all urine and peritoneal fluid samples. IgG showed maximum urine concentration of 205 mg/L and a maximum IgG/creatinine ratio of 0.026 mg/μmoL, while in the peritoneal fluid a maximum IgG concentration of 231 mg/L could be detected. When IgG/creatinine ratios were obtained, we again saw a correlation of IgG and Rituximab excretion both for urine and peritoneal fluid.

3. Discussion

Both patients of this case report received Rituximab not for the reduction of proteinuria as the primary intention. The indication to give Rituximab in the first patient was severe proteinuria resulting from cryoglobulinemia and cryoglobulinemia associated MPGN. Although treatment with Rituximab is well established in hepatitis C associated cryoglobulinemic vasculitis and renal disease [13–16], only case reports exist describing successful utilization of Rituximab in hepatitis B associated cryoglobulinemia [17] and the role of immunosuppression in this disease entity is therefore highly controversial. The second patient received Rituximab as a reserve treatment for Felty syndrome. Successful treatment of Felty syndrome associated neutropenia and synovitis has been described in a series of different case reports [18–20].

Counsilman et al. recently described a case of one pediatric patient with steroid resistant nephrotic syndrome and biopsy proven minimal change nephropathy, who received

Rituximab as second line treatment [21]. The authors used a direct enzyme linked immunosorbent assay to detect high levels of Rituximab in the patients urine and pleural fluid and calculated, following a two-compartment pharmacokinetic model [22], urinary clearance of Rituximab as about 25% of the total clearance and a very short serum half-life of less than one day compared to about 20 days in nonnephrotic patients [21]. While the previous studies used ELISA technology to detect Rituximab, we employed a novel flow cytometry based approach using Daudi cells as a CD20 expressing B-cell line to measure Rituximab concentrations. Another small size case series of pediatric patients with steroid dependant nephrotic syndrome reported a smaller reduction of median serum half-life of about 15 days [23].

A significant amount of Rituximab excretion into the urine could be detected in both patients. While Counsilman et al. reported a maximum excretion of Rituximab into the urine of about 12000 μg/L at a very high proteinuria of 19469 mg albumin/g creatinine, the first patient had a maximum excretion of Rituximab of 3513 μg/L at a proteinuria of 10662 mg/g creatinine, while in the second patient's urine a maximum Rituximab concentration of 2314 μg/L was measured at a proteinuria of 3138 mg/g creatinine. This suggests that the amount of Rituximab excretion into the urine roughly correlates with the degree of proteinuria in these three patients despite different etiologies of the present nephrotic syndromes (steroid resistant nephrotic syndrome, MPGN, and IgA-nephropathy) and despite the different demographic patient characteristics (pediatric versus adult patients). However, due to a great degree of variation in the degree of proteinuria in the first patient (see Figure 1(a)) and since not always proteinuria values have been obtained at the very day of Rituximab administration in this patient, it is not possible to draw a precise conclusion concerning a direct correlation.

We hypothesized that the amount of Rituximab loss into the urine might be largely dependent on the degree of selectivity loss of the glomerular filter. Therefore, we additionally measured IgG excretion in all acquired samples and indeed a substantial amount of IgG secretion was found in all patient urine samples. When Rituximab and IgG urine levels were standardized to the creatinine concentration, we could see a very close correlation of Rituximab/creatinine with the IgG/creatinine ratios. Thus when IgG urine secretion increased, so did Rituximab loss into the urine. Interestingly, the first patient showed clearly a stepwise increasing Rituximab excretion into the urine, despite that his level of proteinuria greatly varied over time (and even was greatest before the first Rituximab administration) and despite that the Rituximab administrations were partly separated a few weeks from each other, which excludes considering the severely reduced serum half-time of less than a day and additive effects. Since IgG excretion into the urine also increased in a stepwise fashion in this patient's case, we speculate that progressive loss of glomerular selectivity may be responsible for this.

In the first case we saw an incomplete B-cell depletion despite the first three Rituximab administrations and a complete B-cell depletion with the higher dose of 1250 mg of Rituximab. Since we measured B-cell count always about 10–14 days after Rituximab administration we cannot exclude temporal complete B-cell depletion followed by a fast rebound due to a severely reduced Rituximab serum half-time as described by Counsilman et al. [21]. High Rituximab excretion into the urine might on the other hand prevent complete CD20+ cell depletion therefore contributing to poor treatment response.

Excretion of Rituximab into the pleural fluid in nephrotic syndrome has been described previously [21]. Interestingly we found in the second case a substantial excretion of Rituximab into the peritoneal fluid. Maximum Rituximab excretion into the peritoneal fluid was with 3518 μg/L significantly higher than the previously reported maximal secretion of Rituximab into the pleural fluid with about 700 μg/L [21]. Surprisingly, when Rituximab and IgG levels in the peritoneal fluid samples were standardized to the corresponding creatinine concentration, again a clear correlation of IgG and Rituximab excretion could be seen. Since this patient received two doses of Rituximab only two days apart, excretion of Rituximab in the peritoneal fluid, when expressed as creatinine ratios, additionally exhibited a time dependent and slightly additive pattern. Rapid loss of Rituximab into the urine and in the third space compartments might have contributed again to poor treatment success in this patient.

To our knowledge, this is the first report describing Rituximab kinetics in two adult nephrotic patients, in one patient, who demonstrates no adequate suppression of CD20+ B-cells despite two applications of Rituximab in short distance from each other, and in the other patient showing excretion of Rituximab in both urine and peritoneal dialysate fluid. We used a novel approach to measure Rituximab applying flow cytometry based detection on a CD20+ cell line. Our data demonstrate a possible close correlation of Rituximab excretion into urine and peritoneal fluid with the amount of IgG secretion suggesting a loss of filter selectivity as the primary determinant of Rituximab urine excretion. The first case shows that high Rituximab excretion into the urine might prevent complete CD20+ cell depletion, therefore contributing to poor treatment response. The second case demonstrates that Rituximab can be lost not only into the urine but also in the third space again causing reduced treatment efficacy.

Future larger scale clinical studies will have to confirm that high nonselective protein loss significantly correlates with an increased excretion of Rituximab into the urine and poor treatment response rate in nephrotic diseases. Evaluating an optimal cut-off value of IgG urinary loss before a possible administration of Rituximab could significantly contribute to a patient individualized treatment approach in refractory nephrotic syndrome.

Disclosure

Klaus Stahl and Michelle Duong share first authorship; Mario Schiffer and Roland Jacobs share last authorship. Michelle Duong present address is Department of Nephrology, Hannover Medical School, Carl Neuberg Strasse 1, 30625 Hannover, Germany.

References

[1] H. M. Gürcan, D. B. Keskin, J. N. H. Stern, M. A. Nitzberg, H. Shekhani, and A. R. Ahmed, "A review of the current use of rituximab in autoimmune diseases," *International Immunopharmacology*, vol. 9, no. 1, pp. 10–25, 2009.

[2] G. L. Plosker and D. P. Figgitt, "Rituximab: a review of its use in non-Hodgkin's lymphoma and chronic lymphocytic leukaemia," *Drugs*, vol. 63, no. 8, pp. 803–843, 2003.

[3] G. M. Keating, "Rituximab: a review of its use in chronic lymphocytic leukaemia, low-grade or follicular lymphoma and diffuse large b-cell lymphoma," *Drugs*, vol. 70, no. 11, pp. 1445–1476, 2010.

[4] V. Guigonis, A. Dallocchio, V. Baudouin et al., "Rituximab treatment for severe steroid- or cyclosporine-dependent nephrotic syndrome: a multicentric series of 22 cases," *Pediatric Nephrology*, vol. 23, no. 8, pp. 1269–1279, 2008.

[5] A. Prytula, K. Iijima, K. Kamei et al., "Rituximab in refractory nephrotic syndrome," *Pediatric Nephrology*, vol. 25, no. 3, pp. 461–468, 2010.

[6] P. Ravan, A. Magnasco, A. Edefonti et al., "Short-term effects of rituximab in children with steroid- and calcineurin-dependent nephrotic syndrome: a randomized controlled trial," *Clinical Journal of the American Society of Nephrology*, vol. 6, no. 6, pp. 1308–1315, 2011.

[7] P. Ravani, A. Bonanni, R. Rossi, G. Caridi, and G. M. Ghiggeri, "Anti-CD20 antibodies for idiopathic nephrotic syndrome in children," *Clinical Journal of the American Society of Nephrology*, vol. 11, no. 4, pp. 710–720, 2016.

[8] K. Iijima, D. M. Sako, K. Nozu et al., "Rituximab for childhood-onset, complicated, frequently relapsing nephrotic syndrome or steroid-dependent nephrotic syndrome: a multicentre, double-blind, randomised, placebo-controlled trial," *The Lancet*, vol. 384, no. 9950, pp. 1273–1281, 2014.

[9] M. Nakayama, K. Kamei, K. Nozu et al., "Rituximab for refractory focal segmental glomerulosclerosis," *Pediatric Nephrology*, vol. 23, no. 3, pp. 481–485, 2008.

[10] U. S. Bayrakci, E. Baskin, H. Sakalli, H. Karakayali, and M. Haberal, "Rituximab for post-transplant recurrences of FSGS," *Pediatric Transplantation*, vol. 13, no. 2, pp. 240–243, 2009.

[11] P. Ruggenenti, P. Cravedi, A. Chianca et al., "Rituximab in idiopathic membranous nephropathy," *Journal of the American Society of Nephrology*, vol. 23, no. 8, pp. 1416–1425, 2012.

[12] A. Gulati, A. Sinha, S. C. Jordan et al., "Efficacy and safety of treatment with rituximab for difficult steroid-resistant and -dependent nephrotic syndrome: multicentric report," *Clinical Journal of the American Society of Nephrology*, vol. 5, no. 12, pp. 2207–2212, 2010.

[13] D. Saadoun, M. Resche-Rigon, D. Sene, L. Perard, A. Karras, and P. Cacoub, "Rituximab combined with Peg-interferon-ribavirin in refractory hepatitis C virus-associated cryoglobulinaemia vasculitis," *Annals of the Rheumatic Diseases*, vol. 67, no. 10, pp. 1431–1436, 2008.

[14] D. Saadoun, A. Delluc, J. C. Piette, and P. Cacoub, "Treatment of hepatitis C-associated mixed cryoglobulinemia vasculitis," *Current Opinion in Rheumatology*, vol. 20, no. 1, pp. 23–28, 2008.

[15] S. De Vita, L. Quartuccio, M. Isola et al., "A randomized controlled trial of rituximab for the treatment of severe cryoglobulinemic vasculitis," *Arthritis and Rheumatism*, vol. 64, no. 3, pp. 843–853, 2012.

[16] D. Saadoun, M. R. Rigon, D. Sene et al., "Rituximab plus Peg-interferon-α/ribavirin compared with Peg-interferon-α/ribavirin in hepatitis C-related mixed cryoglobulinemia," *Blood*, vol. 116, no. 3, pp. 326–334, 2010.

[17] F. Pasquet, F. Combarnous, B. MacGregor et al., "Safety and efficacy of rituximab treatment for vasculitis in hepatitis B virus-associated type II cryoglobulinemia: a case report," *Journal of Medical Case Reports*, vol. 6, article 39, 2012.

[18] N. Weinreb, A. Rabinowitz, and P. F. Dellaripa, "Beneficial response to rituximab in refractory Felty syndrome," *Journal of Clinical Rheumatology*, vol. 12, no. 1, p. 48, 2006.

[19] V. Lekharaju and C. Chattopadhyay, "Efficacy of rituximab in Felty's syndrome," *Annals of the Rheumatic Diseases*, vol. 67, no. 9, article no. 1352, 2008.

[20] A. Salama, U. Schneider, and T. Dörner, "Beneficial response to rituximab in a patient with haemolysis and refractory Felty syndrome," *Annals of the Rheumatic Diseases*, vol. 67, no. 6, pp. 894–895, 2008.

[21] C. E. Counsilman, C. M. Jol-van der Zijde, J. Stevens, K. Cransberg, R. G. M. Bredius, and R. N. Sukhai, "Pharmacokinetics of rituximab in a pediatric patient with therapy-resistant nephrotic syndrome," *Pediatric Nephrology*, vol. 30, no. 8, pp. 1367–1370, 2015.

[22] C. M. Ng, R. Bruno, D. Combs, and B. Davies, "Population pharmacokinetics of rituximab (anti-CD20 monoclonal antibody) in rheumatoid arthritis patients during a phase II clinical trial," *Journal of Clinical Pharmacology*, vol. 45, no. 7, pp. 792–801, 2005.

[23] K. Kamei, S. Ito, K. Nozu et al., "Single dose of rituximab for refractory steroid-dependent nephrotic syndrome in children," *Pediatric Nephrology*, vol. 24, no. 7, pp. 1321–1328, 2009.

New Thrombolytic Infusion Application of Dissolving Renal Artery Embolic Thrombosis: Low-Dose Slow-Infusion Thrombolytic Therapy

Ahmet Karakurt

Department of Cardiology, Faculty of Medicine, Kafkas University, Kars, Turkey

Correspondence should be addressed to Ahmet Karakurt; karakurt38@hotmail.com

Academic Editor: Rumeyza Kazancioglu

Renal artery thromboembolism (RATE) is an uncommon complication of renal arteries from heart chamber. Although there is no treatment protocol prescribed with guidelines, thrombolytic agents such as rt-PA are frequently used. Unfortunately, current thrombolytic agent application protocol in treatment for the RATE is used in acute myocardial infarction or acute pulmonary embolism. In this protocol, 0.9–1.0% cerebral and 4–13% noncerebral hemorrhages are seen. In contrast to this protocol, we aimed to present a case of RATE, in which we applied low-dose, slow-infusion thrombolytic therapy, and we have not observed any complication such as cerebral and noncerebral hemorrhage.

1. Introduction

Although renal artery thromboembolism (RATE) is rarely observed, it is a serious condition that can result in renal infarction. This case is very difficult for physicians to treat. Anticoagulation and thrombolytic and invasive procedure (thrombus aspiration and/or ballooning/stenting) are applied in the treatment of that patient group. If the anticoagulant therapy is administered alone, thrombosis cannot be completely lysed. If the invasive intervention is applied, complete opening cannot be achieved in the occluded region due to multiple thromboembolisms. Moreover, it may lead to slow-flow phenomenon or complete stoppage (no-flow phenomena) in the distal region due to micro- or macroembolism. If a short-durational and high-dose thrombolytic agent (100 mg, for 2 hours), such as recombinant tissue plasminogen activator (rt-PA), is applied, the risk of cerebral or noncerebral hemorrhage may increase [1, 2]. In this study, we aimed to present a case of complete thrombolysis with low-dose slow-infusion thrombolytic therapy (LDSITT) without any complication in a patient with >80% occlusion of the branches of left renal artery due to thromboembolism.

2. Case Report

A 65-year-old male with diagnosed RATE was referred to our Emergency Department complaining of a 1-day history of left upper quadrant and left flank pain from the external center. Complaints occurred after palpitation lasting 45 minutes. The pain started from the left back region as if a knife struck. The intensity of pain increased over time; there was no change in the severity of pain due to the body position changes. He denied recent fever, trauma, chronic atrial fibrillation cardiomyopathy, coagulation disorder, prior history of thromboembolic disease, dysuria, hematuria, or change in bowel pattern. He had been smoking 20 cigarettes per day for 17 years and did not consume alcohol. He had a past medical history of a stent placed in a coronary artery due to acute coronary syndrome three months ago. He did not use prescribed aspirin, metoprolol, clopidogrel, and atorvastatin agents recommended for acute coronary syndrome and stenting.

On physical examination, blood pressure, pulse, and respiratory rates were 144/80 mmHg, 69/min, and 22/min, respectively. Arterial blood oxygen saturation and fever were also 90% and 36.2°C, respectively. The electrocardiogram

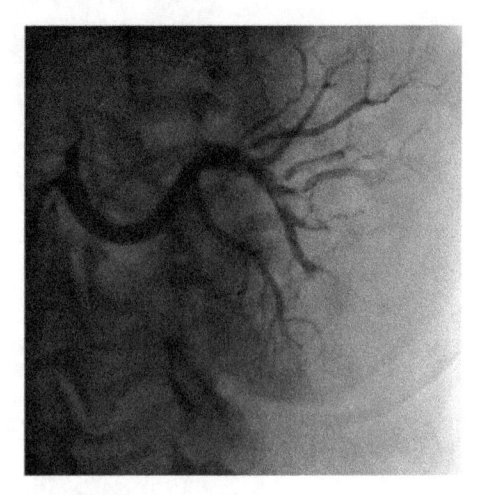

Figure 1: First renal artery angiography showing the multiple thromboembolic materials in the left renal artery branches.

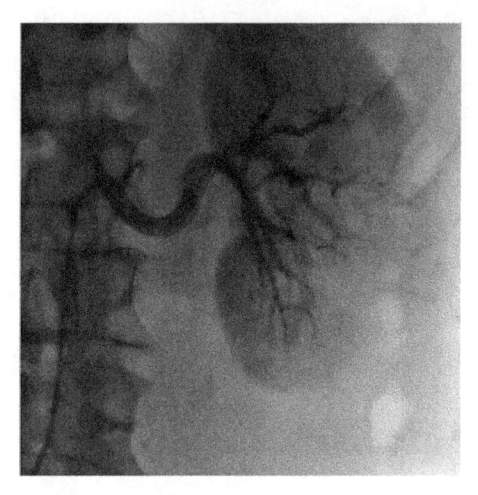

Figure 2: Second renal artery angiography showing residual thromboembolic materials in the left renal artery branches.

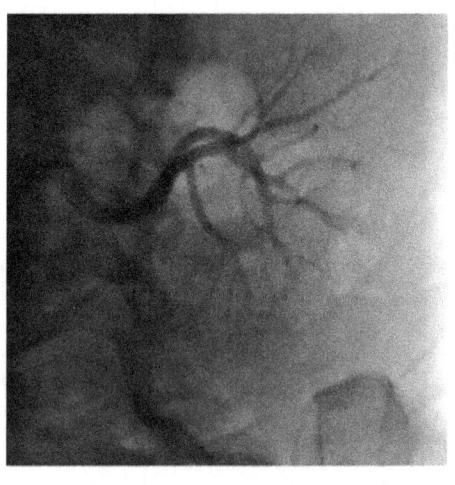

Figure 3: Final renal angiography showing completely lysed thromboembolic materials in the left renal artery branches.

showed normal sinus rhythm. Cardiac examination revealed a fourth heart sound in the apical focus.

Biochemical tests revealed that fasting blood glucose level (182, 70–115 mg/dl), white blood cell (11.9, 3.7–10.4 K/uL), neutrophil count (9.63, 1.8–7.8 K/uL), and C-reactive protein level (18.92, 0–0.5 mg/dl) had increased. There was neutrophil dominance. Platelet count (111, 150–450 K/uL), calcium (7.5, 8.8–10.2 mg/dl), and uric acid levels (2.5, 3.4–7 mg/dl) had decreased. Troponin-I (0.01, <0.3 ng/mL) and creatine kinase-MB isoenzyme levels (51.9, 0–24 U/L) and glomerular filtration rate (70.07) were normal. By urine analysis, +2 glucose, +2 proteinuria, and +2 bloods were detected. Other urine parameters were normal.

A transthoracic echocardiogram revealed hypokinesis of the anterior and anterolateral wall and left ventricular ejection fraction was calculated as 58% by using the modified Simpson technique. There was no thrombus formation in the heart chamber and wall. Lower extremity venous Doppler ultrasonography examination was normal.

The coronary angiography revealed a stent in the left coronary artery and it was open. Other coroner arteries were normal. The renal artery angiography revealed that there were multiple vessel diseases with >80% occlusion with thrombus in right renal artery branches. Figure 1 and Video 1 show the multiple thrombosis in the right renal artery branches.

Depending on clinical, electrocardiographic, biochemical, and angiographic evidence, the patient was diagnosed with the thromboembolic occlusion in the left renal artery branches developing due to unknown origin.

We decided to use LDSITT for the occluded renal artery branches because the patient was not eligible for percutaneous therapy. Antiplatelet agents (aspirin 100 mg and clopidogrel 800 mg) were given prior to invasive process as a premedication from the referral hospital. Neither unfractionated heparin (UFH) (IV bolus end continue infusion) nor low-molecular-weight heparin (LMWH) was given prior to the LDSITT.

2.1. LDSITT Administration. The patient was given an intravenous infusion of 24 ml rt-PA (low dose) in 100 ml normal saline in 48 h (slow infusion time) twice. Following the second dose of fibrinolytic therapy, coronary angiography showed partial regression of the thrombus, leaving a residual thrombus. Figure 2 and Video 2 show residual thrombosis in the right renal artery branches. Therefore, a third dose of 24 ml rt-PA was administered to the patient to completely lyse the thrombus. The third control renal angiography revealed complete lysis of the thrombus with no residue following the third dose of thrombolytic administration. In total, 72 mg rt-PA was administered. Figure 3 and Video 3 show that multiple thrombosis is completely solved.

Although the thrombus was completely lysed after a total of three LDSITT, no complication developed other than minimal ecchymosis at the injection site. On the fifth day of admission, the patient was discharged with the prescription of aspirin 100 mg 1 × 1 and clopidogrel 75 mg 2 × 1 and the recommendation of Internal Medicine Department's outpatient control for diabetes mellitus regulation.

3. Discussion

The true incidence of renal infarction due to renal artery thromboembolism is unknown. Its incidence is reported as 1.4% in an autopsy series of 14411 cases and 0.02/1000 at another series [3, 4]. Depending on the rare occurrence of renal artery thromboembolism due to its rareness and its being less known, a correct diagnosis and a correct treatment are often delayed. If spontaneous renal artery thrombosis is not diagnosed early and is not treated properly, it results in renal insufficiency due to renal infarction.

RATE treatments are antiplatelet, anticoagulant, and/or thrombolytic treatment and/or stent implantation with/without appropriate thrombus aspiration procedures. Thrombolytic therapy is an option of treatment for acute myocardial infarction and pulmonary embolism. Its use in both acute myocardial infarction and pulmonary embolisms has been described in guidelines [1, 2]. Unfortunately, thrombolytic therapy for renal artery thromboembolism causing renal artery infarcts has not been described in current guidelines. Acute myocardial infarction and pulmonary embolism thrombolysis protocols are applied in these patients. For this purpose, rt-PA (total of 100 mg followed by 15 mg intravenous fraction followed by 0.75 mg/kg (not exceeding 50 mg) in 30 minutes and then 0.50 mg/kg (with 35 mg not exceeded) infusion) is one of the most commonly used thrombolytic agents. In this application, rt-PA is given in 90 minutes and high dose [1, 2]. Unfortunately, with this protocol, 0.9–1.0% cerebral and 4–13% noncerebral hemorrhages are observed [1].

Unfortunately, there is no protocol developed to be applied in renal infarction due to the renal artery thromboembolism. According to these protocols, the administration times of this thrombolytic agent are below 90 minutes and the doses are very high. It means that the high rates of cerebral and noncerebral hemorrhages that develop due to both high doses and short treatment times are acceptable. Therefore, unlike the classic thrombolytic administration protocol, LDSITT protocol, which is thought to lower the risk of complications, was applied to this patient and complete dissolution of the thrombus was achieved without any complication.

LDSITT was first used by Özkan et al. [5] in patients with prosthetic valve thrombosis. They performed five different thrombolytic treatment strategies in patients with PVT. These regimens included rapid streptokinase (1.5 MU/3 h), slow streptokinase (1.5 MU/24 h), high-dose rt-PA (100 mg, 10 mg bolus, 90 mg/5 h), half-dose slow-infusion rt-PA (50 mg/6 h), and low-dose slow infusion rt-PA (25 mg/6 h). Treatment success did not differ between the groups. However, the complication rate was found to be significantly lower in the slow-infusion low-dose rt-PA group than in the other groups.

4. Conclusions

Traditional fibrinolytic treatment protocols that are used in the treatment of acute myocardial infarction and pulmonary embolism are associated with high complication rates in patients with RATE. Results of the few single-center, nonrandomized studies consisting of small patient groups showed that LDSITT is associated with low complication rates in patients with thromboembolism. According to our experience and very few literature reports, the LDSITT may be a treatment option in patients with RATE without any contraindication to thrombolytic therapy.

Abbreviations

LDSITT: Low-dose slow-infusion thrombolytic therapy
LWFH: Low-molecular-weight heparin
PVT: Prosthetic valve thrombosis
RATE: Renal artery thromboembolism
rt-PA: Recombinant tissue plasminogen activator
UFH: Unfractionated heparin.

Additional Points

Aim. We aimed to present a case of renal artery thromboembolism in which we applied low-dose slow-infusion thrombolytic therapy (LDSITT), and we have not observed any complication such as cerebral and noncerebral hemorrhage.

Authors' Contributions

Dr. Ahmet Karakurt conceptualized, drafted, reviewed, and revised the manuscript. Also, he contributed to the concept and design of the report and critically reviewed the manuscript. The author approved the final manuscript as submitted and agrees to be accountable for all aspects of the work.

References

[1] B. Ibanez, S. James, S. Agewall et al., "2017 ESC Guidelines for the management of acute myocardial infarction in patients presenting with ST-segment elevation: the Task Force for the management of acute myocardial infarction in patients presenting with ST-segment elevation of the European Society of Cardiology," *European Heart Journal*, pp. 1–66, 2017.

[2] S. V. Konstantinides, A. Torbicki, G. Agnelli et al., "2014 ESC Guidelines on the diagnosis andmanagement of acute pulmonary embolism," *European Heart Journal*, vol. 35, pp. 3033–3080, 2014.

[3] H. J. Hoxie and C. B. Coggin, "Renal infarction: statistical study of two hundred and five cases and detailed report of an unusual case," *JAMA Internal Medicine*, vol. 65, no. 3, pp. 587–594, 1940.

[4] H. Domanovits, M. Paulis, M. Nikfardjam et al., "Acute renal infarction: clinical characteristics of 17 patients," *Medicine*, vol. 78, no. 6, pp. 386–394, 1999.

[5] M. Özkan, S. Gündüz, M. Biteker et al., "Comparison of different TEE-guided thrombolytic regimens for prosthetic valve thrombosis: the TROIA trial," *JACC: Cardiovascular Imaging*, vol. 6, no. 2, pp. 206–216, 2013.

De Novo Atypical Haemolytic Uremic Syndrome after Kidney Transplantation

Arnaud Devresse,[1] Martine de Meyer,[2] Selda Aydin,[3] Karin Dahan,[1,4,5] and Nada Kanaan[1]

[1]Division of Nephrology, Cliniques Universitaires Saint-Luc, Université Catholique de Louvain, Brussels, Belgium
[2]Division of Abdominal Surgery and Transplantation, Cliniques Universitaires Saint-Luc, Université Catholique de Louvain, Brussels, Belgium
[3]Division of Pathology, Cliniques Universitaires Saint-Luc, Université Catholique de Louvain, Brussels, Belgium
[4]Division of Human Genetics, Cliniques Universitaires Saint-Luc, Université Catholique de Louvain, Brussels, Belgium
[5]Center of Human Genetics, Institut de Pathologie et de Génétique, Gosselies, Belgium

Correspondence should be addressed to Nada Kanaan; nada.kanaan@uclouvain.be

Academic Editor: Sophia Lionaki

De novo thrombotic microangiopathy (TMA) can occur after kidney transplantation. An abnormality of the alternative pathway of complement must be suspected and searched for, even in presence of a secondary cause. We report the case of a 23-year-old female patient who was transplanted with a kidney from her mother for end-stage renal disease secondary to Hinman syndrome. Early after transplantation, she presented with 2 episodes of severe pyelonephritis, associated with acute kidney dysfunction and biological and histological features of TMA. Investigations of the alternative pathway of the complement system revealed atypical haemolytic uremic syndrome secondary to complement factor I mutation, associated with mutations in CD46 and complement factor H related protein genes. Plasma exchanges followed by eculizumab injections allowed improvement of kidney function without, however, normalization of creatinine.

1. Background

De novo thrombotic microangiopathy (TMA) has been reported to occur after kidney transplantation [1]. The pathogenic mechanisms are not well understood but are likely multifactorial with implication of specific features attributed to kidney transplantation [2]. However, the implication of a dysregulation in the alternative complement pathway may be underestimated [3].

2. Case Report

A 14-year-old female patient was admitted 9 years ago to our institution for acute pyelonephritis. Massive bilateral ureterohydronephrosis secondary to grade V ureterovesical reflux associated with a trabeculated bladder was evidenced (Figure 1). Neurologic investigations revealed no abnormality, leading to a diagnosis of Hinman syndrome, a very rare entity characterized by all features of a neurogenic bladder with external sphincter dyssynergia, but without evidence of any neurologic alteration [4]. After diagnosis, she had several uncomplicated urinary tract infections, necessitating self-catheterization (importantly never associated with biological thrombocytopenia or haemolytic anemia), and reached end-stage renal disease at age 23 when she underwent preemptive HLA semi-identical living-donor (her mother) kidney transplantation.

Her immunosuppressive regimen included Basiliximab induction, tacrolimus, mycophenolate mofetil, and steroids. She was discharged at day 11 with a normal plasma creatinine (1.26 mg/dl). At day 40, she was admitted for intestinal occlusion due to adhesions requiring adhesiolysis. During hospitalization, she presented a severe pyelonephritis secondary to *Pseudomonas aeruginosa* (colony count > 100,000 colony-forming units of bacteria per mL of urine with negative blood cultures but with increased level of C-reactive protein,

TABLE 1: Laboratory findings.

	Day 11°	Day 40°	Day 120°
C-reactive protein, mg/L ($N < 5.0$)	33.0	117.0	452.0
Plasma creatinine, mg/dL (N: 0.60–1.30)	1.21	2.73	5.5
Lactate dehydrogenase, IU/L ($N < 250$)	376	722	517
Hemoglobin, g/dL (N: 12.2–15.0)	9.6	7.7	7.0
Coombs test	NA	Negative	Negative
Platelets count, per μ/L (N: 150000–450000)	417,000	51,000	96,000
Haptoglobin, g/L (N: 0.3–2.0)	NA	<0.1	<0.1
Schistocytes count, % of red blood cells	NA	4	2
Tacrolimus trough level, ng/mL	9.0	26.5	9.9
Anti-HLA antibody screening*	NA	Negative	Negative
Complement C4, g/L (N: 0.1–0.4)	NA	0.34	0.36
Complement C3, g/L (N: 0.9–1.8)	NA	1.14	1.53
CMV (PCR), copies/mL	Undetected	Undetected	Undetected

°After kidney transplantation. *Class I and class II anti-HLA antibody screening performed by single antigen bead assay. CMV: cytomegalovirus; HLA: human leukocyte antigen; IU: international unit; PCR: polymerase chain reaction; N: normal value; NA: not available.

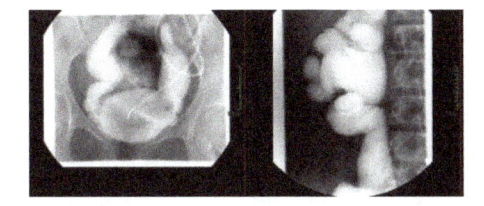

FIGURE 1: Retrograde cystography showing massive ureterovesical reflux and hydronephrosis.

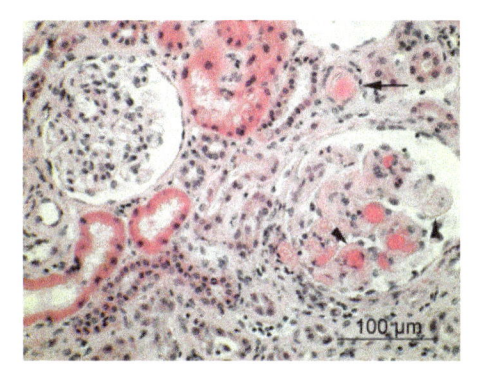

FIGURE 2: Histological examination showing thrombotic microangiopathy in a kidney biopsy from renal allograft at day 120 (hematoxylin and eosin). Microthrombi and lucent deposits (arrowheads) are observed in the glomerulus at the right side, with obstruction of a nearby arteriole by eosinophilic material (arrow). Notice the unaffected glomerulus on the left side of the microphotograph. There is no evidence of acute antibody-mediated rejection according to the 2015 Banff classification (g0, ptc0, and no C4d deposit by immunofluorescence (not shown)).

features consistent with acute pyelonephritis), associated with acute renal failure (creatinine 2.73 mg/dl), increased lactate dehydrogenase level, decreased haptoglobin, haemoglobin, and platelets level. Tacrolimus trough levels were elevated. Complement 3 and 4 levels were normal. Donor-specific antibodies (DSA) were negative (Table 1). She was treated with antibiotics, and a kidney biopsy performed 48 hours later was normal with no sign of acute rejection, acute pyelonephritis, or acute tubular necrosis. Interstitial fibrosis and tubular atrophy (IFTA) was scored 1. Because of the severity of the biological signs of thrombotic microangiopathy (TMA), she was treated with daily plasma exchanges with fresh frozen plasma for one week. Laboratory tests normalized except creatinine that remained elevated (2.1 mg/dl). At day 120, the patient was admitted again for severe pyelonephritis secondary to *Pseudomonas aeruginosa* (>100,000 colony-forming units of bacteria per mL of urine with negative blood cultures) with acute renal failure (creatinine 5.5 mg/dl) and the same biological picture (Table 1). A second kidney biopsy showed pathognomonic features of thrombotic microangiopathy (including a preglomerular arteriole of one glomerulus obstructed by a fresh thrombus and mesangiolysis, without argument for antibody-mediated rejection) (Figure 2). IFTA was scored 1. DSA were absent. Screening for secondary causes of TMA was negative (antiphospholipid syndrome, Shiga toxin, ADMATS13 deficiency or inhibitor, antinuclear factor, Coombs test, disseminated intravascular coagulation, HIV, CMV, pregnancy, hypertension, or occult infection). A genetic screening of the alternative complement pathway revealed a heterozygous mutation in complement factor I *(CFI)* gene c.148C>G (p.(Pro50AIa)), associated with a heterozygous variant of membrane cofactor protein *CD46* (c-366A) and a homozygote deletion of complement factor H *(CFH)* related protein *CFHR1* and *CFHR3* genes. Anti-FH antibody screening was negative. The patient received two plasma exchanges with fresh frozen plasma while waiting to have fast access to anti-C5 antibody. Eculizumab was then started using the recommended doses (900 mg/week for 1 month and then 1200 mg/2 weeks). She was treated for 10 months (the period allowed by our legislation).

Creatinine level stabilized around 2 mg/dl. An allograft biopsy performed 3 months after initiation of eculizumab showed no sign of TMA but a progression of IFTA score to 2. She did not experience any infectious event or biological signs of TMA under eculizumab and is currently doing fine 3 months after treatment cessation.

Screening of the mother revealed the same mutations in *CFI* and *CFHR1–CFHR3*. Her pre-kidney-donation workup was normal and the postnephrectomy evolution was uneventful. Genetic screening was proposed to other members of family (patient's father and brother) but has not been performed yet.

3. Discussion

TMA is a pathologic description, clinically characterized by an association of thrombocytopenia, microangiopathic haemolytic anemia and organ injury [1]. After solid organ transplantation (including kidney, liver, pancreas, lung, and heart) or bone marrow transplantation, de novo TMA had been reported to occur [1, 5, 6]. In the kidney transplantation setting, de novo TMA classically occurred in the 6 first months after kidney transplantation [7] with an incidence between 0.8% to 14% [3, 7]. If the pathogenic mechanisms of de novo TMA are not well understood, they are likely to be multifactorial with ischemia-reperfusion injury, antibody-mediated rejection, viral infection such as cytomegalovirus and immunosuppressant drugs, especially calcineurin inhibitors (CNI), contributing to an "endothelial damaging milieu" [2]. In many cases, supportive treatment and addressing the precipitating factors (CNI dose reduction, CNI withdrawal, treatment of acute antibody-mediated rejection, and viral infections) are sufficient to stop TMA [1]. However, for some patients, this strategy does not lead to an improvement of TMA. For those patients, a complement-mediated TMA secondary to a dysregulation of the alternative complement pathway, classically called atypical haemolytic and uremic syndrome (a-HUS), should be suspected. a-HUS is a rare disorder due to genetic mutation of the alternative complement pathway [8]. These mutations can be found in the regulatory genes *(CFH, CD46, CFI, Thrombomodulin)* or in the activatory genes *(factor B, C3)*. a-HUS can also be secondary to anti-CFH antibodies [8]. A trigger event such as infection or pregnancy is believed to precipitate a-HUS in a susceptible individual. Making the genetic diagnosis of a-HUS before kidney transplantation is crucial: first, the risk of recurrence after kidney transplantation depends on whether the mutant complement factor is membrane-bound (low risk) or circulating (high risk) [9]; second, the introduction of eculizumab, a terminal complement inhibitor, as preventive treatment, has dramatically improved the risk of a-HUS recurrence after kidney transplantation leading to a huge improvement in the allograft survival in these patients [10–12].

In the setting of de novo TMA after kidney transplantation, the implication of a dysregulation in the alternative complement pathway may be underestimated as suggested by one series of de novo TMA after kidney transplantation published by le Quintrec et al. [3]. In a cohort of 24 deceased-donor kidney transplant recipients who experienced de novo TMA after kidney transplantation and who had systematic screening for mutations in genes encoding CFH, CFI, and CD46, 7/24 patients were found to have a mutation: 1 CFH, 4 CFI, and 2 CFH and CFI. Mutations in *CFI* are heterozygous in most patients. Interestingly, 30% of patients with *CFI* mutation were found to have an additional mutation in genes known to be susceptible risk factors for a-HUS. The diagnosis of a-HUS in our patient before transplantation was not suspected. Indeed, she did not show any signs of TMA despite several episodes of urinary tract infections. Her mother also never experienced signs of TMA neither before transplantation (despite 2 pregnancies) nor after kidney donation. The genetics of these mutations is highly complex with a penetrance around 50% [13]. Familial studies suggest a monoallelic autosomal or pseudoautosomal mode of inheritance [14, 15]. Moreover, within families, affected persons may also show different symptoms and ages at onset of the disease [13]. This highly suggests that most a-HUS-associated genetic variants predispose to rather than cause the disease and that triggers are necessary to develop symptoms as for our patient who exacerbated a-HUS symptoms only in the presence of several pathologic conditions: kidney transplantation, immunosuppression, and infection.

Our patient improved her allograft renal function after eculizumab initiation suggesting that, besides preventing recurrence after transplantation, it can be efficient to reverse the fate of renal function in de novo a-HUS occurring after kidney transplantation as demonstrated in a-HUS occurring in the nontransplant setting [11]. Treatment duration of eculizumab is controversial. Despite early recommendations for a lifelong therapy, there is no evidence supporting this attitude [16]. Recently, reports have suggested that, in native kidneys, eculizumab therapy may be discontinued after remission has been achieved, with a prompt resumption of therapy in cases of relapse. Wijnsma et al. reported 20 non-kidney-transplant patients, in whom a restrictive treatment in time followed by a TMA monitoring appeared safe and effective [17]. In kidney transplant recipients, Duineveld et al. reported recently a case series including 17 patients with a-HUS who underwent living kidney transplantation without prophylactic eculizumab. A monitoring strategy was applied and was successful, as only one patient experienced recurrence, which was successfully treated [18]. The good outcomes in this report may be due to the fact that (1) all living donors were genotyped, (2) cold ischemia time was short, and (3) low targets of tacrolimus were used [19]. In our patient, eculizumab was discontinued after 10 months due to limitations imposed by our national reimbursement policy. Currently, 3 months after therapy cessation, she is doing fine with a monthly biological screening. Prospective studies including larger cohorts of kidney transplant recipients with a long follow-up are required to assess whether eculizumab prophylaxis should be restricted to specific profiles and to assess treatment duration.

In conclusion, our case highlights the importance of the following: (1) a genetic screening in de novo TMA after kidney transplantation, (2) identifying the underlying mutation allowing treatment that can potentially reverse the fate of renal function, (3) familial screening and counselling in the context of living donation in case of suspected biological TMA in the donor and/or the recipient.

References

[1] V. Brocklebank, K. M. Wood, and D. Kavanagh, "Thrombotic microangiopathy and the kidney," *Clinical Journal of the American Society of Nephrology*, 2017.

[2] J. Zuber, M. Le Quintrec, H. Morris, V. Frémeaux-Bacchi, C. Loirat, and C. Legendre, "Targeted strategies in the prevention and management of atypical HUS recurrence after kidney transplantation," *Transplantation Reviews*, vol. 27, no. 4, pp. 117–125, 2013.

[3] M. le Quintrec, A. Lionet, N. Kamar et al., "Complement mutation-associated de novo thrombotic microangiopathy following kidney transplantation," *American Journal of Transplantation*, vol. 8, no. 8, pp. 1694–1701, 2008.

[4] S. B. Bauer, "The Hinman Syndrome," *The Journal of Urology*, vol. 197, no. 2, pp. S132–S133, 2017.

[5] A. Verbiest, J. Pirenne, and D. Dierickx, "De novo thrombotic microangiopathy after non-renal solid organ transplantation," *Blood Reviews*, vol. 28, no. 6, pp. 269–279, 2014.

[6] C. Ponticelli and G. Banfi, "Thrombotic microangiopathy after kidney transplantation," *Transplant International*, vol. 19, no. 10, pp. 789–794, 2006.

[7] A. A. Satoskar, R. Pelletier, P. Adams et al., "De novo thrombotic microangiopathy in renal allograft biopsies—role of antibody-mediated rejection," *American Journal of Transplantation*, vol. 10, no. 8, pp. 1804–1811, 2010.

[8] M. Noris and G. Remuzzi, "Atypical hemolytic-uremic syndrome," *The New England Journal of Medicine*, vol. 361, no. 17, pp. 1676–1687, 2009.

[9] M. Okumi and K. Tanabe, "Prevention and treatment of atypical haemolytic uremic syndrome after kidney transplantation," *Nephrology*, vol. 21, pp. 9–13, 2016.

[10] F. Fakhouri, J. Zuber, V. Frémeaux-Bacchi, and C. Loirat, "Haemolytic uraemic syndrome," *The Lancet*, vol. 390, no. 10095, pp. 681–696, 2017.

[11] C. M. Legendre, C. Licht, P. Muus et al., "Terminal complement inhibitor eculizumab in atypical hemolytic-uremic syndrome," *The New England Journal of Medicine*, vol. 368, no. 23, pp. 2169–2181, 2013.

[12] A. Kumar, Z. Stewart, A. Reed et al., "Successful prophylactic use of eculizumab in ahus kidney transplant patients: a report of 9 cases," *American Journal of Transplantation*, vol. 16, supplement 3, 2016.

[13] F. Bu, N. Borsa, A. Gianluigi, and R. J. H. Smith, "Familial atypical hemolytic uremic syndrome: a review of its genetic and clinical aspects," *Clinical and Developmental Immunology*, vol. 2012, Article ID 370426, 9 pages, 2012.

[14] J. Caprioli, M. Noris, S. Brioschi et al., "Genetics of HUS: the impact of MCP, CFH, and IF mutations on clinical presentation, response to treatment, and outcome," *Blood*, vol. 108, no. 4, pp. 1267–1279, 2006.

[15] D. Kavanagh, A. Richards, and J. Atkinson, "Complement regulatory genes and hemolytic uremic syndromes," *Annual Review of Medicine*, vol. 59, pp. 293–309, 2008.

[16] T. H. Goodship, H. T. Cook, F. Fakhouri et al., "Atypical hemolytic uremic syndrome and C3 glomerulopathy: conclusions from a "Kidney Disease: improving Global Outcomes" (KDIGO) Controversies Conference," *Kidney International*, vol. 99, no. 3, pp. 539–551, 2017.

[17] K. L. Wijnsma, C. Duineveld, E. B. Volokhina, L. P. van den Heuvel, N. C. van de Kar, and J. F. Wetzels, "Safety and effectiveness of restrictive eculizumab treatment in atypical haemolytic uremic syndrome," *Nephrology Dialysis Transplantation*, 2017.

[18] C. Duineveld, J. C. Verhave, S. P. Berger, N. C. A. J. van de Kar, and J. F. M. Wetzels, "Living donor kidney transplantation in atypical hemolytic uremic syndrome: a case series," *American Journal of Kidney Diseases*, vol. 70, no. 6, pp. 770–777, 2017.

[19] M. Noris, P. Ruggenenti, and G. Remuzzi, "Kidney transplantation in patients with atypical hemolytic uremic syndrome: a therapeutic dilemma (or not)?" *American Journal of Kidney Diseases*, vol. 70, no. 6, pp. 754–757, 2017.

In Acute IgA Nephropathy, Proteinuria and Creatinine Are in the Spot, but Podocyturia Operates in Silence: Any Place for Amiloride?

H. Trimarchi,[1] M. Paulero,[1] R. Canzonieri,[2] A. Schiel,[2] A. Iotti,[3] C. Costales-Collaguazo,[4] A. Stern,[2] M. Forrester,[1] F. Lombi,[1] V. Pomeranz,[1] R. Iriarte,[1] T. Rengel,[1] I. Gonzalez-Hoyos,[1] A. Muryan,[2] and E. Zotta[3]

[1]Nephrology, Hospital Británico de Buenos Aires, Buenos Aires, Argentina
[2]Biochemistry, Hospital Británico de Buenos Aires, Buenos Aires, Argentina
[3]Pathology Services, Hospital Británico de Buenos Aires, Buenos Aires, Argentina
[4]IFIBIO Houssay-UBA CONICET, Facultad de Medicina, Universidad de Buenos Aires, Argentina

Correspondence should be addressed to H. Trimarchi; htrimarchi@hotmail.com

Academic Editor: Yoshihide Fujigaki

IgA nephropathy is the most frequent cause of primary glomerulonephritis, portends erratic patterns of clinical presentation, and lacks specific treatment. In general, it slowly progresses to end-stage renal disease. The clinical course and the response to therapy are usually assessed with proteinuria and serum creatinine. Validated biomarkers have not been identified yet. In this report, we present a case of acute renal injury with proteinuria and microscopic hematuria in a young male. A kidney biopsy disclosed IgA nephropathy. Podocyturia was significantly elevated compared to normal subjects. Proteinuria, renal function, and podocyturia improved promptly after steroids and these variables remained normal after one year of follow-up, when steroids had already been discontinued and patient continued on valsartan and amiloride. Our report demonstrates that podocyturia is critically elevated during an acute episode of IgA nephropathy, and its occurrence may explain the grim long-term prognosis of this entity. Whether podocyturia could be employed in IgA nephropathy as a trustable biomarker for treatment assessment or even for early diagnosis of IgA nephropathy relapses should be further investigated.

1. Introduction

IgA nephropathy is the most frequent cause of primary glomerulopathies worldwide. It can clinically emerge with a wide variety of presentations, ranging from asymptomatic microhematuria to nephrotic syndrome or rapidly progressive glomerulonephritis. It is an autoimmune disease diagnosed by immunofluorescent positive IgA mesangial deposits in the kidney biopsy [1]. Hypogalactosylated IgA molecules evoke the synthesis of IgG autoantibodies that form circulating immune complexes that end up entrapped in the mesangial area due to interactions between CD89 and mesangial cell receptors like CD71. Finally, this abnormal deposition of immune complexes in the glomerulus causes local inflammation, mesangial proliferation, matrix expansion, and eventually fibrosis, while endocapillary proliferation and extracapillary proliferation are more rare findings [2]. All these histologic alterations correlate with hematuria and proteinuria, the latter being the main culprit of chronic kidney disease progression. Finally, protein trafficking in the kidney interstitium results in interstitial fibrosis and tubular atrophy. Renal function decline is mainly due to glomerular obliteration and interstitial changes, which generally occur in a chronic progressive course.

The only usual markers that physicians count on to assess the above morphologic derangements in routine clinical practice are proteinuria, dysmorphic hematuria, and creatinine creeping. Like in most glomerulopathies, in IgA nephropathy, there are no specific validated biomarkers. When matrix expansion is observed in a glomerulus in the kidney biopsy, it is estimated that approximately 20% of the podocyte population of that glomerulus has already been detached and forever lost in the urine, as podocytes are not capable of undergoing mitosis [3, 4]. This phenomenon is named podocyturia [4]. When the glomerulus loses between 20 and 40% of the podocyte population, usually associated with morphologic changes as focal adhesions between the glomerular tuft and Bowman capsule and/or focal and segmental glomerulosclerosis, it is rendered to be obliterated [3]. We present a case of acute renal failure with proteinuria and microhematuria in a young male whose biopsy disclosed IgA nephropathy. Concurrent significant podocyturia was observed. After immunosuppressive therapy, proteinuria became negative, renal function was recovered, and podocyturia remained similar to controls. When renal function improved, valsartan and amiloride were prescribed and steroids discontinued. We believe that the loss of podocytes in IgA nephropathy could be the reason why this entity shows a relentless progressive course in most of these patients. Podocyturia could be employed to guide the type of therapy to be employed and also as a follow-up tool for nephrologists.

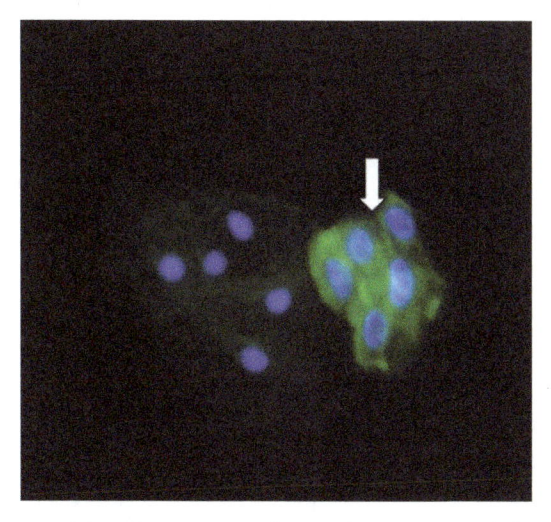

FIGURE 1: The white arrow indicates the presence of clustered podocytes, as bright green fluorescent cells. A tubular cell is observed to the left. Fluorescent microscopy, ×200.

2. Case Presentation

A healthy 18-year-old male was admitted due to kidney failure (serum creatinine: 3 mg/dL), proteinuria (1.89 g/day), and recent past episodes of intermittent macrohematuria. Urine smear disclosed 30–50 red blood cells per high power field (Table 1). Four months before admission, a routine blood exam had been within normal limits, except for a urinalysis that had shown 10 red blood cells per high power field. Past medical history was negative for prior upper respiratory tract infections or any infections of clinical relevance. At the time of admission, physical examination was normal; blood pressure was 110/70 mmHg. A renal ultrasound showed kidneys with normal shape and measurements with echogenic alterations, while all complementary serologic studies were noncontributory: blood, urine, and throat cultures, HIV, hepatitis B and C serologies, complement levels, p- and c-ANCA antibodies, antiglomerular basement membrane antibodies, and electrophoretic proteinogram. Podocyturia was performed as described previously [5]. Briefly, the podocyte count was assessed by counting in urinary smears the number of cells in 10 microscopy fields of ×20. The podocyte count was 2.1 cells per ×20 field and the number of podocytes per gram of urinary creatinine was 166 (Figure 1). Podocytes were identified by tagging synaptopodin (ab109560 Alexa Fluor®, Abcam, Cambridge, UK), an specific marker of podocytes, to establish their identity by immunofluorescence techniques using a secondary antibody (Alexa Fluor 488, Abcam, Cambridge, Uk). The smears were analyzed employing an epifluorescence microscopy, Nikon Eclipse E200. This result was compared with 10 controls (6 males and 4 females; mean age: 20 ± 2.1 years, with no past history of morbidities: serum creatinine, 0.7 ± 0.1 mg/dL; mean 24-hour urinary albumin excretion, 66 ± 12 mg/day. The mean podocyte count was 0.11 ± 0.3 cells per ×20 field, while the mean number of podocytes per gram of urinary creatinine was 8.3. One day after admission, a kidney biopsy was performed and was consistent with IgA nephropathy, with the following Oxford score over 14 glomeruli: M1E0S0T0. The immunofluorescence was positive for IgA and mesangial C3 deposits +++/4 y C3. Due to the rapidly progressive course of the altered kidney function, oral methyl prednisone 1 mg/kg/day was started. Two weeks later when creatinine was 1.2 mg/dL, amiloride was started at 5 mg/day. Four weeks after initiation of therapy, proteinuria and hematuria were negative and serum creatinine dropped to 0.7 mg/dL (Table 1). Two consecutive podocyturia tests were similar to controls after one year of follow-up. Current therapy consists of amiloride 5 mg/day and valsartan 80 mg/day.

3. Discussion

In our opinion, this case report illustrates several aspects of IgA nephropathy which deserve special consideration. From the clinical point of view, an acute episode of renal injury due to IgA nephropathy may not necessarily be associated with endocapillary proliferation or extracapillary proliferation. However, it must be borne in mind that, due to limitations inherent to a biopsy sample size factor, areas of endocapillary proliferation or extracapillary proliferation may have well been missed. In addition, in IgA nephropathy, endocapillary proliferation is not easily identified, even by trained pathologists [6]. Although the previous episodes of macrohematuria might have well contributed to transient creeping of serum creatinine, as described previously [7], creatinine continued to rise long after macrohematuria had disappeared.

Certainly, a prompt therapeutic intervention may have stopped the potential development of a more proliferative histologic pattern. Macroscopic hematuria was the one sign that alerted the patient for a quick medical consult. In this regard, it is interesting to contrast our findings with the ones published by Asao et al. who reported the relationships between podocyturia marked with podocalyxin, the level of urinary podocalyxin, and the histologic findings in 51 patients with

TABLE 1: Clinical, biochemical, and interventional data.

Variables	Days							
	0	1	2	3	4	15	30	365
	Interventions							
	Admission	Biopsy steroids		Biopsy result	Hospital discharge	Amiloride	Valsartan	
Blood pressure (mmHg)	110/70	124/76	120/70	120/72	110/76	126/72	116/78	110/66
Serum creatinine	3	3.1	2.6	2.2	1.6	1.2	0.7	0.9
CKD-EPI (mL/min)	29	28	34	42	62	88	138	124
Podocytes/gram urinary creatinine (cells/g)	166	NP	NP	NP	NP	110	0.8	0.7
Proteinuria (g/day)	1.89	NP	NP	NP	1.1	0.5	0.07	0.09
Dysmorphic red blood (%)	95	NP	NP	NP	89	40	15	20
Serum potassium (mEq/L)	4.9	4.8	4.3	4.1	3.8	3.7	4.1	4.3

NP, not performed.

IgA nephropathy [8]. Our urinary podocyte number adjusted to grams of urinary creatinine was lower when compared to their results, and a control cohort of 10 patients was employed. This observation could have many explanations: our Oxford score was only positive for M1, while their patients included many different Oxford scores. In addition, their findings underscored the noteworthy observation that higher levels of podocyturia correlated with glomerulosclerosis and extracapillary proliferation, histologic findings that our patient did not present. In addition, our case represents an early clinical event, while their work included 51 patients, many with advanced lesions, and no control group was included. Finally, different markers were employed, which assess different podocyte compartments. Asao et al. have clearly stated that podocalyxin, a sialomucin that is located in the glycocalyx, is not specific for podocytes [8]. Synaptopodin is a postmitotic cytoplasmic podocyte protein that has been proven by many authors to be a reliable and specific marker of podocytes [5, 9, 10]. As Maestroni et al. have shown and as we have addressed in our previous publications, there are different podocyte subpopulations that may be missed if only one biomarker is employed, as is the case in our case report and Asato's elegant work [4, 5, 9].

Advantages and disadvantages of measuring podocyturia emerge in clinical practice. As we have previously reported, the methods employed to assess podocyturia are time-consuming, are laborious, and must be performed by skilled professionals [5]. However, it offers many advantages as a biomarker for early stages of glomerular injury and can be employed to unravel the pathophysiologic pathways of podocyte detachment [submitted work]. We believe that as detached podocytes may be released intermittently, serial podocyturia employing several markers would be a more reliable way to assess podocyte loss (group ongoing study).

Another controversial aspect of the present case is the therapy employed. As the patient was with renal failure and serum creatinine worsened after admission until the biopsy was performed, renin-angiotensin blockade was not initiated. As proteinuria was >1 g/day, the patient was started on steroids [11, 12]. However, this prescription may be questioned by the fact that the Oxford score, based on a validated histologic classification with proposed standardization of diagnosis and also with impact in clinical outcomes, was low in aggressiveness [13]. Moreover, in the recently published STOP-IGAN trial, the addition of immunosuppressants to renin-angiotensin blockade and supportive care would not provide substantial kidney-related benefits in patients with high-risk IgA nephropathy, due to the fact that there are no differences in the rate of decrease in renal function, although corticosteroid/immunosuppressive therapy induced complete remission of proteinuria more frequently than supportive care alone. Side effects were more common in those who had received immunosuppression. Finally, immunosuppressed patients had a worse outcome than those treated with renin-angiotensin inhibition. Noteworthy, in this important prospective study, kidney biopsies were not included [14]. Recent data support that patients with preserved renal function and proteinuria > 1 g/day or subjects with E1 lesions or with apparent isolated nonaggressive M1 lesion in the Oxford score plus proteinuria < 0.75 g/day may benefit from steroid therapy [11]. Steroids were indicated due to acute renal injury in a young adult with >1 gram of proteinuria. In our opinion, as has been shown by numerous studies, we believe that there is no question that angiotensin converting enzyme inhibitors and/or angiotensin receptor blockers are the first-line drugs to be employed in IgA nephropathy patients. However, from the physiopathological point of view, we treated the patient with amiloride, as podocyturia was elevated, due to the fact that we and others have demonstrated that, in the podocyte detachment that occurs in IgA nephropathy, podocyte urokinase-type plasminogen activator receptor (uPAR) may be involved, with potential coupling of basal membrane integrins, such as $\alpha V\beta 3$ or $\alpha 3\beta 1$ [15]. We have also assessed the use of amiloride without steroids in patients with other glomerulopathies, and amiloride was successful to decrease podocyturia in the long term as maintenance therapy [16, 17]. Amiloride blocks the synthesis of uPAR and the consequent coupling to β subunits of integrins [18]. This would result in a decreased interaction of uPAR with podocyte actin and with integrins, diminishing podocyte contraction and motility and the risk of detachment and proteinuria [15–18]. In summary, the rationale of our therapeutic approach was to start the patient on amiloride first so as to decrease the podocyte loss, and after a more clinical steady state, valsartan, a proven drug that improves IgA nephropathy prognosis, was added [12, 16, 17]. It could be argued that amiloride ought not to have been prescribed. However, as the patient was hemodynamically stable, no hyperkalemia was present, and serum creatinine had decreased from 3 mg/dL to 1.2 mg/dl after two weeks, we assumed the initial creatinine creep to be due to IgA nephropathy activity, based on the urinary findings, clinical picture, and presumably also the steroid response. In this setting, amiloride could be employed at the acute phase of the disease to potentially intervene on podocyte loss, as addressed above.

We believe that if podocyturia is identified, targeted, and decreased, particularly at early stages of a glomerulopathy as IgA nephropathy, the consequent progression of these entities to chronic kidney disease may be at least delayed. In this respect, IgA nephropathy lacks any specific treatment [19]. Podocyturia has been previously addressed in IgA nephropathy [15, 19, 20]. Hara et al. have demonstrated that podocyte loss reflected disease progression [20]. Renin-angiotensin blockade plays a critical role in nephroprotection in IgA nephropathy [11, 12, 14]. This benefit may be due to the effects angiotensin converting enzyme inhibitors and angiotensin receptor blockers exert not only on the interference of angiotensin actions but also on the stabilization they play on the podocyte [21]. The identification of validated biomarkers for the early identification of this disease or for follow-up purposes is mandatory in IgA nephropathy. Podocyturia could be an available tool to count on in patients with this progressive disease. Amiloride is a drug that could be assessed in clinical trials in IgA nephropathy based on the role podocyturia plays in IgA nephropathy and the potential inhibition of podocyte detachment on this entity.

References

[1] I. S. D. Roberts, "Pathology of IgA nephropathy," *Nature Reviews Nephrology*, vol. 10, no. 8, pp. 445–454, 2014.

[2] H. Suzuki, K. Kiryluk, J. Novak et al., "The pathophysiology of IgA nephropathy," *Journal of the American Society of Nephrology*, vol. 22, no. 10, pp. 1795–1803, 2011.

[3] R. C. Wiggins, "The spectrum of podocytopathies: a unifying view of glomerular diseases," *Kidney International*, vol. 71, no. 12, pp. 1205–1214, 2007.

[4] H. Trimarchi, "Podocyturia: what is in a name?" *Journal of Translational Internal Medicine*, vol. 3, no. 2, pp. 51–56, 2015.

[5] H. Trimarchi, R. Canzonieri, A. Schiel et al., "Podocyturia in Fabry adult untreated and treated patients. A controlled study," *Journal of Nephrology*, vol. 6, pp. 791–797, 2016.

[6] R. Coppo, D. D. Lofaro, R. R. Camilla et al., "Risk factors for progression in children and young adults with IgA nephropathy: an analysis of 261 cases from the VALIGA European cohort," *Pediatric Nephrology*, vol. 32, pp. 139–150, 2017.

[7] R. Magistroni, V. D. D'Agati, G. B. Appel, and K. Kiryluk, "New developments in the genetics, pathogenesis, and therapy of IgA nephropathy," *Kidney International*, vol. 88, no. 5, pp. 974–989, 2015.

[8] R. Asao, K. Asanuma, F. Kodama et al., "Relationships between levels of urinary podocalyxin, number of urinary podocytes, and histologic injury in adult patients with IgA nephropathy," *Clinical Journal of the American Society of Nephrology*, vol. 7, no. 9, pp. 1385–1393, 2012.

[9] S. Maestroni, A. Maestroni, G. Dell'Antonio et al., "Viable podocyturia in healthy individuals: implications for podocytopathies," *American Journal of Kidney Diseases*, vol. 64, no. 6, pp. 1003–1005, 2014.

[10] P. Mundel, P. Gilbert, and W. Kriz, "Podocytes in glomerulus of rat kidney express a characteristic 44 KD protein," *Journal of Histochemistry and Cytochemistry*, vol. 39, no. 8, pp. 1047–1056, 1991.

[11] R. Coppo, "Corticosteroids in IgA nephropathy: lessons from recent studies," *Journal of the American Society of Nephrology*, vol. 28, no. 1, pp. 25–33, 2016.

[12] Kidney Disease: Improving Global Outcomes (KDIGO) Glomerulonephritis Work Group, "KDIGO clinical practice guideline for glomerulonephritis," *Kidney International Supplements*, vol. 2, pp. 139–274, 2012.

[13] Working Group of the International IgA Nephropathy Network, the Renal Pathology Society, I. S. Roberts et al., "The Oxford classification of IgA nephropathy: pathology definitions, correlations, and reproducibility," *Kidney International*, vol. 76, no. 5, pp. 546–556, 2009.

[14] T. Rauen, F. Eitner, C. Fitzner et al., "Intensive supportive care plus immunosuppression in IgA nephropathy," *New England Journal of Medicine*, vol. 373, no. 23, pp. 2225–2236, 2015.

[15] N. Kobayashi, T. Ueno, K. Ohashi et al., "Podocyte injury-driven intracapillary plasminogen activator inhibitor type 1 accelerates podocyte loss via uPAR-mediated β_1- integrin endocytosis," *American Journal of Physiology—Renal Physiology*, vol. 308, no. 6, pp. F614–F626, 2015.

[16] H. Trimarchi, M. Forrester, F. Lombi et al., "Amiloride as an alternate adjuvant antiproteinuric agent in fabry disease: the potential roles of plasmin and uPAR," *Case Reports in Nephrology*, vol. 2014, Article ID 854521, 6 pages, 2014.

[17] H. Trimarchi, R. Canzonieri, A. Muryan et al., "Podocyturia: a clue for the rational use of amiloride in Alport renal disease," *Case Reports in Nephrology*, vol. 2016, Article ID 1492743, 4 pages, 2016.

[18] B. Zhang, S. Xie, W. Shi, and Y. Yang, "Amiloride off-target effect inhibits podocyte urokinase receptor expression and reduces proteinuria," *Nephrology, Dialysis, Transplantation*, vol. 27, no. 5, pp. 1746–1755, 2012.

[19] K. V. Lemley, R. A. Lafayette, M. Safai et al., "Podocytopenia and disease severity in IgA nephropathy," *Kidney International*, vol. 61, no. 4, pp. 1475–1485, 2002.

[20] M. Hara, T. Yanagihara, and I. Kihara, "Cumulative excretion of urinary podocytes reflects disease progression in IgA nephropathy and Schönlein-Henoch purpura nephritis," *Clinical Journal of the American Society of Nephrology*, vol. 2, no. 2, pp. 231–238, 2007.

[21] A. Fukuda, L. T. Wickman, M. P. Venkatareddy et al., "Angiotensin II-dependent persistent podocyte loss from destabilized glomeruli causes progression of end stage kidney disease," *Kidney International*, vol. 81, no. 1, pp. 40–55, 2012.

Rhabdomyolysis Induced by Coadministration of Fusidic Acid and Atorvastatin: A Case Report

Dimitrios Patoulias,[1] **Theodoros Michailidis,**[1] **Thomas Papatolios,**[2] **Rafael Papadopoulos,**[2] **and Petros Keryttopoulos**[1]

[1]Department of Internal Medicine, General Hospital of Veria, Veria, Greece
[2]Department of Nephrology, General Hospital of Veria, Veria, Greece

Correspondence should be addressed to Dimitrios Patoulias; dipatoulias@gmail.com

Academic Editor: Yoshihide Fujigaki

Statins are among the most widely prescribed medications worldwide. Acute rhabdomyolysis constitutes a potentially life-threatening side effect regardless of whether statins are administered alone or in combination. The potentially fatal combination of a statin and fusidic acid has been well described in the literature. Acute renal failure can be a direct consequence of this drug-drug interaction. We present a case of a 79-year-old woman who presented to our Emergency Department with a one-week history of limb weakness, myalgia, and inability to stand and walk. The patient had been given fusidic acid to treat Methicillin-Sensitive *Staphylococcus Aureus* (MSSA) positive dermatitis in the 3 weeks prior to admission, while she continued to take her complete therapeutic regimen, which included atorvastatin. Thus, she developed rhabdomyolysis due to the interaction between fusidic acid and atorvastatin. Herein, we report a life-threatening complication of coadministration of fusidic acid and a statin, which is preventable and predictable. The exact mechanism of the interaction is not fully understood, but coadministration of these two medications must be avoided in clinical practice.

1. Purpose

The purpose of the present case study is to highlight rhabdomyolysis as a potentially life-threatening consequence after coadministration of fusidic acid and a statin. Although the exact mechanism of interaction is not fully understood, the coadministration must be avoided in clinical practice. We present a case of rhabdomyolysis after prescription of fusidic acid in a patient previously treated with atorvastatin who developed rhabdomyolysis early after the coadministration.

2. Case Report

A 79-year-old female patient was admitted to the Emergency Department on 21 September 2016 complaining of one-week history of diffuse limb myalgia and inability to stand or walk. Her medical history was notable for arterial hypertension, type 2 diabetes mellitus, chronic kidney disease, and dyslipidemia over the last 25, 15, 6, and 10 years, respectively. She underwent a right nephrectomy in 2013 for renal oncocytoma.

She had a three-month history of MSSA positive dermatitis of the right knee, which was initially treated with topical antibiotics. Due to inadequate response to treatment, she was prescribed a 3-week course of fusidic acid 250 mg four times daily and clindamycin 300 mg three times daily. At the same time, the patient remained on her therapeutic regimen, which included atorvastatin 20 mg once daily.

During the initial assessment of the patient, her vital signs were within normal range. Her physical examination was unremarkable, except for the significant decrease in muscle strength of the proximal leg muscles. Abnormal laboratory values were as follows: SGOT, 635 U/L; SGPT,

TABLE 1

	1st day	2nd day	4th day	5th day	6th day	7th day	8th day	11th day	14th day	17th day	21st day
CPK (U/L)	17263	11632	12094	9835	13287	9104	4491	2231	987	556	227
Urea (mg/dl)	121	99	96	90	85	86	79	74	72	71	70
Crea. (mg/dl)	2.6	1.86	1.4	1.69	1.58	1.58	1.58	1.53	1.51	1.52	1.51
SGOT (U/L)	635	541	552	524	574	440	251	117	94	65	44
SGPT (U/L)	317	284	318	356	401	391	322	163	123	87	57

TABLE 2: Summary of the published case reports highlighting the discussed drug-drug interaction.

Authors	Statin	Fusidic acid in therapeutic dosage	Indication for fusidic acid administration	Outcome
Bachoumas et al. [10]	Pravastatin	✓	MSSA positive abscess of the tibial plate	Death
Wenisch et al. [11]	Atorvastatin	✓	S. aureus and E. coli-infected gangrenous foot lesion	Discharged home with restored mobility
Gabignon et al. [12]	Atorvastatin	✓	MSSA positive hip prosthetic joint infection	Discharged home with restored mobility
Nandy and Gaïni [13]	Atorvastatin	✓	Infected aortic aneurysm, with involvement of the endovascular stent and para-aortic abscesses	Discharged home with improved mobility
Cowan et al. [4]	Atorvastatin/rosuvastatin	✓	MSSA positive hip prosthesis	Death
Burtenshaw et al. [14]	Simvastatin	✓	Isolation of MRSA from aneurysmal sac after elective AAA repair	Death
Teckchandani et al. [5]	Atorvastatin	✓	Infected hip prosthesis	Discharged home with restored mobility
O'Mahony et al. [15]	Atorvastatin	✓	NP	Discharged home with restored mobility
Saeed and Azam [6]	Atorvastatin	✓	Postarthroscopy MRSA right knee infection	Discharged home with improved mobility

NP: not provided.

317 U/L; LDH, 1335 U/L; CPK, 17263 U/L; CK-MB, 534 U/L; TBIL, 1.54 mg/dl; DBIL, 0.91 mg/dl; IBIL, 0.63 mg/dl; urea, 121 mg/dl; and Crea., 2.6 mg/dl. Air blood gases test revealed the following: Ph, 7.45; PO_2, 79.7 mmHg; PCO_2, 37.9 mmHg; and HCO_3, 26.0 mmol/l. Electrolytes were all within the normal range. Myoglobinuria was also present, while there was no hematuria. Abdominal ultrasonography did not reveal any pathology. Computerized tomography of the brain was also unremarkable.

She had no history of trauma, significant exertion, or immobilization. Screening for autoimmune diseases, including ANA, anti-dsDNA, c-ANCA, p-ANCA, and anti-Jo-1, was negative. The patient did not give a written consent for the performance of a muscle biopsy in order to confirm the diagnosis histologically. She was finally diagnosed with acute rhabdomyolysis due to coadministration of fusidic acid and atorvastatin.

Intravenous hydration and diuresis were the only therapeutic intervention, while sodium bicarbonate was administered only on the first day of hospitalization. Antibiotic treatment and statin therapy were discontinued.

The range of the main laboratory values of the patient during hospitalization is shown in Table 1.

The patient gradually regained muscle strength and was able to stand and walk before being discharged home. Ten days later, her CPK, SGOT, and SGPT values had normalized, while her serum creatinine level was at baseline. During her follow-up on a 3-month basis, she remains asymptomatic without issues.

3. Discussion

Few case reports highlighting the potentially life-threatening drug-drug interaction between statins and fusidic acid have been published (Table 2).

Magee et al. [1] published a series of 4 cases of acute rhabdomyolysis after coadministration of fusidic acid and atorvastatin. All patients were on long-term therapy with atorvastatin before administration of fusidic acid. Fusidic acid was prescribed due to osteomyelitis in three patients and septic arthritis in one patient. Two out of three patients suffered previously from end-stage renal disease and diabetes mellitus type 2. They died after admission to ICU due to multiple organ dysfunction syndrome (MODS). The third patient suffered from diabetes mellitus type 1. He developed acute kidney injury in the term of rhabdomyolysis. The 4th patient developed acute kidney injury due to rhabdomyolysis, but aggressive measures led to normalization of his renal function. It is notable that he was the younger patient in this case series, with no significant medical history. The authors emphasize on the need of avoidance of coadministration of the two agents.

In the largest available case series including 8 patients who developed rhabdomyolysis due to interaction of statin and fusidic acid, Kearney et al. [2] conclude the following: (a) the risk of rhabdomyolysis is 50-fold higher in patients receiving both statin and fusidic acid compared with patients receiving only a statin, (b) admission to ICU in those cases may be required, especially in patients with subject diseases, (c) MODS is the typical cause of death, and (d) long-term follow-up of those patients is usually required, with emphasis on their renal function. The authors suggest that, in cases of short-term therapy with fusidic acid, statin should be temporarily withdrawn, while when long-term therapy is required statin should be replaced by another lipid-lowering agent.

Another case series of rhabdomyolysis induced by interaction of fusidic acid and statin was presented by Collidge et al. [3]. The authors report 4 cases of patients suffering from diabetes mellitus type 2 who were prescribed the discussed combination. Three of them received simvastatin, and one received atorvastatin. Rhabdomyolysis was diagnosed at least two weeks after initiation of fusidic acid (18–32 days). The authors emphasize upon the potential mimicry between rhabdomyolysis and Guillain-Barré Syndrome (GBS). All 4 patients were initially diagnosed with GBS due to clinical presentation, nerve conduction studies, and needle electromyogram. The combination was discontinued 0–2 days after notice of elevated serum CK levels. Long rehabilitation and gradual restoration of patients' mobility were required.

The exact mechanism of interaction between the two agents remains unclear. According to previous reports, fusidic acid serves as a CYP450 3A4 enzyme inhibitor [4–7]. However, the latter has been questioned [1]. Based on the fact that the main metabolite of fusidic acid is a glucuronide conjugate, interference with the glucuronidation system potentially leads to increased serum levels of statins and thus significant risk of myotoxicity. According to Eng et al. [8], fusidic acid inhibits significantly organic anion transporting polypeptides OATP1B1 and OATP1B3, modifying hepatic uptake of statins, leading to increased serum concentration and, thus, increased risk of rhabdomyolysis. In the same study, fusidic acid was recognized as a weak, reversible, and time-dependent inhibitor of CYP450 3A4, while it did not affect breast cancer resistance protein (BCRP). In the study performed by Gupta et al. [9], the researchers confirmed that fusidic acid inhibits BCRP and OATP1B1 mediated liver and intestinal uptake of statins, while it also inhibits hepatic metabolism of statins. According to the authors, single dosing of fusidic acid leads to unbound plasma or hepatic inlet levels high enough to inhibit OATP1B1 and P450s, while multiple dosing of fusidic acid, as in all cases described above, inhibits BCRP as well. Despite the interesting findings of Eng et al. and the perspective of Gupta et al., it is clear that further studies are required in order to elucidate the mechanisms of this drug-drug interaction.

4. Conclusions

We conclude the following:

(1) The mechanism of interaction between statins and fusidic acid is under discussion. Further investigation is required.

(2) Acute kidney injury is the main cause of morbidity and mortality in patients with rhabdomyolysis after coadministration of fusidic acid and a statin. Certain factors (medical history, other medications, etc.) may worsen the clinical outcome.

(3) Coprescription of the two agents must be avoided in clinical practice. This drug-drug interaction is preventable and predictable.

References

[1] C. N. Magee, S. A. Medani, S. F. Leavey, P. J. Conlon, and M. R. Clarkson, "Severe Rhabdomyolysis as a Consequence of the Interaction of Fusidic Acid and Atorvastatin," *American Journal of Kidney Diseases*, vol. 56, no. 5, pp. e11–e15, 2010.

[2] S. Kearney, A. S. Carr, J. McConville, and M. O. McCarron, "Rhabdomyolysis after co-prescription of statin and fusidic acid," *BMJ*, vol. 345, pp. e6562–e6562, 2012.

[3] T. A. Collidge, S. Razvi, C. Nolan et al., "Severe statin-induced rhabdomyolysis mimicking Guillain-Barré syndrome in four patients with diabetes mellitus treated with fusidic acid," *Diabetic Medicine*, vol. 27, no. 6, pp. 696–700, 2010.

[4] R. Cowan, P. D. Johnson, K. Urbancic, and M. L. Grayson, "A Timely Reminder About the Concomitant Use of Fusidic Acid With Statins," *Clinical Infectious Diseases*, vol. 57, no. 2, pp. 329–330, 2013.

[5] S. Teckchandani, S. Robertson, A. Almond, K. Donaldson, and C. Isles, "Rhabdomyolysis following co-prescription of fusidic acid and atorvastatin," *The Journal of the Royal College of Physicians of Edinburgh*, vol. 40, no. 1, pp. 33–36, 2010.

[6] N. T. Saeed and M. Azam, "'Rhabdomyolysis secondary to interaction between atorvastatin and fusidic acid," *BMJ Case Reports*, 2009.

[7] Y. Khaliq, K. Gallicano, R. Leger, B. Foster, and A. Badley, "A drug interaction between fusidic acid and a combination of ritonavir and saquinavir," *British Journal of Clinical Pharmacology*, vol. 50, no. 1, pp. 83-84, 2000.

[8] H. Eng, R. J. Scialis, C. J. Rotter et al., "The Antimicrobial Agent Fusidic Acid Inhibits Organic Anion Transporting Polypeptide-Mediated Hepatic Clearance and May Potentiate Statin-Induced Myopathy," *Drug Metabolism and Disposition*, vol. 44, no. 5, pp. 692–699, 2016.

[9] A. Gupta, J. J. Harris, J. Lin, J. P. Bulgarelli, B. K. Birmingham, and S. W. Grimm, "Fusidic acid inhibits hepatic transporters and metabolic enzymes: potential cause of clinical drug-drug interaction observed with statin coadministration," *Antimicrobial Agents and Chemotherapy*, vol. 60, no. 12, pp. 5986–5994, 2016.

[10] K. Bachoumas, M. Fiancette, J. Lascarrou, J. Lacherade, F. Leclair, and J. Reignier, "Fatal rhabdomyolysis following the co-prescription of fusidic acid and pravastatin," *Médecine et Maladies Infectieuses*, vol. 45, no. 10, pp. 417–419, 2015.

[11] C. Wenisch, R. Krause, P. Fladerer, I. El Menjawi, and E. Pohanka, "Acute rhabdomyolysis after atorvastatin and fusidic acid therapy," *The American Journal of Medicine*, vol. 109, no. 1, p. 78, 2000.

[12] C. Gabignon, V. Zeller, N. Le Guyader, N. Desplaces, O. Lidove, and J. Ziza, "Interaction atorvastatine et acide fusidique : une cause de rhabdomyolyse sévère," *La Revue de Médecine Interne*, vol. 34, no. 1, pp. 39–41, 2013.

[13] A. Nandy and S. Gaïni, "Severe Rhabdomyolysis as Complication of Interaction between Atorvastatin and Fusidic Acid in a Patient in Lifelong Antibiotic Prophylaxis: A Dangerous Combination," *Case Reports in Medicine*, vol. 2016, Article ID 4705492, 4 pages, 2016.

[14] A. J. Burtenshaw, G. Sellors, and R. Downing, "Presumed interaction of fusidic acid with simvastatin," *Anaesthesia*, vol. 63, no. 6, pp. 656–658, 2008.

[15] C. O'Mahony, V. L. Campbell, M. S. Al-Khayatt, and D. J. Brull, "Rhabdomyolysis with atorvastatin and fusidic acid," *Postgraduate Medical Journal*, vol. 84, no. 992, pp. 325–327, 2008.

A Report of Two Cases of Hazards Associated with High Flow Arteriovenous Fistula in ESRD Patients

Vipuj Shah,[1] Rakesh Navuluri,[2] Yolanda Becker,[3] and Mary Hammes[1]

[1]Department of Medicine, Section of Nephrology, University of Chicago, Chicago, IL, USA
[2]Department of Interventional Radiology, University of Chicago, Chicago, IL, USA
[3]Department of Transplant Surgery, University of Chicago, Chicago, IL, USA

Correspondence should be addressed to Mary Hammes; mhammes@medicine.bsd.uchicago.edu

Academic Editor: Władysław Sułowicz

High flow arteriovenous fistulas are a common clinical entity affecting patients with end-stage renal failure receiving hemodialysis. Given the difficulty in predicting who will develop a high flow arteriovenous fistula the exact prevalence is unclear. We present two cases of patients with high flow arteriovenous fistula that developed clinical cardiac failure at a time point after the fistula was placed with findings of significant cephalic arch stenosis. Both patients required treatment of cephalic arch stenosis with balloon angioplasty with subsequent surgical aneurism resection. Accurate and timely diagnosis of high flow arteriovenous hemodynamics by prospective monitoring of volumetric flow and cardiac function is required to halt this process prior to cardiac compromise.

1. Introduction

The long term outcome of autologous arteriovenous fistulas (AVF) remains poor, contributing to patient morbidity and immense economic burden. In a recent large meta-analysis of 12,383 patients with AVF, the primary failure rate was found to be 23%; at one year 40% of patients either had a failed access or required at least one intervention to maintain patency [1]. Guidelines support a peripheral-to-central sequence of AVF construction beginning with a lower arm AVF so as preserve as many sites as possible for future access creation [2]. Unfortunately, the primary failure rate of AVF is most marked in the lower arm [3]. Because of this higher failure rate, many upper arm AVFs are being placed. Upper arm AVF, especially brachiocephalic fistulas (BCF), have a number of long term complications, including higher flow rates and greater incidence of cephalic arch stenosis (CAS), compared with lower arm AVF [4, 5]. A high flow AVF is defined when the volumetric flow is greater than 1,500 mL/min [6]. We review two cases of high flow AVF with complications of CAS, cardiac failure and aneurysms. The discussion that follows reviews important clinical considerations and treatment options for high flow AVF.

2. Case Reports

Case 1. A 36-year-old African American female, with PMH of systemic lupus erythematosus, hypertension, seizures, hypothyroidism, and end-stage renal disease (ESRD) had been receiving hemodialysis for 5 years as a result of end-stage disease secondary to lupus nephropathy. Hemodialysis was started in 2012 via a right IJ permcath with right brachiocephalic (BCF) creation later that same year. The patient received hemodialysis three days a week and began developing access complications in 2015. She was referred to vascular surgery on two occasions because of prolonged bleeding postdialysis. Venograms performed on both occasions showed marked tortuosity of the venous outflow with focal CAS that was treated with angioplasty using a standard 7 mm balloon. In February 2016 she was admitted from the pulmonary hypertension clinic with hypervolemia in the setting of volume overload. Her chief complaint at admission was fatigue and orthopnea, causing her to sleep sitting in a chair for the past two days, and edema. The patient had been unable to obtain her dry weight at dialysis due to hypotension and cramping. In addition she had been having prolonged bleeding postdialysis from her AVF. The

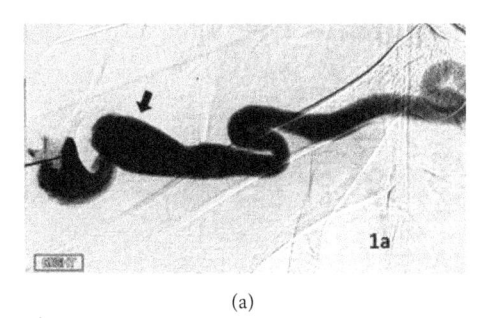

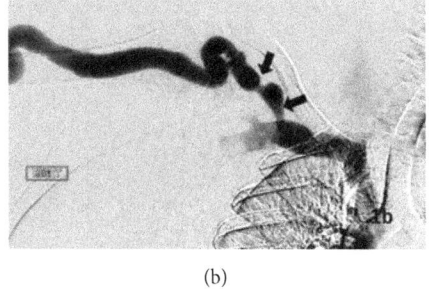

FIGURE 1: Venogram for Case 1 of venous outflow with tortuosity and aneurysms (arrow) (a). Venogram for Case 1 of cephalic arch with marked tortuosity and tight short segment stenosis (arrows) (b).

patient had been adherent to a dialysis treatment schedule of three days a week and complex medication regime which included amlodipine, clonidine, hydralazine, lasix, labetalol, levetiracetam, levothyroxine, simvastatin, topiramate, and renvela. On physical exam vitals showed a blood pressure of 159/94 with a pulse of 83. Cardiac exam showed normal rate and rhythm, 4/6 systolic ejection murmur heard best at the RUSB with radiation to the carotids which increased with inspiration, and a loud S2. Jugular venous distension was present to the mid neck as was hepatojugular reflex to the anterior ear. Lungs were clear; however 2+ lower leg edema was present. Transthoracic echo showed elevated right ventricular systolic pressure consistent with pulmonary hypertension. The patient was diagnosed with heart failure with preserved ejection fraction (HFpEF) due to diastolic dysfunction and high flow state. The patient was treated with aggressive ultrafiltration with hemodialysis to establish lower dry weight. In March 2016, the patient was again referred to access surgery for prolonged bleeding, difficulty with cannulation and expansile aneurysms. An AVF venous Duplex ultrasound showed volumetric flow measured mid upper arm to be 5180 ml/min. Venogram done at this time showed large aneurysms and tortuous venous outflow (Figure 1(a)) with multiple short tight stenoses in the cephalic arch (Figure 1(b)). This outflow narrowing at the cephalic arch was presumed to be the causative factor for the presenting history of prolonged bleeding and the decision was made to pursue angioplasty. Initial angioplasty was performed using a Mustang 8 mm × 40 mm standard pressure balloon catheter (Boston Scientific, Marlborough, MA) rated up to 20 atm. Postangioplasty imaging demonstrated only moderate improvement. Thus a second angioplasty was performed using a Conquest 8 mm × 40 mm high-pressure angioplasty balloon catheter (C.R. Bard, Murray Hill, NJ) rated up to 40 atm. The more peripheral stenosis opened to 5.5 mm from 4 mm, which equated to a 27% improvement in stenosis. The more central stenosis opened to 5 mm diameter from 2 mm and equated to a 60% improvement in stenosis. Postangioplasty venography demonstrated subjectively improved flow and satisfactory resolution of the stenoses. Due to the high flow state and aneurysms the patient was taken to the OR in April 2016 and the two aneurysms were resected and brought together with end to side anastomosis. Over the following months, the patient returned for angioplasty of the cephalic arch stenosis on two occasions but had marked improvement in symptoms of heart failure, with follow-up venous Duplex ultrasound on Jan 30, 2017, which showed volumetric flow measured mid upper arm to be 1244 ml/min.

Case 2. A 53-year-old African American male with PMH of hypertension and drug use had been receiving hemodialysis for 6 years as a consequence of end-stage renal disease secondary to hypertension. After failed attempts at a left lower nondominate arm AVF, a left BCF was placed in 2011. Over the years the BCF developed large aneurysms at sites of repeated cannulation. In 2015, the patient presented to the Emergency Room with chief complaint of altered mental status. Symptoms at presentation included disorientation to place and time and missed medication and inability to care for himself. He had been receiving hemodialysis three days a week. Clinically during the preceding weeks, the patient was experiencing marked dyspnea with exertion and lower extremity edema, cramping with hemodialysis and inability to achieve prescribed dry weight. Medications on admission included amlodipine, sensipar, hydralazine, megace, pantoprazole, thiamine, and renvela. Physical exam showed a blood pressure of 198/110 a pulse of 106. He was oriented only to person. Lungs were clear, cardiac exam normal S1, S2, 2+ edema. Left AVF was very dilated from the anticubital area to the mid arm. There were multiple large aneurysms which were nontender, thinning skin, but there is no evidence of excoriation. The workup including CT was negative for an intracerebral event. Blood cultures were drawn and came back positive with growth of alpha hemolytic strep treated with intravenous vancomycin and cefepime for 6 weeks. The source of the bacteremia was unclear and a venous Duplex of the access and an echo was done. The AVF Duplex ultrasound study showed a volumetric flow of 10,731 mL/min measured in the mid venous outflow. An echocardiogram done showed moderate LVH, moderate dilation of the right atrium, and marked increase in left atrial volume. Patient was discharged and at subsequent hemodialysis the patient was found to have elevated venous pressures which prompted interrogation via a fistulogram. The venogram study was done in June 2016 with findings of long segment tight CAS (Figure 2(a)) and two large aneurysms (Figure 2(b)). The outflow narrowing at the cephalic arch was presumed to be the causative factor for the presenting history of elevated venous pressures at dialysis

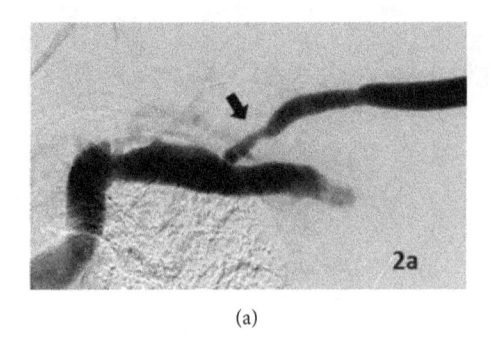

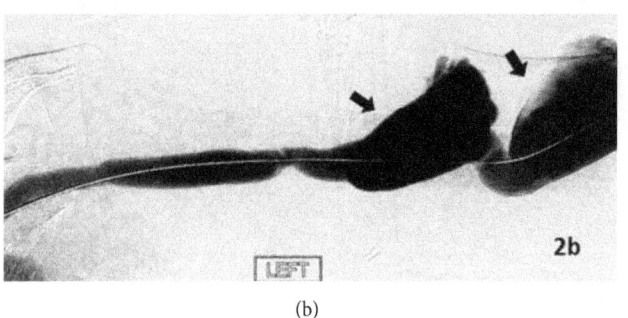

Figure 2: Venogram for Case 2 of cephalic arch with long segment stenosis (arrow) (a). Venogram for Case 2 of venous outflow with marked aneurysms (arrows) (b).

and the decision was made to pursue angioplasty. Initial angioplasty was performed using a Mustang 7 mm × 40 mm standard pressure balloon catheter (Boston Scientific, Marlborough, MA) rated up to 20 atm. Postangioplasty imaging demonstrated only moderate improvement. Thus a second angioplasty was performed using a larger Mustang 9 mm × 40 mm standard pressure angioplasty balloon catheter (Boston Scientific, Marlborough, MA) rated up to 18 atm. The cephalic arch stenosis opened up to 6 mm from 3.5 mm, which equated to a 42% improvement in stenosis. Postangioplasty venography demonstrated subjectively improved flow and satisfactory resolution of the stenosis. In August 2016 the patient underwent revision of the left upper extremity AVF with a jump graft inserted, followed by interval ligation and excision of two large pseudo aneurysms. After surgery, the AVF was able to be used with hemodialysis delivered at a 450 mL/min blood flow without the need for central venous catheter access. The patient's volume status was better managed after the AVF revision and subsequently went on to receive a renal transplant in May 2017.

3. Discussion

The two cases reported summarize characteristics and complex clinical complications of heart failure, aneurisms, and CAS. These three problems occur commonly together and while a cause and effect are not clearly defined, we are concerned that the high flows diagnosed in upper arm AVF contribute to pulmonary hypertension and high output heart failure and ultimately contribute to CAS. Cephalic arch stenosis once it develops is very difficult to treat often requires repeat angioplasty and stents and may lead to access failure [5].

The diagnosis of a high flow AVF is complicated [7]. One needs to have a high index of suspicion and then determine the volumetric flow in the AVF and the cardiac output. When determining the volumetric flow of the AVF, it is commonly measured in the proximal, mid, and distal venous outflow which may differ dramatically. The volumetric flow should be measured at the feeding brachial artery as it is most reproducible, there is ease of brachial artery imaging and there is less turbulent blood flow when compared to Doppler flow measured throughout the venous conduit [8]. Ko et al.

have devised a "Fast, 5-min Dialysis Duplex Scan" which correlates with brachial artery volume flow as a predictor of dialysis access flow maturation and successful hemodialysis [8]. While we acknowledge the limitation of not having brachial artery volume flow available for our case reports, we recommend that the brachial artery be used in future Duplex studies when evaluating an AVF for volumetric flow. High output heart failure may be diagnosed with a transthoracic echo but may require a right heart catheterization for definitive diagnosis [9]. A simple clinical maneuver that can easily aide in the diagnosis is the Nicoladoni-Branham sign [10]. This is performed by occluding the AVF for 30 seconds which may cause bradycardia and increased blood pressure which occurs as a result of the normalization of the cardiac output with AVF compression. Nonetheless, the diagnosis must be confirmed as if high output heart failure is left untreated; it will contribute to cardiovascular and access complications.

High flow within a vascular access for hemodialysis develops over time. As an AVF ages, increased flow within the artery and vein induces dilation, resulting in a gradual reduction in resistance. The resultant high flow circuit leads to altered hemodynamics causing intimal hyperplasia. Intimal hyperplasia results in venous stenosis which causes increased venous pressure, aneurysms, eventual decreased blood flow rate, and venous thrombosis. This, in turn, results in the need for a multitude of access procedures to maintain patency and ultimately may result in access failure. High flow in an AVF will lead to pathological accelerated access growth and cardiac overload. In the BCF all blood flow is committed to traversing the cephalic arch unless there are penetrating veins that communicate with the basilica system. Flows as great as 2,000 mL/min may enter the axillary vein and high flow of over 1000 mL/min predict CAS [11, 12]. BCF access have an increase in cross-sectional area and a dramatic increase in blood flow (mean 1,983 ± 1,199 ml/min) when compared to lower arm AVF [13]. The cases presented illustrate the detrimental sequelae of high flow in an upper arm BCF.

Previous studies have shown that wall shear stress (WSS) plays a significant role in regulating the function of endothelial cells [14]. High and laminar WSS is related to normal endothelial function which has anti-inflammatory and anti-neointimal hyperplasia activity [15]. With high flow, there are low flow pockets that occur in the curves of vessels as evident in the cephalic arch [16]. Low flow causes disturbed WSS which is associated with vascular endothelial dysfunction resulting in neointimal hyperplasia and a predisposition to the development of CAS [17]. Occurrence of neointimal hyperplasia has an inverse relationship with WSS and is also related to flow patterns [18]. The physiology proposed is that, after arteriovenous fistula creation, high flows cause increased pressure and wall shear stress necessary for AVF maturation. With time low shear stress, described as recirculation zones, develops in the curve of the arch which causes endothelial cell dysfunction and resultant cephalic arch stenosis [16]. As the venous stenosis impedes flow, pressures rise. CAS creates a vicious cycle of high pressure causing tortuous veins and aneurysms. Over time, these extremes cause an abnormal complex interplay between biologic factors that induce outward remodeling and physical factors of wall tension with the end result of the mega-fistula [7].

Cardiovascular disease remains the number one cause of death in ESRD patients. Both traditional risk factors such as diabetes, peripheral vascular disease, and hypertension and nontraditional risk factors such as increased inflammatory markers, homocysteine, anemia, hyperparathyroidism, endothelial dysfunction, and abnormal lipoprotein B are commonly found in hemodialysis patients and can increase cardiovascular mortality [19]. Studies have shown that a 15% increase in cardiac output occurs early after AVF creation by the seventh day [20]. There is a relationship between cardiac output and high flow in an AVF leading to late complications such as high output heart failure manifest as increased left ventricular end-diastolic volume and pulmonary hypertension [21–26].

According to K/DOQI guidelines, asymptomatic aneurysms do not require intervention and should be managed by avoiding cannulation of the aneurysmal areas [2]. Careful cannulation techniques using rope and ladder or area cannulation are best practice when the AVF is mature for use to prevent aneurysms. Management of AVF aneurysms is generally based on clinical signs and symptoms, assessment of overlying skin, ease of cannulation, and functionality of AVF. The diameter of the aneurysm is not an indication for treatment. Venography can define anatomic anatomy of the aneurysm and the presence of upstream venous stenosis such as CAS. The main indication for treatment is based on clinical presentation. Bleeding from an AV aneurysm can be severe and life-threatening. It can occur spontaneously, after hemodialysis treatment when needles are removed or secondary to trauma. Some of the predisposing risk factors to bleeding are thinning or erosion of overlying skin layer, rapidly expanding aneurysm, anticoagulation, prolonged bleeding time after removal of hemodialysis needles, and increased intra-access pressure. In patient with prolonged active bleeding with the above-mentioned signs, immediate surgery is essential. Inadequate dialysis in the setting of aneurysms may be due to as impaired arterial flow or venous outflow stenosis. The treatment is that such cases should be focused on the lesion responsible for low flow and angioplasty would be recommended. However, if there is a risk of bleeding from the aneurysm with associated stenosis, recommended treatments are either an open surgical approach or a covered stent with or without angioplasty. Aneurysmorrhaphy has been an approach to treat high flow AVF resulting in high output congestive heart failure [27]. Multiple surgical treatment techniques have been described in the literature but it is difficult to compare treatment modalities due to lack of randomized control trials.

Any ESRD patient with a history of congestive heart failure or progressive left ventricular hypertrophy should have vascular access flow measured. Access flow may be measurement monthly in the clinical setting using a saline ultrasound dilution method (Transonic Hemodialysis Monitor HDO2 Transonic Systems Incorporated, Ithaca, NY, USA) [28]. We acknowledge the limitation of not providing intradialytic measurements of cardiac output in the present study. The transonic device provides a wealth of longitudinal information that would help to identify and prevent high output AVF and cardiac failure. The ultrasound dilution technique can be used to determine both the access flow (greater than 2 L/min) and the cardiac output (greater than 5 L/min). An access flow to cardiac output ratio greater than 25% may be associated with increased risk of high output cardiac failure [22, 26]. When high access flow is detected and correlated with adverse outcomes such as CAS, high output heart failure, and steal syndrome a difficult decision must be made and every attempt to salvage the AVF. Banding has been shown to be an effective intervention to decrease flow and treat steal syndrome in high flow AVF [29–31].

High flow AVF is a common clinical problem that has been loosely defined, but no doubt contributes to cardiac risk and access complications. Prospective trials to follow the volumetric flow in AVF access and its relationship to cardiac dysfunction are needed. We need to define and then optimize blood flow to prevent these long term complication associated with AVF access.

Acknowledgments

This publication was made possible in part by the National Institute of Diabetes and Digestive Diseases (NIDDK) and the National Institutes of Health (NIH) under Award no. RO1DK090769.

References

[1] A. A. Al-Jaishi, M. J. Oliver, S. M. Thomas et al., "Patency rates of the arteriovenous fistula for hemodialysis: a systematic review and meta-analysis," *American Journal of Kidney Diseases*, vol. 63, no. 3, pp. 464–478, 2014.

[2] Vascular Access Work Group, "Clinical practice guidelines for vascular access," *American Journal of Kidney Diseases*, vol. 48, supplement 1, pp. S248–S273, 2006.

[3] P. P. G. M. Rooijens, J. H. M. Tordoir, T. Stijnen, J. P. J. Burgmans, A. A. E. A. de Smet, and T. I. Yo, "Radiocephalic wrist arteriovenous fistula for hemodialysis: Meta-analysis indicates

a high primary failure rate," *European Journal of Vascular and Endovascular Surgery*, vol. 28, no. 6, pp. 583–589, 2004.

[4] M. Hammes, B. Funaki, and F. L. Coe, "Cephalic arch stenosis in patients with fistula access for hemodialysis: Relationship to diabetes and thrombosis," *Hemodialysis International*, vol. 12, no. 1, pp. 85–89, 2008.

[5] D. K. Rajan, T. W. I. Clark, N. K. Patel, S. W. Stavropoulos, and M. E. Simons, "Prevalence and treatment of cephalic arch stenosis in dysfunctional autogenous hemodialysis fistulas," *Journal of Vascular and Interventional Radiology*, vol. 14, no. 5, pp. 567–573, 2003.

[6] P. Bourquelot and J. Stolba, "Vascular access surgery for hemodialysis and central venous stenosis," *Nephrologie*, vol. 22, no. 8, pp. 491–494, 2001.

[7] G. A. Miller and W. W. Hwang, "Challenges and Management of High-Flow Arteriovenous Fistulae," *Seminars in Nephrology*, vol. 32, no. 6, pp. 545–550, 2012.

[8] S. H. Ko, D. F. Bandyk, K. D. Hodgkiss-Harlow, A. Barleben, and J. Lane, "Estimation of brachial artery volume flow by duplex ultrasound imaging predicts dialysis access maturation," *Journal of Vascular Surgery*, vol. 61, no. 6, pp. 1521–1528, 2015.

[9] A. B. Stern and P. J. Klemmer, "High-output heart failure secondary to arteriovenous fistula," *Hemodialysis International*, vol. 15, no. 1, pp. 104–107, 2011.

[10] H. B. Burchell, "Observations on bradycardia produced by occlusion of an artery proximal to an arteriovenous fistula (Nicoladoni-Branham sign)," *Medical Clinics of North America*, vol. 42, no. 4, pp. 1029–1035, 1958.

[11] R. H. Vaes, J. H. Tordoir, and M. R. Scheltinga, "Systemic effects of a high-flow arteriovenous fistula for hemodialysis," *Journal of Vascular Access*, vol. 15, no. 3, pp. 163–168, 2014.

[12] A. Jaberi, D. Schwartz, R. Marticorena et al., "Risk factors for the development of cephalic arch stenosis," *Journal of Vascular Access*, vol. 8, no. 4, pp. 287–295, 2007.

[13] R. Albayrak, S. Yuksel, M. Colbay et al., "Hemodynamic changes in the cephalic vein of patients with hemodialysis arteriovenous fistula," *Journal of Clinical Ultrasound*, vol. 35, no. 3, pp. 133–137, 2007.

[14] P. F. Davies, "Hemodynamic shear stress and the endothelium in cardiovascular pathophysiology," *Nature Clinical Practice Cardiovascular Medicine*, vol. 6, no. 1, pp. 16–26, 2009.

[15] C. Hahn and M. A. Schwartz, "Mechanotransduction in vascular physiology and atherogenesis," *Nature Reviews Molecular Cell Biology*, vol. 10, no. 1, pp. 53–62, 2009.

[16] M. Hammes, M. Boghosian, K. Cassel et al., "Increased inlet blood flow velocity predicts low wall shear stress in the cephalic arch of patients with brachiocephalic fistula access," *PLoS ONE*, vol. 11, no. 4, Article ID e0152873, 2016.

[17] L. Jia, L. Wang, and F. Wei, "Effects of wall shear stress in venous neointimal hyperplasia of arteriovenous fistulae," *Nephrology*, vol. 20, no. 5, pp. 335–342, 2015.

[18] A. Remuzzi, B. Ene-lordache, and L. Moscomi, "Radial artery wall shear stress evaluation in patients with arteriovenous fistula hemodialysis access," *Biorheology*, vol. 40, no. 1-3, pp. 423–430, 2003.

[19] J. M. MacRae, "Vascular access and cardiac disease: Is there a relationship?" *Current Opinion in Nephrology and Hypertension*, vol. 15, no. 6, pp. 577–582, 2006.

[20] Y. Iwashima, T. Horio, Y. Takami et al., "Effects of the creation of arteriovenous fistula for hemodialysis on cardiac function and natriuretic peptide levels in CRF," *American Journal of Kidney Diseases*, vol. 40, no. 5, pp. 974–982, 2002.

[21] A. A. Beigi, A. M. M. Sadeghi, A. R. Khosravi, M. Karami, and H. Masoudpour, "Effects of the arteriovenous fistula on pulmonary artery pressure and cardiac output in patients with chronic renal failure," *Journal of Vascular Access*, vol. 10, no. 3, pp. 160–166, 2009.

[22] C. Basile, C. Lomonte, L. Vernaglione, F. Casucci, M. Antonelli, and N. Losurdo, "The relationship between the flow of arteriovenous fistula and cardiac output in haemodialysis patients," *Nephrology Dialysis Transplantation*, vol. 23, no. 1, pp. 282–287, 2008.

[23] C. Kariyawasam, R. Gajanayaka, R. Raut, P. Lisawat, and W. Shih, "Pulmonary hypertension develops following arteriovenous fistula placement for hemodialysis," *Am J Kidney Disease*, vol. 65, no. 4, p. A132, 2015.

[24] Z. Abassi, F. Nakhoul, E. Khankin, S. A. Reisner, and M. Yigla, "Pulmonary hypertension in chronic dialysis patients with arteriovenous fistula: Pathogenesis and therapeutic prospective," *Current Opinion in Nephrology and Hypertension*, vol. 15, no. 4, pp. 353–360, 2006.

[25] S. Yilmaz, M. Yetim, B. Yilmaz et al., "High hemodialysis vascular access flow and impaired right ventricular function in chronic hemodialysis patients," *Indian Journal of Nephrology*, vol. 26, no. 5, pp. 352–356, 2016.

[26] J. M. MacRae, C. Dipchand, M. Oliver et al., "Arteriovenous access: Infection, neuropathy, and other complications," *Canadian Journal of Kidney Health and Disease*, vol. 3, no. 1, article no. 9127, 2016.

[27] P. Balaz and M. Björck, "True aneurysm in autologous hemodialysis fistulae: Definitions, classification and indications for treatment," *Journal of Vascular Access*, vol. 16, no. 6, pp. 446–453, 2015.

[28] N. M. Krivitski, "Theory and validation of access flow measurement by dilution technique during hemodialysis," *Kidney International*, vol. 48, no. 1, pp. 244–250, 1995.

[29] F. Van Hoek, M. Scheltinga, M. Luirink, H. Pasmans, and C. Beerenhout, "Banding of hemodialysis access to treat hand ischemia or cardiac overload," *Seminars in Dialysis*, vol. 22, no. 2, pp. 204–208, 2009.

[30] M. R. Scheltinga, F. van Hoek, and C. M. A. Bruyninckx, "Surgical banding for refractory hemodialysis access-induced distal ischemia (HAIDI)," *Journal of Vascular Access*, vol. 10, no. 1, pp. 43–49, 2009.

[31] G. A. Miller, N. Goel, A. Friedman et al., "The MILLER banding procedure is an effective method for treating dialysis-associated steal syndrome," *Kidney International*, vol. 77, no. 4, pp. 359–366, 2010.

Clinical Relapses of Atypical HUS on Eculizumab: Clinical Gap for Monitoring and Individualised Therapy

Chia Wei Teoh,[1,2,3] Kathleen Mary Gorman,[2] Bryan Lynch,[4] Timothy H. J. Goodship,[5] Niamh Marie Dolan,[2] Mary Waldron,[6] Michael Riordan,[2] and Atif Awan[2]

[1]Division of Nephrology, The Hospital for Sick Children, Toronto, ON, Canada
[2]Department of Paediatric Nephrology & Transplantation, The Children's University Hospital, Temple Street, Dublin 1, Ireland
[3]Department of Paediatrics, University of Toronto, Toronto, ON, Canada
[4]Department of Neurology, The Children's University Hospital, Temple Street, Dublin 1, Ireland
[5]Institute of Genetic Medicine, Newcastle University, International Centre for Life, Central Parkway, Newcastle upon Tyne, UK
[6]Department of Paediatric Nephrology, Our Lady's Children's Hospital, Crumlin, Dublin 12., Ireland

Correspondence should be addressed to Chia Wei Teoh; chiawei.teoh@sickkids.ca

Academic Editor: Salih Kavukcu

Atypical hemolytic uremic syndrome (aHUS) is caused by dysregulation of the complement system. A humanised anti-C5 monoclonal antibody (eculizumab) is available for the treatment of aHUS. We present the first description of atypical HUS in a child with a coexistent diagnosis of a POL-III leukodystrophy. On standard eculizumab dosing regime, there was evidence of ongoing C5 cleavage and clinical relapses when immunologically challenged. Eculizumab is an effective therapy for aHUS, but the recommended doses may not be adequate for all patients, highlighting the need for ongoing efforts to develop a strategy for monitoring of treatment efficacy and potential individualisation of therapy.

1. Introduction

Atypical hemolytic uremic syndrome (aHUS) is a rare disorder characterised by thrombotic microangiopathy and renal failure. It is a disease of complement dysregulation associated with poor prognosis and high mortality with up to 50% progressing to end-stage renal disease [1]. It accounts for 5–10% of children presenting with HUS and approximately 60% of cases are associated with an inherited and/or acquired abnormality of complement [2].

In 2011, a humanised anti-C5 monoclonal antibody (eculizumab) was licenced for treating aHUS in the USA and Europe. The efficacy and safety of its use were demonstrated in adults and children with aHUS, with and without identified pathogenic variants in complement activating/regulating factors or CFH-autoantibodies [3–6]. Eculizumab therapy in aHUS caused by a gain-of-function pathogenic variant of complement factor B (CFB) is described [7]. Despite excellent clinical response with standard recommended dosage, there was laboratory evidence of ongoing excessive complement activation.

POL-III [4H leukodystrophy (4H)] leukodystrophy is characterised by a triad of hypomyelination, hypodontia, and hypogonadotropic hypogonadism [8]. First described in 2003, it consists of 5 overlapping phenotypes, which were initially presented as similar but distinct disease entities [8]. Pathogenic variants in 2 genes coding for subunits of RNA polymerase III, *POLR3a* (10q22.3) and *POLR3b* (12q23.3), were identified with genotype-phenotype correlation. Variants in *POL3a* are more severely affected with a later onset, faster regression, and shorter life [9].

We provide the first report of aHUS in a patient with POL-III leukodystrophy. There were clinical relapses when immunologically challenged and laboratory evidence of excessive complement activation on eculizumab therapy. This case emphasises the need to develop a strategy for monitoring treatment efficacy and potential individualisation of anticomplement therapy. It also highlights the need to consider alternative diagnoses should there be discordant genotype-phenotype features.

2. Case Report

A previously well male infant born to nonconsanguineous Irish parents presented at 9 months old with a two-day history of fever, vomiting, nonbloody diarrhea, irritability, and poor feeding. This was preceded by an upper respiratory tract infection (URTI) a week prior to presentation. He received a second dose of H1N1 vaccine two weeks previously. At presentation, he was pale and irritable with petechial rash, had microscopic hematuria and proteinuria, and was hypertensive (systolic blood pressure of 140 mmHg). He developed hypertensive encephalopathy with seizures requiring labetalol, sodium nitroprusside, and phenytoin infusions.

Investigations at presentation revealed thrombotic microangiopathy (hemoglobin, 105 g/L; platelets 77×10^9/L; lactate dehydrogenase (LDH) 4795 U/L, blood film showed numerous red cell fragments) and impaired renal function (urea 8.5 mmol/L, creatinine 90 μmol/L). Stools were positive for rotavirus but negative for E. coli 0157 and verotoxin. Urinary protein/creatinine ratio (PCR) was 2851 mg/mmol. The patient's ADAMTS13 activity, complement C3 and C4 were normal. A diagnosis of aHUS was suspected, direct sequencing of the entire coding regions for CFH, CFI, CD46, DGKε, and C3 did not reveal any disease causing variant and multiplex ligation-dependant probe amplification analysis for deletions, and duplications of CFH, CFHR1, and CFHR3 exons were negative. Sequencing of CFB identified a missense heterozygous variant of c.724A>C (Chr 6:31915584 (p.Ile242Leu, rs144812066)), a benign variant as it was identified in his phenotypically normal mother, common in ExAC control database and predicted to be benign by in silico programs.

He received eight daily sessions of plasma exchanges (PE) with clinical improvement and subsequently relapsed on day 15 leading to resumption of daily PE. He required at least twice weekly PE but was gradually weaned over the course of 6 months, until eventual discontinuation at 15 months old (total 64 sessions of PE). Although LDH remained persistently elevated (620–925 U/L), full blood count (FBC), plasma creatinine, and haptoglobin levels normalised. Urinary PCR fell to <50 mg/mmol. He remained in clinical remission for 18 months.

The first clinical relapse of aHUS occurred at 33 months of age, preceded by an URTI (hemoglobin 102 g/L, platelets 39×10^9/L, LDH 1785 U/L, haptoglobin 0.06 g/L, and creatinine 35 μmol/L). He received the first dose of eculizumab 600 mg, which led to clinical, haematological, and biochemical improvement within two days, and was maintained on fortnightly doses (300 mg) thereafter. On fortnightly eculizumab regimen, he presented with three relapses, in the setting of immunological challenges (vaccination and URTI). Clinical, haematological, and biochemical improvement occurred within 2-3 days of eculizumab infusion with each relapse (Figure 1).

Since the first relapse, he remained hypertensive requiring captopril, amlodipine, and carvedilol. On fortnightly

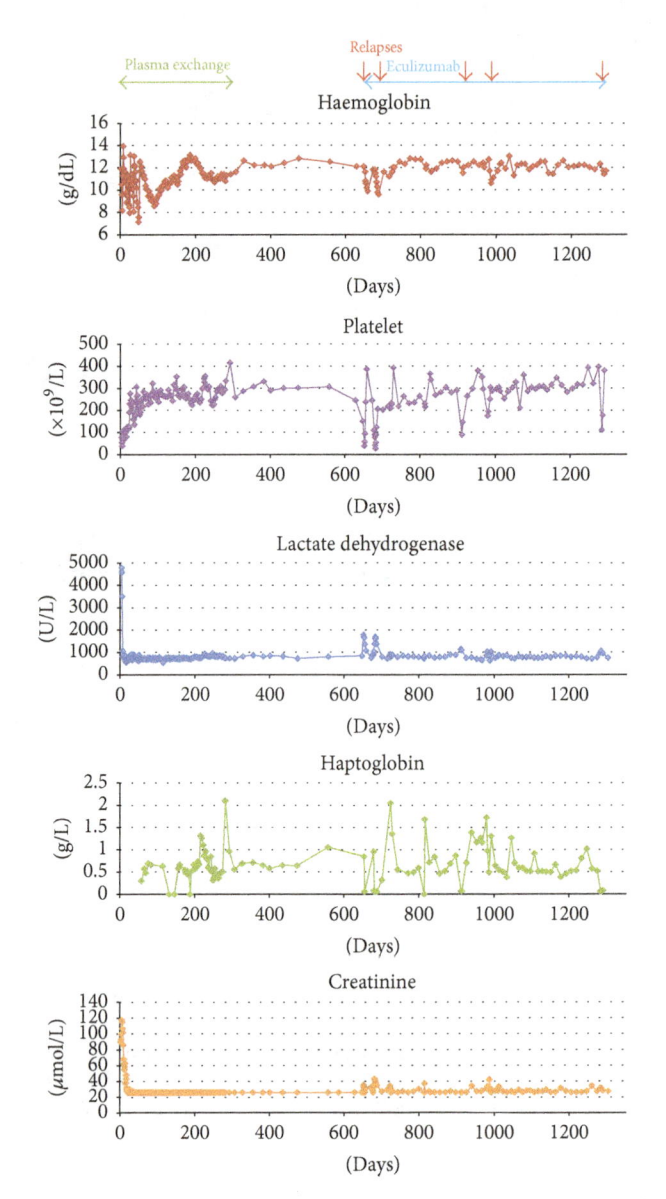

FIGURE 1: Graphical illustration of aHUS patient's clinical course and treatment. Clinical relapses depicted by red arrows.

eculizumab, FBC, plasma creatinine, haptoglobin, and C3/C4 levels remained within normal limits, with persistently elevated LDH (630–881 U/L). The alternative and classical complement pathways were suppressed confirming drug action (CH50 and AP50 hemolytic assays < 10%). Although clinically in remission (Hb 122 g/L, platelets 380×10^9/L, LDH 707 U/L, haptoglobin 1.16 g/L, and creatinine 26 μmol/L), plasma sC5b-9 concentrations measured 14 days after eculizumab dose were high at 240 ng/ml. The high sC5b-9 was interpreted as ongoing dysregulated complement activation and his maintenance eculizumab dose was changed to 300 mg every 10 days. Eight weeks after decreasing the interdose interval, sC5b-9 concentration remained elevated at 227 ng/ml (10 days after eculizumab dose) despite clinical remission (Hb 125 g/L, platelet 309×10^9/L, LDH 756 U/L, haptoglobin 0.51 g/L, and creatinine 27 μmol/L) and adequate trough eculizumab levels (>600 μg/ml) with levels >99 μg/ml considered to be therapeutic.

During follow-up, it became evident that he had global developmental delay. Careful review of his history demonstrated subtle gross and fine motor delays were present prior to his initial presentation with aHUS (sat with support at 9 months, not reaching for objects/transferring). He made slow developmental progress, without regression. At 4 years, he could stand with support, had palmar but no pincer grip, and only two words with meaning. He had good understanding, could follow 4-step commands, and was sociable and interactive. Examination at 4 years showed occipitofrontal circumference less than the 0.2nd centile, bilateral optic nerve pallor, hypodontia, truncal ataxia, upper limb tremor, and hypotonia. Therefore, an alternate pathology to the aHUS and associated hypertensive encephalopathy was required to explain the preexisting developmental delay and neurological deficits.

A MRI brain performed at 10 months following initial presentation showed subtle changes in the basal ganglia. He underwent extensive genetic and metabolic work-up including karyotype, microarray, PLP gene, very long chain fatty acids, paired serum and CSF glucose and amino acids, CSF neurotransmitters, urinary organic acids, and skin and muscle biopsy, all of which were negative. Two subsequent MRI brain scans at 2.25 and 3.5 years showed very delayed myelination with no progression since the original scan showing hypomyelination, increased T2 signal in the basal ganglia with volume loss, and cerebellar atrophy. Based upon these findings, he was diagnosed with 4H syndrome with subsequent confirmation of compound heterozygous mutation of *POL3B* (c.1568T>A, p. Val523Glu and c. 1464+1 G>A), reported previously [10].

Eculizumab treatment was discontinued after careful consideration with his parents due to ongoing relapses and the diagnosis of a progressive severe neurological condition.

3. Discussion

Pathogenic variants in *CFB* result in the formation of C3bBb (C3 convertase) which is resistant to decay by CFH and decay accelerating factor, resulting in increased quantities of active convertase [7]. Eculizumab is an anti-C5 monoclonal antibody, which prevents cleavage of C5 by C5 convertase, preventing the assembly of the membrane attack complex and generation of C5a. It is effective in treating aHUS associated with a variety of complement disorders [3–6, 11–13], including CFB mutation [7].

In our patient, a persistent, mildly elevated LDH and clinical relapses while on eculizumab prompted further investigations which showed that although the classical and alternative pathways were fully suppressed (CH50 and AP50 levels < 10%), plasma sC5b-9 concentration remained elevated, a finding which persisted despite reducing the interdose interval to 10 days, with high trough drug levels. This finding has been previously reported [14, 15], suggesting ongoing C5 cleavage that may explain the relapses. Volokhina et al. reported normalisation of sC5b-9 levels during remission [16]. The use of soluble complement profile as diagnostic and/or prognostic biomarkers remains debatable as highlighted by Noris et al. who reported inconsistent complement profiles in patients with aHUS regardless of whether they had any complement genetic mutations [17]. In that study, up to 64% of patients had markers of complement activation which persisted in a subgroup of patients despite clinical remission with treatment [17]. These discrepancies emphasise the need to develop a strategy for monitoring treatment efficacy that can be used to individualise eculizumab therapy in patients with aHUS [18].

The heterozygous variant in CFB did not explain our patient's phenotype. Whole exome sequencing did not identify any other disease causing variant. Up to 40% of patients with aHUS have no identified disease-causing variant [2]. Our patient also had a clinical and genetically confirmed diagnosis of 4H leukodystrophy. To date, there are no reports of any association with aHUS or defects in the complement system. 4H leukodystrophy is a spectrum of disorders with genotype-phenotype correlations [9]. The variant in our patient has been described previously but no further information is available on his clinical course [10]. This case emphasises the importance of considering separate diagnoses in a patient with a complex medical history. The clinical picture in this setting could have been assumed to be due to his prolonged illness and ICU admission at presentation. However, identification of preceding neurodevelopmental delay, clinical examinations, and recognition of typical MRI features of 4H leukodystrophy were key to the diagnosis [9].

4. Conclusion

We report an aHUS patient with no identified pathogenic variant, who responded to eculizumab therapy, but with ongoing clinical relapses during periods of immunological challenges, despite adequate drug levels. To our knowledge, he is the only patient with aHUS to be diagnosed with 4H leukodystrophy, which became apparent on follow-up with neurodevelopmental delay that was not in keeping with the initial diagnosis. Our case highlights the importance of maintaining a high index of suspicion for a separate diagnosis in a patient with a complex medical history, especially with discordant genotype-phenotype features. Further studies are necessary to reconcile these conflicting results (absent CH50/AP50 activity with elevated sC5b-9 concentration), to ascertain the best method for monitoring adequacy of eculizumab therapy to inform future individualisation of aHUS therapy.

Authors' Contributions

Drs. Teoh and Gorman conceptualized, drafted, reviewed, and revised the manuscript. Drs. Lynch, Dolan, Riordan, Waldron, and Awan and Professor Goodship contributed to the concept and design of the report and critically reviewed the manuscript. All authors approved the final manuscript as submitted and agree to be accountable for all aspects of the work.

References

[1] M. Noris and G. Remuzzi, "Atypical hemolytic-uremic syndrome," *The New England Journal of Medicine*, vol. 361, no. 17, pp. 1676–1687, 2009.

[2] C. Loirat and V. Frémeaux-Bacchi, "Atypical hemolytic uremic syndrome," *Orphanet Journal of Rare Diseases*, vol. 6, article 60, 2011.

[3] C. M. Legendre, C. Licht, P. Muus et al., "Terminal complement inhibitor eculizumab in atypical hemolytic-uremic syndrome," *The New England Journal of Medicine*, vol. 368, no. 23, pp. 2169–2181, 2013.

[4] C. Licht, L. A. Greenbaum, P. Muus et al., "Efficacy and safety of eculizumab in atypical hemolytic uremic syndrome from 2-year extensions of phase 2 studies," *Kidney International*, vol. 87, no. 5, pp. 1061–1073, 2015.

[5] L. A. Greenbaum, M. Fila, G. Ardissino et al., "Eculizumab is a safe and effective treatment in pediatric patients with atypical hemolytic uremic syndrome," *Kidney International*, vol. 89, no. 3, pp. 701–711, 2016.

[6] F. Fakhouri, M. Hourmant, J. M. Campistol et al., "Terminal complement inhibitor eculizumab in adult patients with atypical hemolytic uremic syndrome: a single-arm, open-label trial," *American Journal of Kidney Diseases*, vol. 68, no. 1, pp. 84–93, 2016.

[7] R. D. Gilbert, D. J. Fowler, E. Angus, S. A. Hardy, L. Stanley, and T. H. Goodship, "Eculizumab therapy for atypical haemolytic uraemic syndrome due to a gain-of-function mutation of complement factor B," *Pediatric Nephrology*, vol. 28, no. 8, pp. 1315–1318, 2013.

[8] S. Atrouni, A. Darazé, J. Tamraz, A. Cassia, C. Caillaud, and A. Mégarbané, "Leukodystrophy associated with oligodontia in a a large inbred family: fortuitous association or new entity?" *American Journal of Medical Genetics*, vol. 118, no. 1, pp. 76–81, 2003.

[9] N. I. Wolf, A. Vanderver, R. M. van Spaendonk et al., "Clinical spectrum of 4H leukodystrophy caused by POLR3A and POLR3B mutations," *Neurology*, vol. 83, no. 21, pp. 1898–1905, 2014.

[10] M. Tétreault, K. Choquet, S. Orcesi et al., "Recessive mutations in POLR3B, encoding the second largest subunit of Pol III, cause a rare hypomyelinating leukodystrophy," *American Journal of Human Genetics*, vol. 89, no. 5, pp. 652–655, 2011.

[11] N. Besbas, B. Gulhan, D. Karpman et al., "Neonatal onset atypical hemolytic uremic syndrome successfully treated with eculizumab," *Pediatric Nephrology*, vol. 28, no. 1, pp. 155–158, 2013.

[12] F. S. Cayci, N. Cakar, V. S. Hancer, N. Uncu, B. Acar, and G. Gur, "Eculizumab therapy in a child with hemolytic uremic syndrome and CFI mutation," *Pediatric Nephrology*, vol. 27, no. 12, pp. 2327–2331, 2012.

[13] S. I. Al-Akash, P. S. Almond, V. H. Savell Jr., S. I. Gharaybeh, and C. Hogue, "Eculizumab induces long-term remission in recurrent post-transplant HUS associated with C3 gene mutation," *Pediatric Nephrology*, vol. 26, no. 4, pp. 613–619, 2011.

[14] E. Goicoechea de Jorge, C. L. Harris, J. Esparza-Gordillo et al., "Gain-of-function mutations in complement factor B are associated with atypical hemolytic uremic syndrome," *Proceedings of the National Acadamy of Sciences of the United States of America*, vol. 104, no. 1, pp. 240–245, 2007.

[15] R. Vilalta, E. Lara, A. Madrid et al., "Long-term eculizumab improves clinical outcomes in atypical hemolytic uremic syndrome," *Pediatric Nephrology*, vol. 27, no. 12, pp. 2323–2326, 2012.

[16] E. B. Volokhina, D. Westra, T. J. A. M. van der Velden, N. C. A. J. van de Kar, T. E. Mollnes, and L. P. van den Heuvel, "Complement activation patterns in atypical haemolytic uraemic syndrome during acute phase and in remission," *Clinical & Experimental Immunology*, vol. 181, no. 2, pp. 306–313, 2015.

[17] M. Noris, M. Galbusera, S. Gastoldi et al., "Dynamics of complement activation in aHUS and how to monitor eculizumab therapy," *Blood*, vol. 124, no. 11, pp. 1715–1726, 2014.

[18] C. W. Teoh, M. Riedl, and C. Licht, "The alternative pathway of complement and the thrombotic microangiopathies," *Transfusion and Apheresis Science*, vol. 54, no. 2, pp. 220–231, 2016.

Fatal Pneumococcus Sepsis after Treatment of Late Antibody-Mediated Kidney Graft Rejection

Gunilla Einecke,[1] Jan Hinrich Bräsen,[2] Nils Hanke,[1] Hermann Haller,[1] and Anke Schwarz[1]

[1]Department of Nephrology and Hypertension, Hannover Medical School, Hannover, Germany
[2]Department of Pathology, Hannover Medical School, Hannover, Germany

Correspondence should be addressed to Gunilla Einecke; einecke.gunilla@mh-hannover.de

Academic Editor: Władysław Sułowicz

Antibody-mediated rejection (ABMR) is a major cause of late renal allograft dysfunction and graft loss. Risks and benefits of treatment of late ABMR have not been evaluated in randomized clinical trials. We report on a 35-year-old patient with deterioration in renal function and progressive proteinuria 15 years after transplantation. Recurrent infections after a splenectomy following traumatic splenic rupture 3 years earlier had led to reduction of immunosuppression. Renal transplant biopsy showed glomerular double contours, 40% fibrosis/tubular atrophy, peritubular capillaritis, and positive C4d staining indicating chronic-active ABMR. ABMR treatment was initiated with steroids, plasmapheresis, and rituximab. Fourteen days later, she presented to the emergency department with fever, diarrhea, vomiting, and hypotension. Despite antibiotic treatment she deteriorated with progressive hypotension, capillary leak with pleural effusion, peripheral edema, and progressive respiratory insufficiency. She died due to septic shock five days after admission. Blood cultures showed *Streptococcus pneumoniae*, consistent with a diagnosis of overwhelming postsplenectomy infection syndrome, despite protective pneumococcus vaccination titers. We assume that the infection was caused by one of the strains not covered by the Pneumovax 23 vaccination. The increased immunosuppression with B cell depletion may have contributed to the overwhelming course of this infection.

1. Introduction

Antibody-mediated renal allograft rejection (ABMR) is a major cause of late allograft dysfunction and graft loss [1–3]. The clinical impact of ABMR has been increasingly appreciated since the recognition of C4d negative antibody-mediated rejection, which can be diagnosed in the absence of C4d staining, based on microcirculation lesions and the presence of circulating donor specific antibodies alone [4]. This modification of the diagnostic classification has resulted in a higher incidence of the diagnosis of ABMR [5], especially in late deterioration of graft function, and supported the recognition of the contribution of late ABMR to graft loss [6].

Clinical presentation and course of disease are heterogeneous, with rapid graft loss (within months after diagnosis) in some patients and slow progression of disease over years in others [5, 7]. There are no reliable factors to predict the natural clinical course or response to treatment for an individual patient [8]. Treatment options include increase in maintenance immunosuppression, antibody removal, and B cell depleting strategies. In contrast to early ABMR, where benefit of treatment has been shown in clinical trials, there are no large randomized trials to evaluate the benefits and side effects of treatment of late ABMR. Therefore, treatment strategies are not standardized, and decisions regarding type and intensity of treatment have to be made on an individual basis, trying to weigh the chances of treatment success with prolongation of graft survival against the risks of increased immunosuppression. In the absence of systematic evaluation of side effects of ABMR treatment with plasma exchange and rituximab, the clinical impression in many centers is that treatment with plasma exchange does "little harm" and that rituximab therapy is generally well tolerated with few side effects (personal communication). Thus, in many cases of ABMR, the perceived threat of graft loss outweighs the perceived risks of increased immunosuppression, and the decision is made in favor of active treatment of rejection.

Here, we report on a young patient with chronic-active ABMR in whom the decision was made for treatment with steroids, plasma exchange, and rituximab (despite severely impaired graft function and chronic changes by histology) in an attempt to stabilize kidney function and prolong the time before her return to dialyses, but in whom our treatment resulted in fatal outcome.

2. Case Presentation

We report on a 36-year-old female patient who presented to our clinic fifteen years following kidney transplantation with deterioration in renal allograft function.

The patient had been diagnosed in 05/1992 with rapid progressive, severe diffuse necrotizing intra- and extracapillary proliferative glomerulonephritis (p-ANCA positive). In 06/1995 she received a kidney transplant. Initial immunosuppression consisted of steroids and cyclosporine. Due to early steroid-resistant vascular rejection, she received treatment with OKT3, and maintenance immunosuppression was switched from cyclosporine to tacrolimus. Renal function improved slowly, and she reached a baseline creatinine of ~180 μmol/l (~2.0 mg/dl).

During the following years, the clinical course was complicated by recurrent infections: CMV reactivation (07/1996), upper respiratory infections with otitis media, and tympanoplasty of the right ear (1996); recurrent urinary tract infections and recurrent axillary and inguinal abscess formation (since 2004), which resulted in repeated prolonged periods of antibiotic prophylaxis; anogenital condyloma (09/2003); HSV-II infection (02/2009). In 12/2003 a bone marrow biopsy was performed for evaluation of prolonged leukocytosis; hematologic disorder was ruled out. In 07/2006 the patient had a splenectomy following traumatic splenic rupture. Subsequently, she was vaccinated with pneumococcus polyvalent vaccine (Pneumovax 23).

Renal function was largely stable over a course of 15 years, with intermittent deterioration in function (Figure 1) which led to several biopsies. The first biopsy (04/2003) showed borderline rejection with interstitial edema and mild vascular rejection, but the following biopsies showed mainly chronic changes with signs of nephrosclerosis, arteriolar hyalinosis, and increasing interstitial fibrosis and tubular atrophy (07/2003, 11/2005, and 08/2009). Because these changes were consistent with calcineurin inhibitor toxicity, immunosuppression with tacrolimus was discontinued and switched to dual therapy with prednisolone plus mycophenolate mofetil 3 × 500 mg/day.

A year later (10/2010), the patient presented with severe decline in renal function (creatinine 332 μmol/l (3.8 mg/dl), eGFR 40 ml/min) and increased proteinuria (1.85 g/l). Renal biopsy was performed; however, the biopsy core was not representative. Histology was suspicious for rejection, but formal criteria for this diagnosis were not met. Due to intercurrent infection (fever (>39°C) with signs of otitis media and urinary tract infection (*E. faecalis* and *Proteus mirabilis*)), no changes

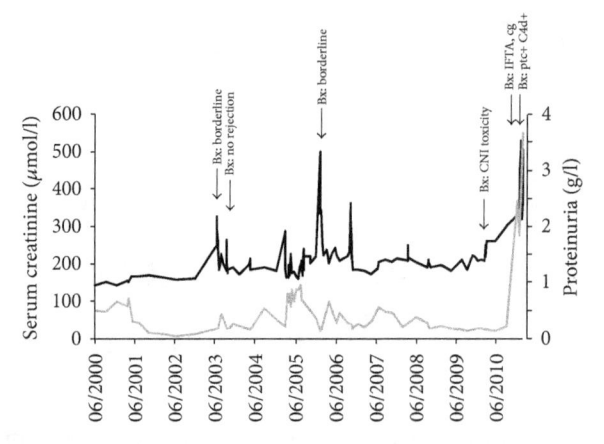

FIGURE 1: *Renal function and proteinuria over time*. Renal function remained largely stable over 15 years, with intermittent decreases in renal function that led to transplant biopsies.

to the immunosuppression were made at this time. Antibiotic therapy with Ampicillin/Sulbactam was initiated and resulted in resolution of clinical and laboratory signs of infection. Renal function continued to decline (creatinine 452 μmol/l (5.1 mg/dl), eGFR < 20 ml/min). Considering the histologic changes suggestive of rejection in the biopsy performed 10 days earlier, steroid bolus therapy was initiated (3 × 500 mg) but did not result in improvement of renal function (creatinine 530 μmol/l (6.0 mg/dl), proteinuria 3.5 g/l). Repeat transplant biopsy was performed and showed signs of chronic-active ABMR (peritubular capillaritis with positive C4d staining, glomerular double contours, and severe atrophy/fibrosis) (Figure 2). Circulating HLA antibodies were detected (PRA I 24%, PRA II 30%), which were donor specific (HLA-A*24 (MFI 16422); HLA-DQ*05 (MFI 21521)). After critical discussion of risks and benefits of ABMR treatment, the decision was made for active treatment of ABMR, which was initiated with 3 cycles of plasma exchange, followed by rituximab (375 mg/m^2). With this treatment, renal function stabilized with a creatinine of 320 μmol/l (3.6 mg/dl) and the patient was discharged.

2.1. Follow-Up and Outcome. Fourteen days later she presented to the emergency department with acute onset of nausea, vomiting, diarrhea, and fever (39°C) which had begun a few hours earlier. She had noted decreasing urinary output over the last few days with peripheral edema and therefore had taken increased doses of diuretic medication. At presentation, temperature was 39.5°C, blood pressure 76/40 mmHg, heart rate 140/min, and oxygen saturation 95%. She felt weak but was able to walk. Lab results showed leukopenia (2.3 × 10^3/μl), anemia (hemoglobin 9.1 g/dl), and decreased renal function (creatinine 408 μmol/l = 4.6 mg/dl) but were otherwise unremarkable (normal range for platelet count, coagulation, liver function tests, and C-reactive protein). Urinalysis was not possible due to oliguria. Chest X-ray showed no indication for pneumonia but small pleural effusion. Oxygen saturation was initially 83% but stabilized at 97% with 3 l/min. The initial clinical presentation was

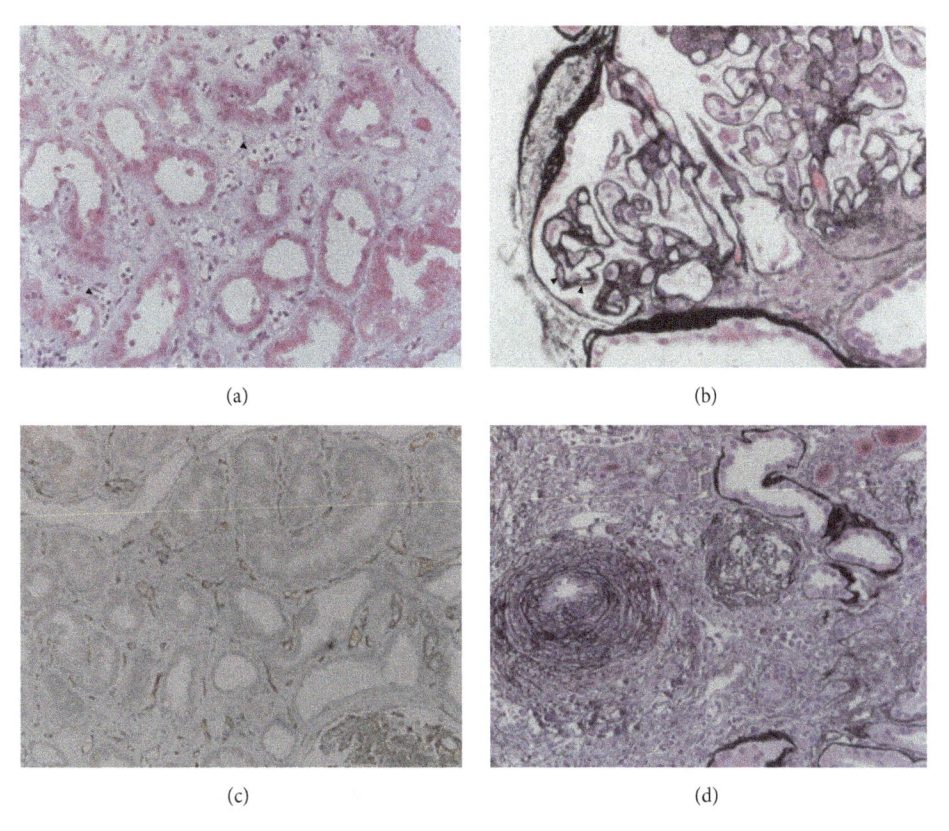

Figure 2: *Histologic assessment of renal transplant biopsy.* The biopsy showed signs of chronic-active antibody-mediated rejection with severe tubular damage, interstitial edema, and peritubular capillaritis ((a) arrowheads); glomerulitis with double contours ((b) arrowheads); diffuse positive C4d staining in peritubular capillaries (c); and interstitial fibrosis with severe arteriosclerosis (d). ((a) H&E, (b) and (d) Jones methenamine, and (c) C4d immunohistochemistry; original magnification: (a) and (b) ×60, (c) ×20, and (d) ×40).

suggestive of acute gastroenteritis with volume depletion, and volume substitution was initiated. However, the peripheral edema and pleural effusion were suspicious of capillary leakage, suggesting alternative disease mechanisms. Considering the immunosuppressed state, empiric antibiotic therapy was initiated with levofloxacin despite lack of strong evidence of bacterial infection.

Over the next few hours, continuous volume substitution was necessary to stabilize the blood pressure; the patient became anuric and showed progressive respiratory insufficiency. She was transferred to the intensive care unit 8 hours after admission. Vasopressor therapy was initiated, and the patient was intubated 3 hours later. Laboratory evaluation showed metabolic acidosis (HCO3 11 mmol/l, pH 7.18, lactate 9.8 mmol/l), thrombopenia (53 Tsd/μl), disturbed coagulation (PTT 118 s, INR 2.66), CRP (53 mg/l), and procalcitonin (337 μg/l). Antibiotic therapy was escalated (switch to Piperacillin/Tazobactam and Moxifloxacin plus Caspofungin). Dialysis treatment was initiated. Microbiology results from blood cultures drawn at time of admission revealed infection with *Streptococcus pneumoniae*. The antibiogram confirmed susceptibility to the current antibiotic treatment. Nevertheless, the patient could not be stabilized and showed progressive multiorgan failure with capillary leak, respiratory failure (PaO2 50 mmHg with 100% FiO2), circulatory failure, renal failure, and disseminated intravascular coagulation. Despite all supportive measures, she died 5 days after admission.

3. Discussion

The clinical course of our patient, together with detection of *Streptococcus pneumoniae* in the blood cultures, is consistent with a diagnosis of overwhelming postsplenectomy infection (OPSI) syndrome. In patients after splenectomy, the incidence of the OPSI syndrome is 0.4–7.2 cases/1000 patient-years [9, 10]. Mortality in patients with OPSI is high (50–70%) [9–13]. The risk for OPSI syndrome is highest in the first 2-3 years after splenectomy but remains lifelong [9, 14]. Vaccination against pneumococcus is recommended in all patients with splenectomy. Indication for daily use of prophylactic antibiotics in patients after splenectomy is a gray zone. In adult patients there is no clear recommendation for such prophylaxis [15]; however, the clinical course of our patient would support use of such prophylactic treatment with increased immunosuppression.

Our patient had been vaccinated with pneumococcus polyvalent vaccine (Pneumovax 23) following the splenectomy three years earlier. Our initial suspicion was that the ABMR treatment with plasma exchange plus rituximab had resulted in depletion of the vaccination titer, thereby enhancing the patient's susceptibility to infection with *Streptococcus pneumoniae*. The effect of therapeutic apheresis on specific antibody levels against bacterial antigens is not well documented and has been investigated only in small patient groups. A significant reduction of total IgG and IgM levels including reduction of antibodies against pneumococcus and *Haemophilus* polysaccharide antigens has been reported following immunoadsorption [16, 17]. After plasma exchange, no data is available for total IgG or pneumococcus antibodies; however a reduction of anti-measles antibody by 40% has been shown after plasma exchange [18]. Rituximab treatment has not been proven to have significant impact on serum immunoglobulin G levels, probably because CD20 negative long-lived plasma cells maintain antibody production [19]. We retrospectively assessed immunoglobulin levels and vaccination titers before and after ABMR treatment in our patient. Immunoglobulins were removed with plasma exchange (demonstrated by significant concentrations in the waste bag), and serum IgG levels decreased significantly after treatment (7.99 g/l before treatment, 1.02 g/l after the second plasma exchange) (Figure 3). Similarly, the pneumococcus vaccination titer was significantly decreased after treatment (9.9 mg/l) compared to the titer before initiation of ABMR therapy (34.2 mg/l). However, even the titer after therapy remains in the range considered to be protective against pneumococcus infection (laboratory reference values). Thus we assume that the infection in our patient was caused by one of the few *Streptococcus pneumoniae* strains not covered by the Pneumovax 23 vaccination. The distribution of serotypes (Germany, 2009/2010) shows that ~90% of capsular polysaccharides in invasive pneumococcal disease are contained in the 23-valent polysaccharide vaccine and ~10% of polysaccharides are not [20].

However, regardless of the effect of the treatment on IgG levels or vaccination titers, it must be considered that the B cell depletion induced by treatment with rituximab may have contributed to the increased susceptibility to infection and the overwhelming course of disease in our patient. Few data are available regarding the association of rituximab with infection in organ transplant recipients. A retrospective study by Grim et al. observed no increased risk of infectious complications following rituximab therapy in renal transplant recipients [21]. In another study of 77 kidney transplant patients who received rituximab therapy, the incidence of bacterial infection was similar between these patients and another kidney transplant control group who did not receive rituximab, whereas the viral infection rate was significantly lower and the rate of fungal infection was significantly higher in the rituximab group [22]. Scemla et al. reported bacterial, viral, and fungal infection rates at 55.3%, 47.4%, and 13.2%, respectively, in kidney transplant patients who received rituximab therapy; however, no control group was included in this study [23]. Thus, there is some evidence that the use of rituximab after kidney transplantation is associated with a risk of infectious disease; but randomized controlled trials to confirm this association are lacking. The increased susceptibility to infection with encapsulated bacteria in patients after splenectomy is probably due to a defect in B cell function, that is, lack or reduction of memory B cells

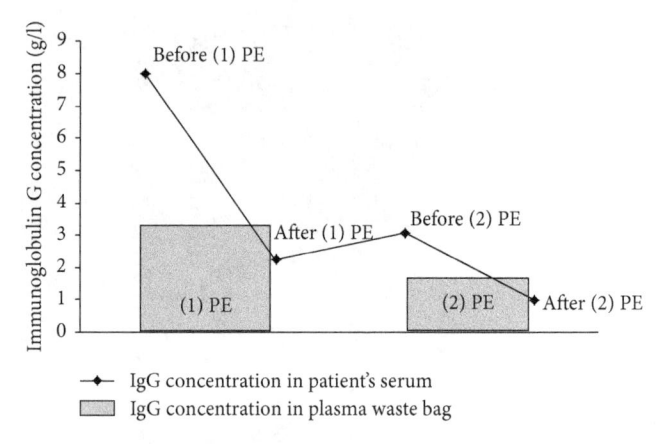

FIGURE 3: *Effect of plasmapheresis on immunoglobulin concentration.* We measured the concentration of immunoglobulin G in the patient's serum before and after the first and second plasma exchanges and in the plasma waste bag. Serum concentration dropped significantly during the course of treatment.

which reside in the spleen [24]. Our patient had responded to the vaccination with adequate titers indicating sufficient B cell function to maintain a certain level of humoral response. However, treatment with rituximab probably depleted those remaining B cells, making it impossible for her to mount a humoral immune response against an infection with strains containing unknown polysaccharides.

Since no data from prospective randomized clinical trials are available to guide treatment decisions in late ABMR, the decision has to be made on an individual basis, trying to weigh the potential benefits with improvement or at least stabilization of renal function against the risks of increased immunosuppression. Standard treatment protocols are based on removal of antibodies (plasmapheresis, immunoadsorption), suppression of new antibody production (rituximab, bortezomib), and immune modulation with intravenous immunoglobulin (IVIG), which has immunomodulatory effects on B and T cells at high dose. New therapeutic opportunities may arise with treatments targeting the complement cascade (eculizumab), interleukin 6 (tocilizumab), or immunoglobulin G-degrading enzyme of *Streptococcus pyogenes* (called IdeS), an endopeptidase that cleaves human IgG into $F(ab')_2$ and Fc fragments, inhibiting complement-dependent cytotoxicity and antibody-dependent cellular cytotoxicity. However, these are experimental strategies whose treatment benefit will need to be assessed in the future and that were not available at the time we were treating our patient. The alternative options in our patient would have been a less aggressive approach to treatment of ABMR. These options include (1) avoiding apheresis in this splenectomized patient, optimizing maintenance immunosuppression, and preparing patient for dialysis; (2) optimizing maintenance immunosuppression, treat ABMR with multiple infusions of small doses of IvIg, and prepare patient for dialysis. However, in many cases, as in our patient, the perceived threat of graft loss with return to dialysis outweighs the perceived risks of increased immunosuppression, and the decision is made in favor of active treatment of rejection. The course of our patient should be kept in mind to remember how severe the side effects of these treatments can be. That the splenectomy in our patient did not prevent formation of antibodies and development of ABMR is of interest. Some protocols for treatment or prevention of ABMR in sensitized patients include splenectomy as a strategy to reduce or prevent antibody production. However, considering the course of our patient, the splenectomy seems to have had no protective effect regarding development of DSA or the clinical course of ABMR.

Considering these severe side effects with no documented benefit of treatment of late ABMR, management of renal transplant patients should focus on avoiding development of this disease. It should be remembered that too much lowering of maintenance immunosuppression may put the patient at risk for ABMR, resulting overall in a higher total burden of immunosuppression which may be harmful to the patient. In retrospect, it has to be questioned whether the discontinuation of tacrolimus after the biopsy in 2009 was the right decision in our patient. Renal function had been reasonably stable until then and showed rapid decline a year later with histologic and serologic signs of antibody-mediated rejection. This decision was based on a histologic diagnosis of CNI toxicity. However, it has to be kept in mind that the histologic lesions that are used to diagnose CNI toxicity are nonspecific. In multivariate analysis, the presence of arteriolar hyalinosis (one of the key lesions used to diagnose CNI toxicity) is not associated with graft loss [3, 25]. In many cases, the presence of arteriolar hyalinosis represents CNI effects (not toxicity) and may simply be an indication of adequate immunosuppression [26]; therefore, presence of arteriolar hyalinosis should not automatically result in discontinuation of CNI. However, whether an alternative immunosuppressive regimen would have delayed deterioration in renal function in our patient remains speculative.

As long as we lack information from prospective trials that identify reliable factors to predict the response to treatment and potential for recovery in individual patients and inform us about the risks and benefits of different treatment regimens, our decisions regarding type, intensity, and duration of treatment of late ABMR remain subjective and thus suboptimal and unsatisfactory.

4. Conclusions

As a result of our experience with this patient, we have modified our ABMR treatment to improve the safety of our protocol and to avoid unnecessary risks. Our consequences are the following:

(i) We do not routinely discontinue CNI therapy with declining renal function since it is one of the most effective immunosuppressants for prevention of ABMR.

(ii) We continue to use rituximab as treatment of ABMR as part of a structured treatment protocol with structured and detailed follow-up. The published data on ABMR treatment is ambiguous regarding benefit of treatment with rituximab; however we believe it is not proven yet that there is no benefit at all, and more data is needed before a definite recommendation can be made.

(iii) We refrain from treatment with rituximab if interstitial fibrosis is severe (we use an arbitrary cut-off >30%) and/or renal function is marginal (arbitrary cut-off < 25 ml/min). In these patients, we limit our treatment to steroids, plasma exchange, and high dose immunoglobulins and possibly increase maintenance immunosuppression.

(iv) In those patients who do receive B cell depleting therapies, we now have lower thresholds for use of antibiotic prophylaxis during treatment of ABMR.

(v) We substitute a total of 0.5 g/kg immunoglobulins in patients who are treated with plasmapheresis. While most of this substitution is given at the end of the complete plasmapheresis course, a proportion (arbitrary choice of 5 g) is given after each single plasmapheresis treatment in order to avoid complete depletion of immunoglobulins between the treatments.

Abbreviations

ABMR: Antibody-mediated rejection
eGFR: Estimated glomerular filtration rate
OPSI syndrome: Overwhelming postsplenectomy infection syndrome
IVIG: Intravenous immunoglobulins.

Authors' Contributions

Gunilla Einecke was involved in clinical management of this patient and wrote the manuscript; Jan Hinrich Bräsen reviewed the kidney transplant biopsies, prepared the histologic images, reviewed the manuscript, and approved the final version of the manuscript; Nils Hanke was involved in the clinical management of this patient, obtained the data on immunoglobulin concentrations, reviewed the manuscript, and approved the final version of the manuscript; Hermann Haller and Anke Schwarz were involved in clinical management of this patient, reviewed the manuscript, and approved the final version of the manuscript.

Acknowledgments

Several clinical teams were involved in the care of the patients described in this case report, including the transplant team and the teams of the nephrology ward, the emergency ward, and the intensive care unit. They all contributed to the clinical management of this patient.

References

[1] J. Sellarés, D. G. de Freitas, M. Mengel et al., "Understanding the causes of kidney transplant failure: the dominant role of antibody-mediated rejection and nonadherence," *American Journal of Transplantation*, vol. 12, no. 2, pp. 388–399, 2012.

[2] Z. M. El-Zoghby, M. D. Stegall, D. J. Lager et al., "Identifying specific causes of kidney allograft loss," *American Journal of Transplantation*, vol. 9, no. 3, pp. 527–535, 2009.

[3] G. Einecke, B. Sis, J. Reeve et al., "Antibody-mediated microcirculation injury is the major cause of late kidney transplant failure," *American Journal of Transplantation*, vol. 9, no. 11, pp. 2520–2531, 2009.

[4] M. Haas, B. Sis, LC. Racusen, K. Solez, D. Glotz, RB. Colvin et al., "meeting report: inclusion of c4d-negative antibody-mediated rejection and antibody-associated arterial lesions," *American Journal of Transplantation*, vol. 14, no. 2, pp. 272–283, 2013.

[5] S. A. De Serres, R. Noël, I. Côté et al., "2013 Banff Criteria for Chronic Active Antibody-Mediated Rejection: Assessment in a Real-Life Setting," *American Journal of Transplantation*, vol. 16, no. 5, pp. 1516–1525, 2016.

[6] M. Haas, "The revised (2013) Banff classification for antibody-mediated rejection of renal allografts: update, difficulties, and future considerations," *American Journal of Transplantation*, vol. 16, no. 5, pp. 1352–1357, 2016.

[7] R. R. Redfield, T. M. Ellis, W. Zhong et al., "Current outcomes of chronic active antibody mediated rejection - A large single center retrospective review using the updated BANFF 2013 criteria," *Human Immunology*, vol. 77, no. 4, pp. 346–352, 2016.

[8] C. Gosset, C. Lefaucheur, and D. Glotz, "New insights in antibody-mediated rejection," *Current Opinion in Nephrology and Hypertension*, vol. 23, no. 6, pp. 597–604, 2014.

[9] A. di Sabatino, R. Carsetti, and G. R. Corazza, "Post-splenectomy and hyposplenic states," *The Lancet*, vol. 378, no. 9785, pp. 86–97, 2011.

[10] S. Ram, L. A. Lewis, and P. A. Rice, "Infections of people with complement deficiencies and patients who have undergone splenectomy," *Clinical Microbiology Reviews*, vol. 23, no. 4, pp. 740–780, 2010.

[11] N. Bisharat, H. Omari, I. Lavi, and R. Raz, "Risk of infection and death among post-splenectomy patients," *Infection*, vol. 43, no. 3, pp. 182–186, 2001.

[12] R. W. Thomsen, W. M. Schoonen, D. K. Farkas et al., "Risk for hospital contact with infection in patients with splenectomy: A population-based cohort study," *Annals of Internal Medicine*, vol. 151, no. 8, pp. 546–555, 2009.

[13] M. H. Kyaw, E. M. Holmes, F. Toolis et al., "Evaluation of severe infection and survival after splenectomy," *American Journal of Medicine*, vol. 119, no. 3, pp. 276–e7, 2006.

[14] R. J. Holdsworth, A. D. Irving, and A. Cuschieri, "Postsplenectomy sepsis and its mortality rate: actual versus perceived risks," *British Journal of Surgery*, vol. 78, no. 9, pp. 1031–1038, 1991.

[15] C. Theilacker and W. V. Kern, "Sepsisprävention nach Splenektomie," *DMW - Deutsche Medizinische Wochenschrift*, vol. 138, no. 34/35, pp. 1729–1733, 2013.

[16] G. Kumlien, L. Ullström, A. Losvall, L.-G. Persson, and G. Tydén, "Clinical experience with a new apheresis filter that specifically depletes ABO blood group antibodies," *Transfusion*, vol. 46, no. 9, pp. 1568–1575, 2006.

[17] P. V. Valli, G. P. Yung, T. Fehr et al., "Changes of circulating antibody levels induced by ABO antibody adsorption for ABO-incompatible kidney transplantation," *American Journal of Transplantation*, vol. 9, no. 5, pp. 1072–1080, 2009.

[18] U. Schönermarck, T. Kauke, G. Jäger et al., "Effect of Apheresis for ABO and HLA Desensitization on Anti-Measles Antibody Titers in Renal Transplantation," *Journal of Transplantation*, vol. 2011, pp. 1–6, 2011.

[19] M. K. Slifka and R. Ahmed, "Long-lived plasma cells: A mechanism for maintaining persistent antibody production," *Current Opinion in Immunology*, vol. 10, no. 3, pp. 252–258, 1998.

[20] Robert Koch Institut, Pneumoweb-Sentinel (2016) http://www.rki.de/DE/Content/Infekt/Sentinel/Pneumoweb/Pneumoweb_node.html.

[21] S. A. Grim, T. Pham, J. Thielke et al., "Infectious complications associated with the use of rituximab for ABO-incompatible and positive cross-match renal transplant recipients," *Clinical Transplantation*, vol. 21, no. 5, pp. 628–632, 2007.

[22] N. Kamar, O. Milioto, B. Puissant-Lubrano et al., "Incidence and predictive factors for infectious disease after rituximab therapy in kidney-transplant patients," *American Journal of Transplantation*, vol. 10, no. 1, pp. 89–98, 2010.

[23] A. Scemla, A. Loupy, S. Candon et al., "Incidence of infectious complications in highly sensitized renal transplant recipients treated by rituximab: A case-controlled study," *Transplantation*, vol. 90, no. 11, pp. 1180–1184, 2010.

[24] S. Kruetzmann, M. M. Rosado, H. Weber et al., "Human immunoglobulin M memory B cells controlling Streptococcus pneumoniae infections are generated in the spleen," *The Journal of Experimental Medicine*, vol. 197, no. 7, pp. 939–945, 2003.

[25] R. S. Gaston, J. M. Cecka, B. L. Kasiske et al., "Evidence for antibody-mediated injury as a Major determinant of late kidney allograft failure," *Transplantation*, vol. 90, no. 1, pp. 68–74, 2010.

[26] G. Einecke, J. Reeve, and P. F. Halloran, "Hyalinosis Lesions in Renal Transplant Biopsies: Time-Dependent Complexity of Interpretation," *American Journal of Transplantation*, vol. 17, no. 5, pp. 1346–1357, 2017.

Antiglomerular Basement Membrane Disease in a Pediatric Patient: A Case Report and Review of the Literature

Vimal Master Sankar Raj,[1] Diana Warnecke,[1] Julia Roberts,[2] and Sarah Elhadi[1]

[1]Department of Pediatric Nephrology, University of Illinois College of Medicine at Peoria, Peoria, IL, USA
[2]Department of Pediatrics, University of Illinois College of Medicine at Peoria, Peoria, IL, USA

Correspondence should be addressed to Vimal Master Sankar Raj; vraj@uicomp.uic.edu

Academic Editor: Kouichi Hirayama

Goodpasture's syndrome (GPS) remains a very rare disease entity in the pediatric population characterized by the presence of pulmonary hemorrhage and rapidly evolving glomerulonephritis. We hereby describe the case of a 2-year-old girl who presented with renal failure and was diagnosed with GPS. A brief review of the literature in regard to data on demographics, pathogenesis, clinical features, diagnosis, treatment, and prognosis for renal recovery is also provided.

1. Introduction

Goodpasture's syndrome (GPS) is a rare and life threatening autoimmune condition with autoantibodies directed against the glomerular basement membrane (GBM) antigen. The term GPS refers to the triad of pulmonary hemorrhage, glomerulonephritis, and anti-GBM antibodies while Goodpasture's disease (GD) is the preferred terminology in the absence of pulmonary hemorrhage [1, 2]. The term antiglomerular basement membrane antibody disease (aGD) describes a patient with serum antibodies against the basement membrane and includes both Goodpasture's syndrome and disease.

2. Case Report

A 2-year, 11-month-old Hispanic female presented to her primary care physician's office with swelling of the hands and face following one week of fever, sore throat, and malaise. A screening urine analysis (U/A) revealed 3+ protein and blood with numerous red blood cells per high power field. Further work-up also demonstrated anemia (Hb of 8.5 g/dl) and several electrolyte imbalances with azotemia (BUN 116 mg/dl and Cr 7.3 g/dl) prompting immediate transfer to our Children's Hospital for further evaluation and management.

On admission, examination revealed a pale child with bilateral mild pedal edema and blood pressure of 125/71 mm Hg. She was afebrile, mildly tachycardic, and saturating at 100% in room air and parents denied any h/o joint pain/swelling or skin rash. Her urine output was noted to be darker and less frequent over the past few days.

Past medical history was significant for an admission about 7 months back with respiratory distress and presumed pneumonia. Labs at that time were significant for severe anemia (Hb 6.9 g/dl) and iron deficiency. Initial chest X-ray showed bilateral diffuse peribronchial cuffing and nodular opacities with concerns for severe bronchiolitis/bronchopneumonia (Figure 1). Patient was started on empiric antibiotic coverage but respiratory distress worsened to the point of requiring ventilator support. A work-up at that time showed elevated erythrocyte sedimentation rate (113 mm/hr) and negative serology for antinuclear antibody. A respiratory viral pathogen array came back positive for rhino virus. Patient's clinical condition continued to deteriorate and patient was placed on extracorporeal membrane oxygenation (ECMO). During this time patient was also started on high dose methylprednisolone with presumptive exaggerated inflammatory response to her viral pneumonia in a bid to reduce inflammation. Patient had a dramatic response to steroids and was off ECMO in 2 days and off ventilator support within a week time. A U/A done during

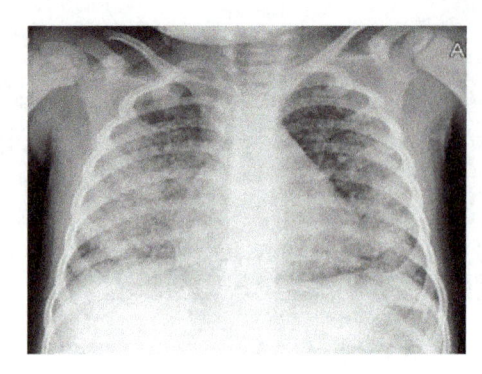

FIGURE 1: Chest X-ray on initial presentation.

TABLE 1: Comparison of lab values between prior and current admission.

Labs	10/2015	5/2016
Sodium (mmol/L)	141	137
Potassium (mmol/L)	4.2	6.0
Chloride (mmol/L)	110	113
Carbon dioxide (mmol/L)	21	8
Glucose (mg/dL)	109	97
BUN (mg/dL)	5	120
Creatinine (mg/dL)	0.41	7.01
Albumin (g/dL)	2.9	2.5
Calcium (mg/dL)	9.3	5.6
Phosphorus (mg/dL)		8.9
White blood cell ($\times 10^3$/mcL)	15.84	10.4
Hemoglobin (g/dL)	6.9	7.8
Hematocrit (%)	22.6	23.7
Platelets ($\times 10^3$/mcL)	616	234
Ferritin (ng/mL)	269	267
Iron (mcg/dL)	6	55
Transferrin (mcg/dL)	130	100
TIBC (mcg/dL)	Not done	125
% saturation	Not done	44
Parathyroid hormone (pg/mL)	Not done	1031
C3 (mg/dL)	166	114
C4 (mg/dL)	30	48
ESR (mm/hr)	113	12.5
CRP (mg/dl)	12.5	Not done

this past hospital stay showed 1+ blood and no protein and a chemistry panel showed normal renal function with a serum creatinine of 0.41 mg/dl.

Work-up during this current admission confirmed anemia (Hb 7.8 g/dl) with a slightly elevated white blood cell count (10,400/mm3) and platelet count (234,000/mm3). Serum chemistry panel was abnormal for hyperkalemia (6 mmol/L), metabolic acidosis (Hco3 of 8 mmol/L), hypocalcemia (5.6 mg/dl), hyperphosphatemia (8.9 mg/dl), and renal failure (BUN 120 mg/dl and Cr 7.01 mg/dl). Further work-up involved evaluation as to identify the cause of glomerulonephritis and showed normal complement levels, normal coagulation profile, negative serology for viral etiology, lupus, and ANCA titers. Parathyroid hormone levels were elevated indicating a state of chronic kidney damage. ESR was elevated at 24 mm/hr but lesser than the prior admission value of 113 mm/hr and a CRP was not checked during the current admission. Urine protein to creatinine ratio was in the nephrotic range and antiglomerular basement membrane (GBM) titers were sent. Urine output recorded was between 1.5 and 2 ml/kg/hr during the initial few days but progressively got oliguric (0.3 to 0.5 ml/kg/hr) from the first week onwards. Renal ultrasound showed normal sized kidneys (right and left kidney around 7.2 cm) with increased cortical echogenicity bilaterally. A comparison of lab values during prior hospital stay and current admission is provided in Table 1.

Patient underwent emergent hemodialysis to correct electrolyte imbalances. We proceeded with a renal biopsy to ascertain a tissue diagnosis for the glomerulonephritis. 12 glomeruli were available for light microscopic examination. 9/12 glomeruli showed global sclerosis (Figure 2). Remaining glomeruli showed cellular to fibrocellular crescents (Figure 3). The interstitium is involved by a dense inflammatory infiltrate composed of lymphocytes, plasma cells, and scattered eosinophils. No definite granulomas were identified. Immunofluorescence showed intense linear glomerular capillary staining with IgG, Kappa, and lambda chains (Figure 4). The renal biopsy findings were consistent with anti-GBM mediated crescentic glomerulonephritis.

Patient was started on high dose methylprednisolone and plasmapheresis once the biopsy results were consistent with anti-GBM disease. Anti-GBM titers (IgG antibody) also came back elevated at 1.1 units (Normal < 1) confirming

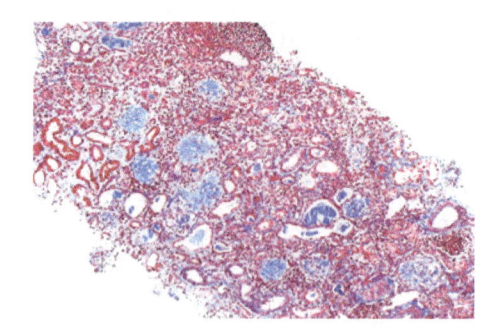

FIGURE 2: Trichrome stain showing global glomerulosclerosis.

the diagnosis. The subtle elevation in anti-GBM titers could be secondary to the possibility of a serological remission though chronic damage to the kidneys has already happened as documented by the amount of fibrosis on renal biopsy. Unfortunately anti-GBM titers were not checked during the initial pneumonia like presentation 7 months back which likely represented the initial acute episode. With every other day plasmapheresis, anti-GBM titers started trending down but renal function did not recover. With the extent of global sclerosis noted in renal biopsy and with the very high PTH levels, chances for renal recovery remained slim. Rituximab was used as an alternate immunosuppressive agent instead

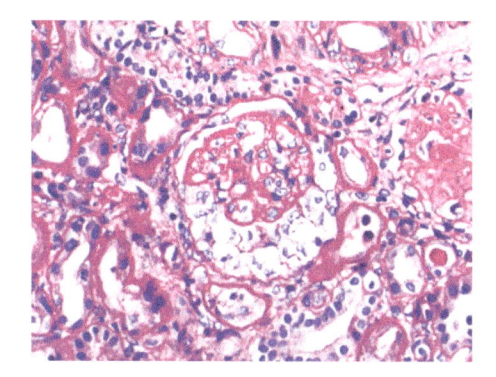

FIGURE 3: Glomerulus showing intraglomerular sclerosis.

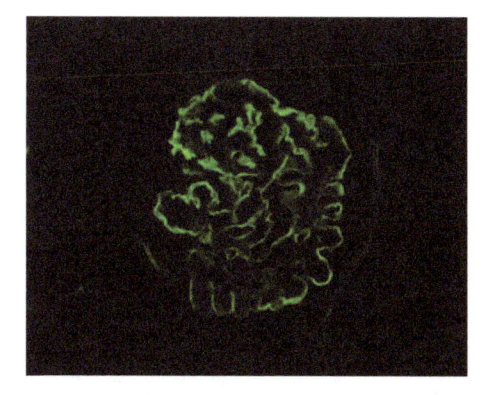

FIGURE 4: Immunofluorescence showing linear IgG deposits.

of cyclophosphamide taking into consideration the amount of chronic damage noted on renal biopsy in an attempt to reduce infectious risk. Patient received a total of 5 sessions of plasmapheresis with no improvement in renal function and was transitioned to peritoneal dialysis. During the inpatient stay she suffered a hypertensive crisis with seizures and the control of blood pressure required multiple antihypertensive agents. Anti-GBM titers were periodically monitored by lab work on a monthly basis and remained negative on maintenance immunosuppression with mycophenolate and low dose prednisone. Patient received a diseased donor kidney transplant, 2 months back, and is currently doing well with normal renal function.

3. Discussion

3.1. Epidemiology. GPS is a rare condition occurring in approximately 0.5 to 1 per million per year in adults and even more rare in children [3]. According to the United States Renal Data Registry, incidence of pediatric end stage renal disease (ESRD) due to this rare entity is only 11-12 per year, accounting for 0.5% of pediatric ESRD in 2009–2013 [4]. It typically has a bimodal distribution with the first peak predominantly affecting males in their teens and twenties. The second peak which happens in older population (>60 years of age) affects male and female equally. GPS is rare in children, with only about 30 cases being reported in the pediatric literature, with the youngest reported child being 11 months of age. The previously reported cases of pediatric Goodpasture's syndrome over the past 25 years are detailed in Table 2 [5–13].

3.2. Pathogenesis. The type IV collagen which provides the backbone for GBM formation is the target for autoantibody formation and damage in GPS. The type IV collagen has six genetically discrete chains ($\alpha 1$ to $\alpha 6$) which are arranged into triple helical protomers ($\alpha 1 \alpha 1 \alpha 2$, $\alpha 3 \alpha 4 \alpha 5$, and $\alpha 5 \alpha 5 \alpha 6$) of varying composition. The protomer has a 7S domain at the N-terminal, a collagenous part in the middle, and a noncollagenous (NC1) domain at the C-terminal [14]. The final collagen IV network in the GBM is a polymerized mesh such that the 7S domain forms a tetramer and the NC1 domain forms a hexamer providing the tensile strength to the basement membrane. $\alpha 1 \alpha 1 \alpha 2 - \alpha 1 \alpha 1 \alpha 2$ is the predominant collagen prototype in embryonic GBM and a developmental switch happens to the final adult form of $\alpha 3 \alpha 4 \alpha 5 - \alpha 3 \alpha 4 \alpha 5$ anywhere between 3 months and 3 years of age [15].

The specific target for autoantibody formation in GPS is the NC1 domain of the $\alpha 3$ subunit in the C-terminal. The NC1 domain also acts as the main promoter for collagen polymerization. The common presence of $\alpha 3$ collagen in the basement membrane of both kidneys and lungs explains the predominant organ involvement in this condition. A triggering event (upper respiratory infection, smoking, hydrocarbon exposure, and influenza) in a genetically susceptible individual causes exposure of the $\alpha 3$ NC1 domain and subsequent antibody formation [16, 17]. Strong HLA association with presence of HLA-DR15 and DR 4 allele in about 80% of affected individuals confirms a genetic predisposition as is the case in the majority of autoimmune diseases [18]. The absence of $\alpha 3$ subunit in younger children (before the developmental switch) could be attributed to the lesser incidence of aGD in younger children.

3.3. Clinical Features. Initial presentation of GPS can be nonspecific and often consists of symptoms such as malaise, weight loss, fever, and arthralgia [19]. Kidney disease may occur independently or with pulmonary disease. Renal manifestations vary widely and can range from hematuria and proteinuria to rapidly progressing renal failure with oliguria, fluid overload, and severe hypertension. Pulmonary symptoms may precede renal symptoms by weeks to months with hemoptysis being the most common pulmonary manifestation. Pulmonary bleeding can be occult leading to anemia and iron deficiency but the usual presentation is with profound pulmonary hemorrhage causing respiratory failure and death in a matter of hours. Other organ system involvement is very rare though cerebral vasculitis with confusion, aphasia, and seizures has been reported in the literature [20].

3.4. Pathology. The diagnosis of antiglomerular basement membrane disease is reliant on detection of anti-GBM antibodies either in circulation or in the tissue by means of renal or pulmonary biopsies. Serological testing for anti-GBM antibody titers (IgG1 subclass) usually employs ELISA methodology. The sensitivity of available commercial kits

TABLE 2: Prior reported cases of pediatric Goodpasture's syndrome.

Age in years	Sex	Anti-GBM titers	Initial clinical presentation	Renal biopsy	Renal outcome	Pulmonary outcome	Treatment	Final outcome	Reference
4	F	Positive	Pallor, fatigue oliguria, proteinuria, and microscopic hematuria with dominant renal involvement	End stage glomerulonephritis with crescent formation; linear deposition of IgG along basement membrane	No improvement	Stable	Prednisone, azathioprine, and cyclophosphamide	Died	[5]
10	F	Positive	Gross hematuria, oliguria, and uremia with dominant renal involvement Preceding infection with strep throat	Endocapillary and extracapillary proliferative GN with 80% crescents Immunofluorescence could not be done	Dialysis dependent with no improvement	Stable	Prednisolone, azathioprine, and plasmapheresis	Remained dialysis dependent	[5]
7	F	Positive	Diarrhea, vomiting, oliguria, and pallor with dominant renal involvement	Crescentic nephritis with linear IgG deposition	Initial improvement in urine output and GFR with subsequent decline and dialysis dependence	Stable	Plasmapheresis, prednisolone, and cyclophosphamide	Dialysis dependent	[5]
6	M	Positive	Dominant renal involvement	Diagnostic with crescentic nephritis	Improved	Stable	Steroid, plasmapheresis, and immunosuppression	Regained renal function	[6]
10	M	Positive	Cough, right lower lobe infiltrate, vomiting, and oliguria with dominant pulmonary involvement and pulmonary hemorrhage	Crescentic nephritis with extensive necrosis	Deterioration in renal function with dialysis dependence	Improved	Steroid, plasmapheresis, and immunosuppression	Dialysis dependent	[7]
2.5	F	Positive	Fever, anorexia with E. coli UTI as initial presentation with worsening renal function and oliguria	Extensive crescentic necrotizing nephritis with linear IgG deposits	No improvement	Stable	Steroid, plasmapheresis, and immunosuppression	Dialysis dependent	[8]
11 months	F	Positive	Dominant renal involvement	Diagnostic with crescentic nephritis	No improvement	Stable	Steroid, plasmapheresis, and immunosuppression	Renal transplant	[9]
5.6	F	Positive	Fever, malaise, and gross hematuria with rapid decline in renal function	Diffuse cellular crescentic nephritis with linear IgG deposits	Recovery of renal function	Stable	Plasma exchange, solumedrol, and Cytoxan	CKD with stable renal function	[10]
9	M	Positive	Malaise, anorexia, and oligoanuria with pulmonary hemorrhage	Not done	Not improved	Pulmonary status improved	Plasma exchange, solumedrol, and Cytoxan	Dialysis dependent	[11]

TABLE 2: Continued.

Age in years	Sex	Anti-GBM titers	Initial clinical presentation	Renal biopsy	Renal outcome	Pulmonary outcome	Treatment	Final outcome	Reference
8	F	Positive	Asymptomatic with persistent nephrotic range proteinuria and microhematuria	No crescents but with linear deposits of IgG	Improvement in proteinuria with stable renal function	Stable	Plasma exchange, prednisone, and oral Cytoxan	Asymptomatic	[12]
19 months	M	Positive	Gross hematuria, proteinuria with rapid decline in renal function	Crescentic GN with weak global linear staining of IgG	Improvement in proteinuria and renal function	Stable	Plasma exchange, solumedrol, and Cytoxan	Asymptomatic	[13]

can vary from 63% to 100% underlying the possibility of missed diagnosis if solely reliant on serological testing [21, 22]. Renal biopsy can help confirm the diagnosis of GPS and also provides important clues on the amount of chronicity/activity helping to guide treatment. Light microscopy usually shows crescentic glomerulonephritis but the characteristic linear IgG deposition along the capillary wall is noted in immunofluorescence microscopy clinching the diagnosis. Lung biopsy also shows the linear IgG deposits but this finding is not as constant as in kidney [23].

3.5. Treatment. Early diagnosis is important in terms of ability to recover renal function. Treatment of choice initially is plasmapheresis to remove circulating antibodies. The preferred immunosuppressive therapy includes corticosteroids and cyclophosphamide to reduce antibody production. Alternate immunosuppressive therapy including rituximab has been tried in resistant cases [24]. Anti-GBM antibodies are monitored weekly until two negatives are achieved, at which time levels are monitored monthly for up to 6 months. Low dose prednisone, azathioprine, or mycophenolate may be used for maintenance immunosuppression once remission is established with cessation of antibody production. If the antibody titer levels remain positive, the immunosuppression therapy should be continued [25].

3.6. Prognosis. Unfortunately, many patients die secondary to pulmonary hemorrhage or renal failure before plasmapheresis and immunosuppression can be initiated. Currently the mortality rate is 20% in adults and 30% in children. Prognosis for renal recovery is worse in the presence of oliguria, presenting creatinine >6.8 or renal biopsy showing >50% crescent formation within glomeruli at time of diagnosis [26]. Evidences of chronic damage as documented by moderate or severe interstitial fibrosis and global glomerulosclerosis always carry a worse prognosis. Renal outcome is dependent on timing of diagnosis with improved outcomes if treatment is initiated within 4 weeks of renal involvement [27]. Despite the potential seriousness of lung hemorrhage with increased fatality, no residual pulmonary deficit or fibrosis is noted once patient recovers from the acute presentation. Though rare, recurrence of disease may occur years after initial presentation.

GPS as a cause of pulmonary renal syndrome in childhood remains extremely rare. A review of pediatric cases in the literature (Table 2) shows a female preponderance in children in comparison to majority male involvement in adults. Anti-GBM titers were positive in almost all of the reported cases. Majority of cases also showed dominant renal involvement with gross hematuria and oligoanuria being the most common presentation. Treatment strategies involved using a combination of steroids, plasma exchange, and cyclophosphamide in most of the patients. Renal recovery was noted only in 3/11 patients among whom one had presentation with nephrotic range proteinuria but with normal renal function [8]. The prognosis for renal recovery seems to be better in the absence of interstitial fibrosis and early treatment initiation as is noted in the adult literature.

4. Conclusion

In conclusion, GPS is a rare autoimmune condition presenting with significant mortality and morbidity in children. We report a case of 2-year, 11-month-old child who presented with this condition and the difficulties involved in coming to an accurate diagnosis. In hindsight, her initial presentation with pneumonia was likely an occult pulmonary hemorrhage as documented by the severe anemia and iron deficiency. Her response to steroids during the initial admission likely constituted a partial treatment. GPS though rare should be considered in the differential diagnosis of clinical presentation with lung and kidney involvement and early diagnosis and intervention are essential for a favorable outcome.

References

[1] H. Gallagher, J. T. C. Kwan, and D. R. W. Jayne, "Pulmonary renal syndrome: a 4-year, single-center experience," *American Journal of Kidney Diseases*, vol. 39, no. 1, pp. 42–47, 2002.

[2] R. W. Lee and D. P. D'Cruz, "Pulmonary renal vasculitis syndromes," *Autoimmunity Reviews*, vol. 9, no. 10, pp. 657–660, 2010.

[3] E. G. Fischer and D. J. Lager, "Anti-glomerular basement membrane glomerulonephritis: a morphologic study of 80 cases," *American Journal of Clinical Pathology*, vol. 125, no. 3, pp. 445–450, 2006.

[4] "USRDS U.S. Renal Data System 2015 Annual Data Report: pediatric ESRD. National Institutes of Health, National Institute of Diabetes and Digestive and Kidney Disease, Bethesda," 2015.

[5] M. Levin, S. P. A. Rigden, J. R. Pincott, C. M. Lockwood, T. M. Barratt, and M. J. Dillon, "Goodpasture's syndrome: treatment with plasmapheresis, immunosuppression, and anticoagulation," *Archives of Disease in Childhood*, vol. 58, no. 9, pp. 697–702, 1983.

[6] J. Gilvarry, G. F. Doyle, and D. G. Gill, "Good outcome in antiglomerular basement membrane nephritis," *Pediatric Nephrology*, vol. 6, no. 3, pp. 244–246, 1992.

[7] L. J. McCarthy, J. Cotton, C. Danielson, V. Graves, and J. Bergstein, "Goodpasture's syndrome in childhood: treatment with plasmapheresis and immunosuppression," *Journal of Clinical Apheresis*, vol. 9, no. 2, pp. 116–119, 1994.

[8] K. Boven, H. P. J. Miljoen, K. J. Van Hoeck, E. A. Van Marck, and K. J. Van Acker, "Anti-glomerular basement membrane glomerulopathy in a young child," *Pediatric Nephrology*, vol. 10, no. 6, pp. 745–747, 1996.

[9] S. A. Bigler, W. M. Parry, D. S. Fitzwater, and R. Baliga, "An 11-month-old with anti-glomerular basement membrane disease," *American Journal of Kidney Diseases*, vol. 30, no. 5, pp. 710–712, 1997.

[10] S. A. Bakkaloglu, C. S. Kasapkara, O. Soylemezoglu et al., "Successful management of anti-GBM disease in a 5 1/2-year-old girl," *Nephrology Dialysis Transplantation*, vol. 21, no. 10, pp. 2979–2981, 2006.

[11] B. Poddar, S. Singhal, A. Azim, S. Gulati, and A. Baronia, "Goodpasture's syndrome in children," *Saudi Journal of Kidney Diseases and Transplantation*, vol. 21, no. 5, pp. 935–939, 2010.

[12] C. Nagano, Y. Goto, K. Kasahara, and Y. Kuroyanagi, "Case report: anti-glomerular basement membrane antibody disease with normal renal function," *BMC Nephrology*, vol. 16, p. 185, 2015.

[13] A. Bjerre, K. Hogåsen, J. Grotta, H. Scott, T. Tangeraas, and C. Dörje, "Rescue of kidney function in a toddler with anti-GBM nephritis," *Clinical Kidney Journal*, vol. 5, no. 6, pp. 584–586, 2012.

[14] P. S. Thorner, R. Baumal, A. Eddy, and P. Marrano, "Characterization of the NC1 domain of collagen type IV in glomerular basement membranes (GBM) and of antibodies to GBM in a patient with anti-GBM nephritis," *Clinical Nephrology*, vol. 31, no. 3, pp. 160–168, 1989.

[15] B. G. Hudson, S. T. Reeders, and K. Tryggvason, "Type IV collagen: structure, gene organization, and role in human diseases. Molecular basis of goodpasture and alport syndromes and diffuse leiomyomatosis," *Journal of Biological Chemistry*, vol. 268, no. 35, pp. 26033–26036, 1993.

[16] E. W. Goodpasture, "Landmark publication from The American Journal of the Medical Sciences: the significance of certain pulmonary lesions in relation to the etiology of influenza.," *The American Journal of the Medical Sciences*, vol. 338, no. 2, pp. 148–151, 2009.

[17] M. Donaghy and A. J. Rees, "Cigarette smoking and lung haemorrhage in glomerulonephritis caused by autoantibodies to glomerular basement membrane," *The Lancet*, vol. 322, no. 8364, pp. 1390–1393, 1983.

[18] M. Fisher, C. D. Pusey, R. W. Vaughan, and A. J. Rees, "Susceptibility to anti-glomerular basement membrane disease is strongly associated with HLA-DRB1 genes," *Kidney International*, vol. 51, no. 1, pp. 222–229, 1997.

[19] F. Dammacco, S. Battaglia, L. Gesualdo, and V. Racanelli, "Goodpasture's disease: a report of ten cases and a review of the literature," *Autoimmunity Reviews*, vol. 12, no. 11, pp. 1101–1108, 2013.

[20] N. Gittins, A. Basu, J. Eyre, A. Gholkar, and N. Moghal, "Cerebral vasculitis in a teenager with Goodpasture's syndrome," *Nephrology Dialysis Transplantation*, vol. 19, no. 12, pp. 3168–3171, 2004.

[21] A. D. Salama, T. Dougan, J. B. Levy et al., "Goodpasture's disease in the absence of circulating anti-glomerular basement membrane antibodies as detected by standard techniques," *The American Journal of Kidney Diseases*, vol. 39, no. 6, pp. 1162–1167, 2002.

[22] C. M. Litwin, C. L. Mouritsen, P. A. Wilfahrt, M. C. Schroder, and H. R. Hill, "Anti-glomerular basement membrane disease: Role of enzyme-linked immunosorbent assays in diagnosis," *Biochemical and Molecular Medicine*, vol. 59, no. 1, pp. 52–56, 1996.

[23] W. A. Briggs, J. P. Johnson, S. Teichman, H. C. Yeager, and C. B. Wilson, "Antiglomerular basement membrane antibody-mediated glomerulonephritis and goodpasture's syndrome," *Medicine (United States)*, vol. 58, no. 5, pp. 348–361, 1979.

[24] M. K. Shah and S. Y. Hugghins, "Characteristics and outcomes of patients with Goodpasture's syndrome," *Southern Medical Journal*, vol. 95, no. 12, pp. 1411–1418, 2002.

[25] D. C. Kluth and A. J. Rees, "Anti-glomerular basement membrane disease," *Journal of the American Society of Nephrology*, vol. 10, no. 11, pp. 2446–2453, 1999.

[26] F. Merkel, O. Pullig, M. Marx, K. O. Netzer, and M. Weber, "Course and prognosis of anti-basement membrane antibody (anti-BM-Ab)-mediated disease: report of 35 cases," *Nephrology Dialysis Transplantation*, vol. 9, no. 4, pp. 372–376, 1994.

[27] B. Alchi, M. Griffiths, M. Sivalingam, D. Jayne, and K. Farrington, "Predictors of renal and patient outcomes in anti-GBM disease: clinicopathologic analysis of a two-centre cohort," *Nephrology Dialysis Transplantation*, vol. 30, no. 5, pp. 814–821, 2015.

Sticky Platelet Syndrome: An Unrecognized Cause of Acute Thrombosis and Graft Loss

Fabio Solis-Jimenez[1], Hector Hinojosa-Heredia[2], Luis García-Covarrubias,[2] Virgilia Soto-Abraham,[3] and Rafael Valdez-Ortiz[4]

[1]Internal Medicine Service, General Hospital of Mexico "Dr. Eduardo Liceaga", Mexico City, Mexico
[2]Transplant Service, General Hospital of Mexico "Dr. Eduardo Liceaga", Mexico City, Mexico
[3]Pathological Anatomy Service, General Hospital of Mexico "Dr. Eduardo Liceaga", Mexico City, Mexico
[4]Nephrology Service, General Hospital of Mexico "Dr. Eduardo Liceaga", Mexico City, Mexico

Correspondence should be addressed to Fabio Solis-Jimenez; fabiosolisjimenez@gmail.com and Rafael Valdez-Ortiz; rafavaldez@gmail.com

Academic Editor: Sophia Lionaki

Introduction. Sticky platelet syndrome (SPS) is a prothrombotic disease that is not well recognized and difficult to diagnose. *Case Report.* We present a case of a 49-year-old diabetic woman on ambulatory peritoneal dialysis therapy who underwent a kidney transplant from living-related donor. The donor was her sister with whom she shared one haplotype and absence of donor specific antibodies. The posttransplant evolution was torpid, developing progressive deterioration, which made us suspect a failure in the graft. Doppler ultrasound reported renal vein thrombosis and hypoperfusion of the renal artery. Without clinical improvement, she required a reintervention that ended in graftectomy, in which the histopathological report showed negative C4d with medullary and cortical infarction. Hematological studies were negative for antibodies against phospholipids, with correct levels of proteins C and S and antithrombin. Platelet aggregometry studies were carried out, which were compatible with SPS. *Conclusions.* Recognition of SPS in pretransplant studies is difficult if there is no history of previous thrombotic events. However, we must consider this entity in cases of acute thrombosis and loss of the graft of uncertain origin.

1. Introduction

Primary graft thrombosis occurs in 0.5% and 6% of renal transplants and usually results in graft loss [1]. Risk factors associated with the development of graft thrombosis have been identified, such as the use of peritoneal dialysis, retransplantation, prolonged cold ischemia (greater than 24 hours), and transsurgical hypotension [2–4]. However, in all patients presenting with thrombosis of the graft, an intentional search for possible primary thrombophilias should be carried out [4]. Retrospective studies performed in transplant patients with graft thrombosis have shown a higher incidence of protein C, protein S, factor V Leiden, and antithrombin deficiency [5]. However, in certain cases, the etiology of thrombosis remains uncertain and this is when a possible pattern of platelet hyperaggregation as sticky platelet syndrome (SPS) could be considered as the cause of thrombosis [6].

The SPS was first described in the 80s as a thrombophilia in which qualitative alterations of the platelet function increase its aggregation capacity, favoring in this way thrombosis with described cases of cerebrovascular disease, acute myocardial infarction, and ischemic retinopathy [7]. Below, we present the case of a patient without history of thrombosis who developed a sudden dysfunction of the graft after living kidney transplantation and whose final diagnosis was SPS.

2. Case Report

We report the case of a 49-year-old woman with O RhD positive blood group and a family history of premature death of her father due to cerebrovascular disease. In her surgical history, she underwent transsphenoidal surgery for pituitary adenoma at the age of 40, with replacement therapy with

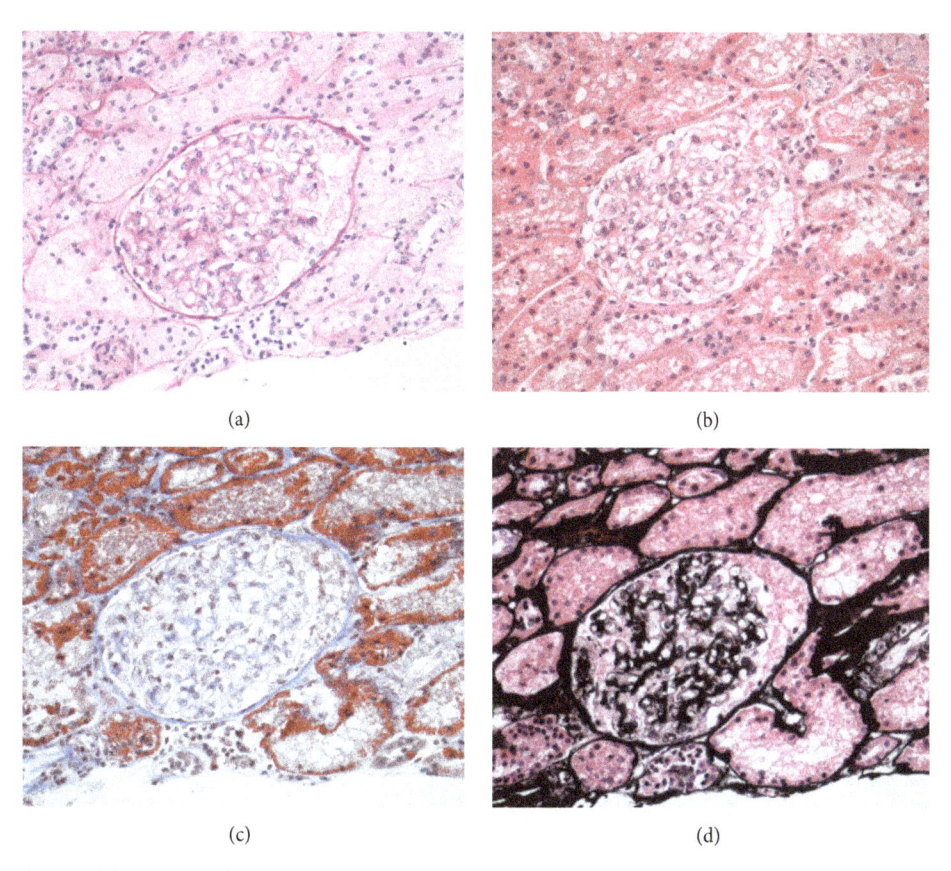

FIGURE 1: *Zero-time biopsy of the renal graft.* (a) Hematoxylin and eosin staining. (b) Periodic acid-Schiff staining. (c) Masson stain. (d) Silver methenamine stain. Renal tissue is visualized without significant vascular, tubular, and glomerular alterations. All photomicrographs are in 40x.

levothyroxine at a dose of 100 mcg per day. The patient was diagnosed with type 2 diabetes mellitus at the age of 29 and has been treated since then with long-acting insulin. She also has a diagnosis of CKD in treatment with automated peritoneal dialysis from 47 years of age. A living-donor kidney transplant protocol was initiated, related to her sister (healthy 39-year-old woman), with whom she shares one haplotype and specific negative anti-donor antibodies.

The induction scheme was performed with basiliximab and methylprednisolone, with a cold ischemia time of 120 minutes. During surgery, arterial anastomosis was observed with progressive decrease of the thrill. For this reason, it was necessary to dismantle the anastomosis followed by exploration, observation, and discharge of a thrombus from the renal artery. The anastomosis was completed with adequate graft perfusion. The renal biopsy at time zero was without significant vascular, glomerular, and interstitial tubule alterations (Figures 1(a)–1(d)). After surgery, the patient remained in oligoanuria. A Doppler ultrasound of the graft was performed, which showed the renal artery throughout its course with high resistance pulsatile flow, with an average systolic flow velocity of 58.7 cm/second and inversion of the diastolic flow. The segmental, interlobar, and arcuate arteries in the upper, lower, and middle poles showed decreased systolic flow with an average of 34.1 cm/second. Meanwhile, the renal vein could not be identified at the time of the study (Figures 2(a) and 2(b)).

Ultrasound diagnosis was a thrombosis of the renal vein with hypoperfusion of the renal artery. The patient was admitted to the operating room and as a macroscopic finding the renal graft showed a purplish coloration and pallor, absence of thrill, complete anastomosis, and the presence of an intrarenal venous clot. Due to the damage, graft transplantectomy was performed and the graft was sent for revision by a pathologist who reported diffuse medullary cortical infarction and acute thrombotic microangiopathy with negative immunohistochemistry for C4d (Figures 3(a)–3(d)). The postsurgical follow-up was performed with the search for potential thrombophilias. The quantification of protein C, protein S, and antithrombin was normal and the profile for anti-phospholipid antibodies was negative. In search of other pathologies, we requested studies of platelet aggregation, which showed platelet hyperaggregability at decreasing doses of epinephrine and normal aggregability associated with the exposure of adenosine diphosphate, compatible with sticky platelet syndrome type II (Figures 4(a) and 4(b)). The patient returned to automated peritoneal dialysis and management with acetylsalicylic acid as an antiplatelet agent was started.

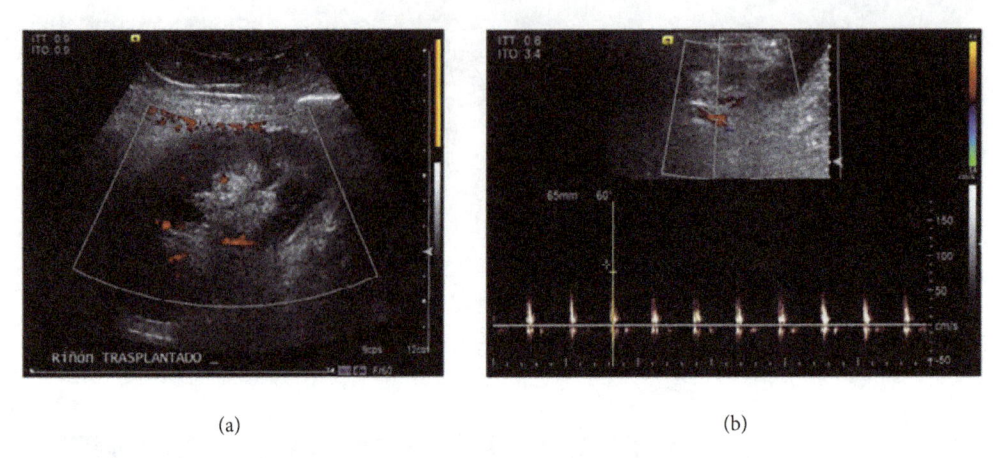

FIGURE 2: *Doppler ultrasound.* (a) Graft of the patient shows the absence of blood flow at the level of the renal cortex, arcuate arteries, interlobular arteries, and arterial anastomosis. (b) Duplex mode shows an arterial biphasic waveform with delayed acceleration, decreased systolic peak, and increased flow in diastole, which is a suggestive pattern of ischemia.

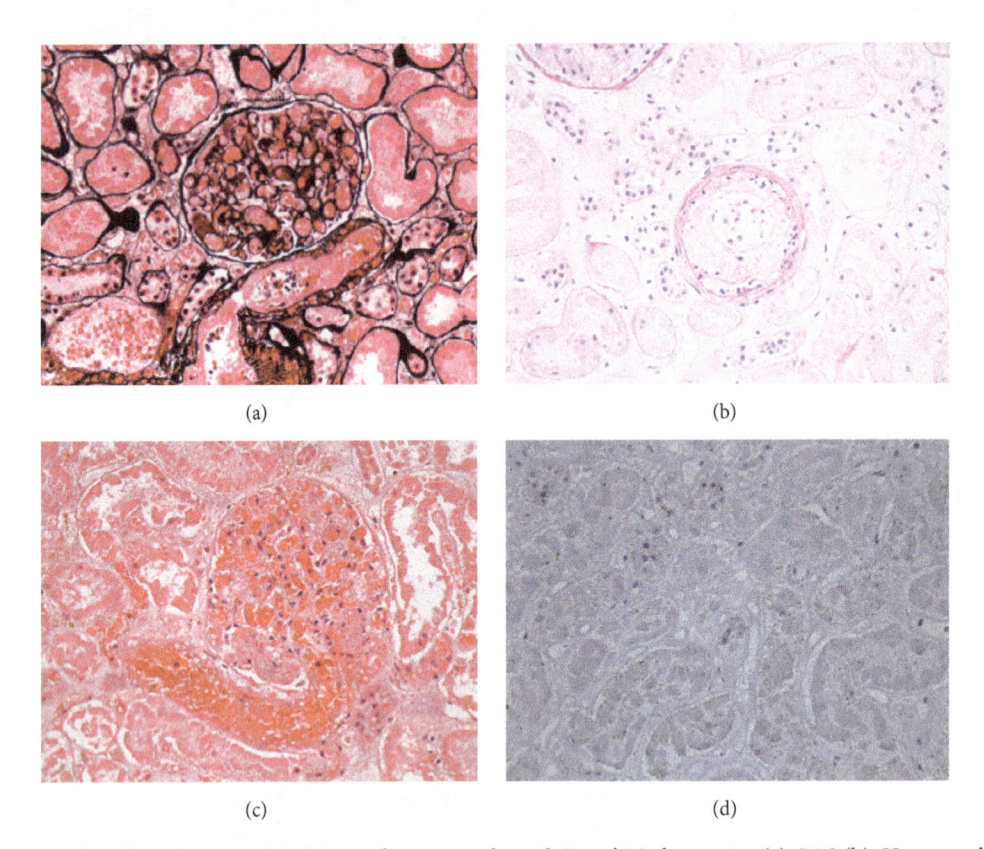

FIGURE 3: *Micrographs of graft nephrectomy (40x).* Stained, respectively, with Jones' Methenamine (a), PAS (b), Hematoxylin and Eosin (c), and indirect peroxidase immunostaining for C4d (d). In all sections, fibrin thrombi adhered to the endothelium of the glomeruli ((a) and (c)) and the arteriolar walls (b) can be observed. C4d (d) was negative. All photomicrographs are in 40x.

3. Discussion

Described for the first time in the Ninth Stroke and Cerebral Circulation Conference by Holiday et al. [8], the sticky platelet syndrome is defined as a qualitative alteration of the platelet function and of autosomal dominant inheritance, characterized by platelet hyperaggregation in vitro with low concentrations of adenosine diphosphate (ADE) and/or epinephrine (EPI) but with normal aggregation in response to collagen, arachidonic acid, ristocetin, and thrombin [9].

Depending on the pattern of platelet aggregation, three different types of sticky platelet syndrome have been described. In type I, hyperaggregation is evidenced with both ADE and EPI. Type II shows hyperaggregation only with

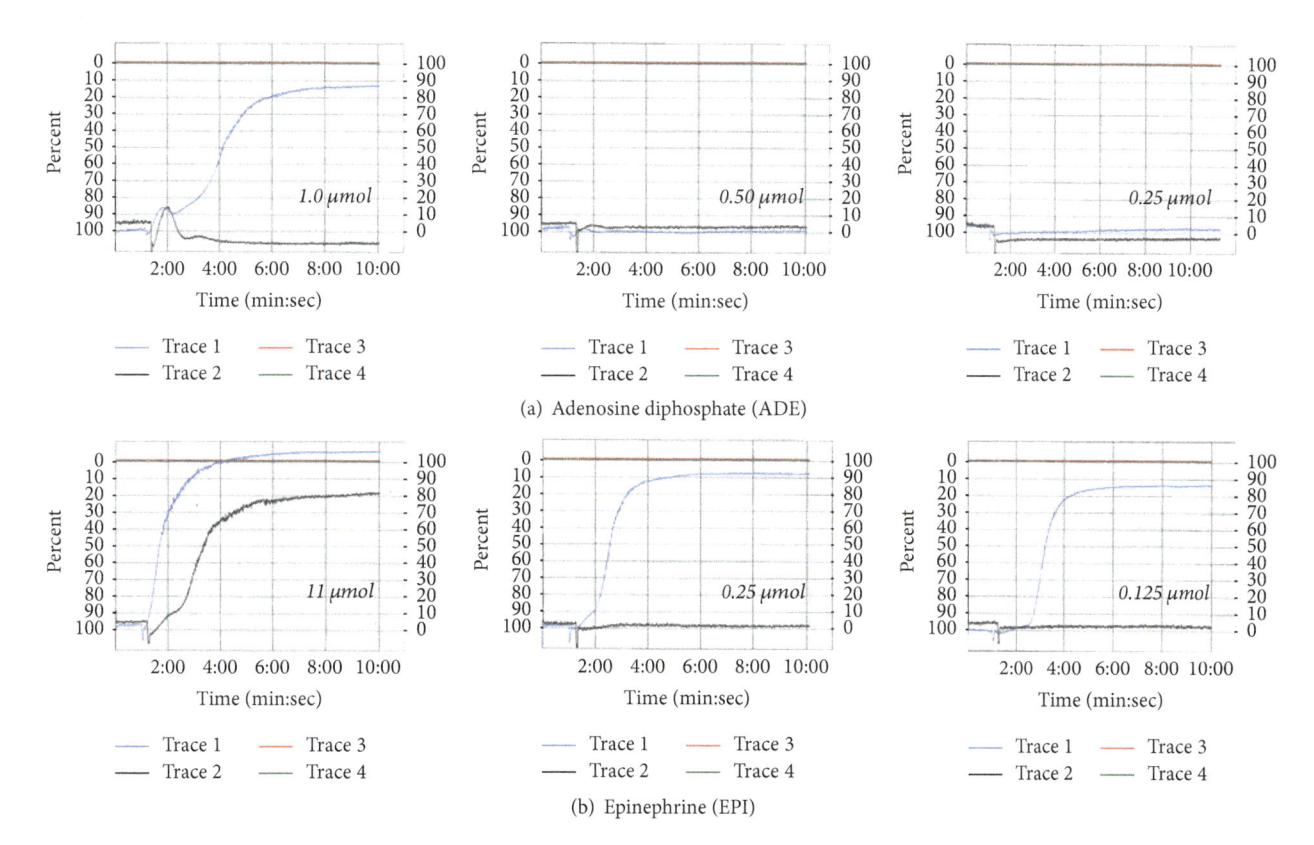

FIGURE 4: *Results of two platelet aggregometry tests: patient (blue line) and control (black line).* (a) From left to right, the percentage of platelet aggregation with decreasing doses of ADE is shown. At 1 μmol, the patient presents platelet aggregation of almost 90% at 10 min. At lower concentrations of ADE, the pattern of aggregation is similar to that of the control (0.5 and 0.25 μmol). (b) From left to right, the percentage of platelet aggregation with decreasing doses of EPI is shown. At 11 μmol, the patient and control present platelet aggregation that reaches more than 80% at 10 min. In contrast to lower concentrations of EPI, while the control stops having platelet aggregation, the patient maintains a pattern of aggregation above 80% at concentrations of 0.25 and 0.125 μmol.

EPI, and in type III, hyperaggregation is seen only with ADE [10]. There are no specific epidemiological data on SPS, because the studies have taken place in very exclusive population groups and in patients with thrombosis without apparent cause. Prevalence has been reported in patients with thrombosis without apparent cause between 17.6 and 28% [7, 11], while in women with miscarriages it has been reported in 20% [12] and in 41% of patients on hemodialysis with recurrent thrombosis of vascular access [13].

Within the clinical picture presented by these patients, arterial thrombosis is the most frequent manifestation of the disease, followed by venous thrombosis [14]. A study conducted by the National Center of Haemostasis and Thrombosis of Slovakia characterized 360 patients with SPS, describing 233 patients (64.7%) with arterial thrombosis and 127 (35.2%) with venous thrombosis [14]. Other characteristic data of SPS are the presentation in young adults with no apparent risk factors, in people with a family history of thrombosis, in women with repeat miscarriages, and in patients who have thrombosis in unusual sites (retinal circulation, cerebral sinuses, etc.) and episodes of thrombosis which occur even in spite of adequate anticoagulation [9].

One of the laboratory tests that help evaluate platelet function is aggregometry, which measures the ability of some substances to induce in vitro platelet activation and aggregation.

The diagnosis of SPS is made through a study of platelet aggregation in which platelet overaggregation is demonstrated when exposed to ADE and/or EPI. The most widely used method is turbidimetry, which measures the average platelet aggregation from the difference in optical density between platelet-rich plasma (PRP) and platelet-poor plasma (PPP), when an agonist is added as ADP, epinephrine, collagen, and ristocetin, to name a few; as the platelets are added, they allow a greater passage of light, decreasing the optical density, yielding the result through the aggregation curves as a function of time. Another method of measurement used is impedance, which measures the increase in resistance to the passage of electrical current through 2 electrodes by placing whole blood in contact with an agonist when platelets begin to aggregate [15].

In 2007, Mühlfeld et al. reported three cases in which patients had presented thrombotic complications after a kidney transplant and were diagnosed with SPS after post-transplant thrombotic episodes. Mühlfeld proposed that the increase in adrenaline secretion due to preoperative stress was likely to induce the typically abnormal aggregation pattern of SPS [6]. However, there is a possibility that other mechanisms may be involved, such as alloimmune vascular damage, postoperative hypertensive episodes, and the use of immunomodulatory drugs such as calcineurin inhibitors [6]. From the description of SPS, Mammen proposed that the underlying cause was in alterations of membrane glycoproteins and their role in platelet activation [16]. Although there have been multiple studies, to date, it has not been possible to find a genetic alteration that explains this syndrome. Different membrane protein polymorphisms have been studied, such as mutations in GPIIIaPlA A1/A2 and in Gas6 c. 834 + 7G>A, in which no statistically significant difference was found between the groups with SPS and controls [17, 18]. However, some polymorphisms of GP6 SNPs have been shown to be present more frequently in cases of SPS [19]. Despite these associations, there is still not enough evidence to define the etiology of SPS, which, due to its different forms of clinical presentation and inducibility characteristics of platelet aggregation, could have a multifactorial origin [9].

Because there are no treatment guidelines for SPS to date, the current recommendations are based on observations that acetylsalicylic acid (ASA) at low doses can normalize the pattern of platelet aggregation [14, 16]. For this reason, it is recommended to start treatment with ASA at doses of 80 to 100 mg every 24 hours [14]. However, for those patients who do not have an adequate response, it is recommended to scale the dose to 325 mg/day. The use of ADP inhibitors such as clopidogrel could be recommended only if, despite the escalation of the ASA dose, there is no normalization of the platelet aggregation pattern or there is any contraindication to the use of ASA [20]. Although monitoring of the efficacy of platelet antiaggregants is not standardized, it is recommended that once the treatment with ASA or clopidogrel has begun, the aggregation tests should be reevaluated in order to achieve adequate efficacy.

A targeted search for SPS should be recommended if there is a history of thrombosis without a specific cause or when the patient on the transplant and hemodialysis waiting list has reports of recurrent thrombosis of vascular access, particularly in renal transplant recipients.

The preoperative treatment of a transplant recipient when they have a proven SPS is controversial. Traditionally, it is described that there is an increased risk of bleeding during a surgical procedure (approximately 20% only with aspirin and up to 50% with aspirin and clopidogrel) [21]. However, there are studies in which it has been proven that the use of aspirin before and after transplantation reduces the risk of graft thrombosis without significantly increasing the risk of bleeding [22, 23]. These studies use low doses of aspirin (75–150 mg), which seems to be a strategy to be used in patients with SPS who will undergo kidney transplantation [24].

In conclusion, SPS is a poorly recognized entity but with an adverse prognosis in patients with kidney transplantation. Its recognition must be done in the pretransplant period to avoid adverse complications in the postoperative period. Its diagnosis requires evidence of platelet aggregation and its treatment is relatively effective with the use of antiplatelet agents.

References

[1] N. Bakir, W. J. Sluiter, R. J. Ploeg, W. J. Van Son, and A. M. Tegzess, "Primary renal graft thrombosis," *Nephrology Dialysis Transplantation*, vol. 11, no. 1, pp. 140–147, 1996.

[2] A. O. Ojo, J. A. Hanson, R. A. Wolfe et al., "Dialysis modality and the risk of allograft thrombosis in adult renal transplant recipients," *Kidney International*, vol. 55, no. 5, pp. 1952–1960, 1999.

[3] J. T. Adler, J. F. Markmann, and H. Yeh, "Renal allograft thrombosis after living donor transplantation: risk factors and obstacles to retransplantation," *Clinical Transplantation*, vol. 30, no. 8, pp. 864–871, 2016.

[4] C. Ponticelli, M. Moia, and G. Montagnino, "Renal allograft thrombosis," *Nephrology Dialysis Transplantation*, vol. 24, no. 5, pp. 1388–1393, 2009.

[5] J. L. Kujovich, "Thrombophilia and thrombotic problems in renal transplant patients," *Transplantation*, vol. 77, no. 7, pp. 959–964, 2004.

[6] A. S. Mühlfeld, M. Ketteler, K. Schwamborn et al., "Sticky platelet syndrome: An underrecognized cause of graft dysfunction and thromboembolic complications in renal transplant recipients," *American Journal of Transplantation*, vol. 7, no. 7, pp. 1865–1868, 2007.

[7] R. L. Bick, "Sticky platelet syndrome: A common cause of unexplained arterial and venous thrombosis," *Clinical and Applied Thrombosis/Hemostasis*, vol. 4, no. 2, pp. 77–81, 1998.

[8] P. L. Holiday, E. Mammen, and J. Gilroy, "Sticky platelet syndrome and cerebral infarction in young adults," in *Proceedings of the Ninth International Joint Conference on Stroke and Cerebral Circulation*, Phoenix, Arizona, 1983.

[9] G. J. Ruiz-Delgado, Y. Cantero-Fortiz, M. A. Mendez-Huerta et al., "Primary thrombophilia in Mexico XII: Miscarriages are more frequent in people with sticky platelet syndrome," *Turkish Journal of Hematology*, vol. 34, no. 3, pp. 239–243, 2017.

[10] P. Kubisz, J. Stasko, and P. Holly, "Sticky platelet syndrome," *Seminars in Thrombosis and Hemostasis*, vol. 39, no. 6, pp. 674–683, 2013.

[11] J. A. Andersen, Report: bleeding and thrombosis in women. Biomed Progress, 12: 40, 1999.

[12] R. L. Bick and D. Hoppensteadt, "Recurrent miscarriage syndrome and infertility due to blood coagulation protein/platelet defects: A review and update," *Clinical and Applied Thrombosis/Hemostasis*, vol. 11, no. 1, pp. 1–13, 2005.

[13] R. Klamroth, F. Seibt, and H. Rimpler, "Recurrent vascular access site thrombosis in patients on hemodialysis a problem of thrombophilia?" *Blood*, vol. 104, p. 300a, 2004.

[14] J. Sokol, M. Skerenova, Z. Jedinakova et al., "Progress in the Understanding of Sticky Platelet Syndrome," *Seminars in Thrombosis and Hemostasis*, vol. 43, no. 1, Article ID 02342, pp. 008–013, 2017.

[15] M. Martínez-Arias, B. López-Martínez, and I. Parra-Ortega, "Pruebas de laboratorio para la evaluación de la función de las plaquetas," *Revista Latinoamericana de Patología Clínica y Medicina de Laboratorio*, vol. 62, no. 4, pp. 245–252, 2015.

[16] E. F. Mammen, "Ten Years' Experience with the "Sticky Platelet Syndrome"," *Clinical and Applied Thrombosis/Hemostasis*, vol. 1, no. 1, pp. 66–72, 1995.

[17] G. J. Ruiz-Argüelles, J. Garcés-Eisele, C. Camacho-Alarcón et al., "Primary thrombophilia in Mexico IX: The glycoprotein IIIa PL A1/A2 polymorphism is not associated with the sticky platelet syndrome phenotype," *Clinical and Applied Thrombosis/Hemostasis*, vol. 19, no. 6, pp. 689–692, 2013.

[18] P. Kubisz, L. Bartošová, J. Ivanková et al., "Is Gas6 protein associated with sticky platelet syndrome?" *Clinical and Applied Thrombosis/Hemostasis*, vol. 16, no. 6, pp. 701–704, 2010.

[19] D. Kotuličová, P. Chudý, M. Škereňová, J. Ivanková, M. Dobrotová, and P. Kubisz, "Variability of GP6 gene in patients with sticky platelet syndrome and deep venous thrombosis and/or pulmonary embolism," *Blood Coagulation & Fibrinolysis*, vol. 23, no. 6, pp. 543–547, 2012.

[20] E. F. Mammen, "Sticky platelet syndrome," *Seminars in Thrombosis and Hemostasis*, vol. 25, no. 4, pp. 361–366, 1999.

[21] P. G. Chassot, C. Marcucci, A. Delabays, and D. R. Spahn, "Perioperative antiplatelet therapy," *American Family Physician*, vol. 82, no. 12, pp. 1484–1489, 2010.

[22] G. J. Murphy, R. Taha, D. C. Windmill, M. Metcalfe, and M. L. Nicholson, "Influence of aspirin on early allograft thrombosis and chronic allograft nephropathy following renal transplantation," *British Journal of Surgery*, vol. 88, no. 2, pp. 261–266, 2001.

[23] A. J. Robertson, V. Nargund, D. W. R. Gray, and P. J. Morris, "Low dose aspirin as prophylaxis against renal-vein thrombosis in renal-transplant recipients," *Nephrology Dialysis Transplantation*, vol. 15, no. 11, pp. 1865–1868, 2000.

[24] J.-M. El-Amm, J. Andersenb, and S. A. Gruber, "Sticky platelet syndrome: A manageable risk factor for posttransplant thromboembolic events [3]," *American Journal of Transplantation*, vol. 8, no. 2, p. 465, 2008.

A Rare Benign Tumor in a 14-Year-Old Girl

Meral Hassan Abualjadayel,[1] Osama Y. Safdar,[2] Maysaa Adnan Banjari,[1] Sherif El Desoky,[2] Ghadeer A. Mokhtar,[3] and Raed A. Azhar[4]

[1]King Abdulaziz University, Jeddah, Saudi Arabia
[2]Center of Excellence in Pediatric Nephrology, King Abdulaziz University, Jeddah, Saudi Arabia
[3]Pathology Department, King Abdulaziz University, Jeddah, Saudi Arabia
[4]Urology Department, King Abdulaziz University, Jeddah, Saudi Arabia

Correspondence should be addressed to Osama Y. Safdar; safderosama@hotmail.com

Academic Editor: Władysław Sułowicz

Background. Oncocytomas are the second most common benign renal neoplasm but, unfortunately, they are difficult to differentiate from renal cell carcinoma. Renal oncocytomas are rare and have mostly been reported in adults. To our knowledge, this is only the sixth pediatric reported case of renal oncocytoma worldwide. *Case Presentation.* A 14-year-old Yemeni girl with a recurrent history of urinary tract infections came to our clinic complaining of left flank pain with a frontal headache. Ultrasound showed a 3 cm, well-defined echogenic lesion with mild vascularity. This lesion increased in size on her subsequent follow-ups. Computed tomography showed no intralesional fat, vessels invasion, or enlarged lymph nodes. The patient underwent laparoscopic radical nephrectomy, and a pathology report confirmed the diagnosis of renal oncocytoma. *Conclusion and Recommendations.* We present the rare occurrence of renal oncocytoma in a pediatric patient and highlight the importance of considering oncocytomas in the diagnosis of a renal mass.

1. Background

Most of the renal oncocytomas have been reported in the Western literature, and only a few cases have been detected in eastern populations. In the present study, we demonstrate the occurrence of renal oncocytoma in a pediatric patient in Saudi Arabia.

Renal oncocytoma was first described by Zippel in 1942 as a malignant entity [1]. However, in 1976, Klein and Valensi were able to demonstrate its benign characters based on their long series of 13 cases [2].

Renal oncocytoma is the second most common benign renal neoplasm after angiomyolipoma, accounting for 3–7% of all renal tumors [3]. Classical macroscopic characteristics of oncocytomas include a brown, well-demarcated lesion that has central stellate scar [4].

Unfortunately, most oncocytomas are difficult to differentiate from chromophobe renal cell carcinoma due to overlapping ultrastructural, immunohistochemical, and morphological characteristics [5]. Moreover, fine needle aspiration is often not diagnostic due to oncocytoma having similar cytological characteristics as renal cell carcinoma [6].

Development of renal oncocytoma in pediatric patients is rare. To our knowledge, this is only the sixth reported pediatric case of renal oncocytoma in a 14-year-old young girl.

2. Case Presentation

An 11-year-old Yemeni young girl presented with a history of recurrent urinary tract infections. Her past medical history was insignificant. Radiological investigations revealed that both kidneys are normal in size, position, and echogenicity, with bilateral renal fullness. Voiding cystourethrography was unremarkable, and follow-up ultrasound showed minimal fullness in the right renal pelvis.

At the age of 14 years old, she developed left flank pain along with a frontal headache. Ultrasound revealed a well-defined echogenic lesion measuring three centimeters at the lower pole of the left kidney, demonstrating mild vascularity,

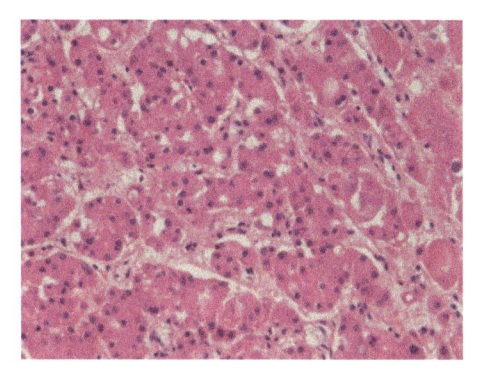

(a) The neoplastic cells have abundant eosinophilic granular cytoplasm and uniform nuclei, arranged in nests and acini (H&E, 200x)

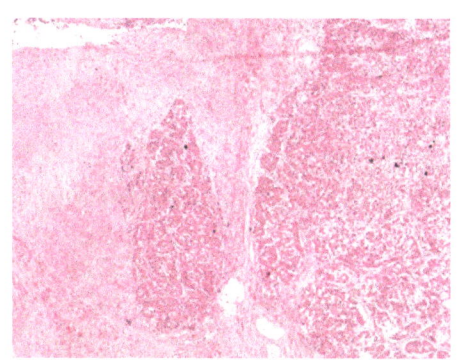

(b) A well-defined tumor mass with focal extension into the renal capsule (H&E, 40x)

Figure 1: Pathology pictures.

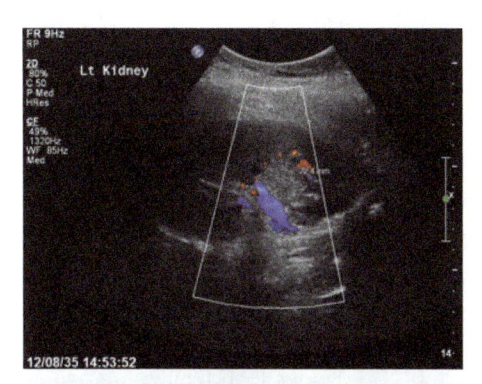

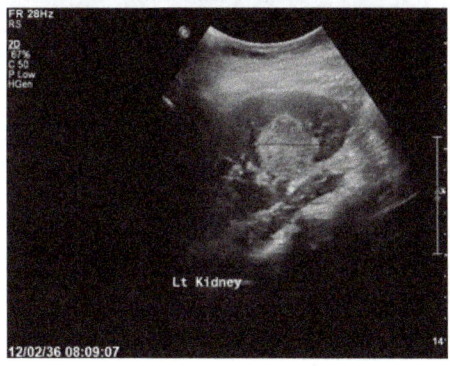

Figure 2: Ultrasound studies.

which was presumed to be angiomyolipoma. Further follow-up after three months revealed an increase in the size of the mass that measured around 3.22 × 3.8 cm with the same degree of vascularity (Figure 2).

A subsequent computed tomography (CT) scan showed an enhancing mass, measuring 4 × 5 cm, arising from the mid- and lower-left renal pelvis. No macroscopic intralesional fat was identified with no invasion of the renal vessels or enlarged lymph nodes (Figure 3).

By magnetic resonance imaging (MRI), we identified a solitary well-circumscribed left renal hilum mass that measured 5 × 3 × 5 cm. No vascular invasion was identified, and the mass showed avid enhancement in the arterial phase and minimal washout in the delay phase (Figure 4).

The patient underwent laparoscopic radical nephrectomy with an uneventful recovery. On regular follow-up, the patient was found to have persistent right kidney hydronephrosis, along with recurrent urinary tract infections, chronic kidney disease (stage three) with an estimated GFR of 58 ml/min/1.73 m^2, and stage 2 hypertension.

A pathology report revealed a well-defined tumor mass measuring 4 × 4 × 4 cm, located at the lower pole of the left kidney, brown, with foci of hemorrhage. No gross invasion of the renal capsule or perinephric fat was identified, and the adrenal glands were unremarkable (Figure 1).

Microscopic examination revealed a well-defined tumor composed of round to polygonal cells with abundant granular eosinophilic cytoplasm and regular, uniform nuclei, arranged in nests, acini, and tubules. Foci of hemorrhage were noted, and rare mitotic figures were identified. There was no evidence of necrosis. The nonneoplastic renal parenchyma shows only glomerular congestion and focal dilatation of the renal calyces. Hale colloidal iron histochemical staining was negative in the tumor cells. The neoplastic cells were also negative for vimentin and CK7 immunohistochemical stains.

3. Discussion

Renal oncocytoma is a rare benign tumor that has unexpectedly occurred in our young patient regardless of the known mean age of this tumor, which strongly influenced the quality of her life.

Oncocytoma usually occurs during the seventh decade of life, varying from 20 to 86 years of age with a predominance in males [7]. Most oncocytomas are single and unilateral, although, occasionally, they can be bilateral and multifocal [8]. The size of these tumors typically varies from 0.6 to 14 cm [9].

Most oncocytomas are diagnosed incidentally when the patients are assessed for nonurological complaints. However, symptomatic patients usually manifest with gross hematuria, flank pain, or a palpable mass [10]. Even though renal

TABLE 1: Review of case reports of the occurrence of renal oncocytoma in pediatric patients.

Sex	Age	Presentation	Treatment	Genetic association
Male (20)	13 years old	Left flank pain	Partial nephrectomy	None
Male (21)	17 years old	Viral illness, abdominal mass	Nephrectomy	None
Male (22)	10 years old	Recurrent abdominal pain, malaise, anorexia, macroscopic hematuria and dysuria	Nephrectomy	None
Female (23)	12 years old	Left sided abdominal fullness	Nephrectomy	None
Female (19)	12 years old	Right flank pain	Nephrectomy	None
Female (this case)	14 years old	Left flank pain	Nephrectomy	None

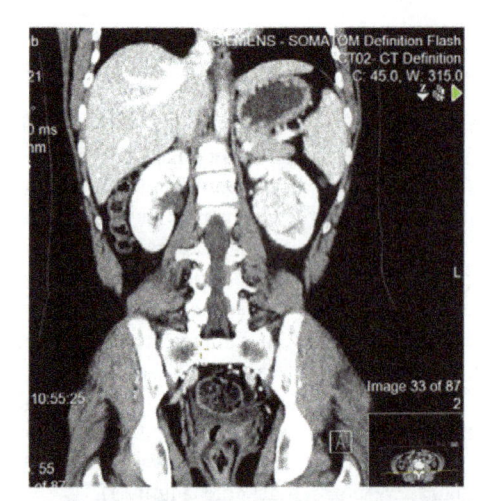

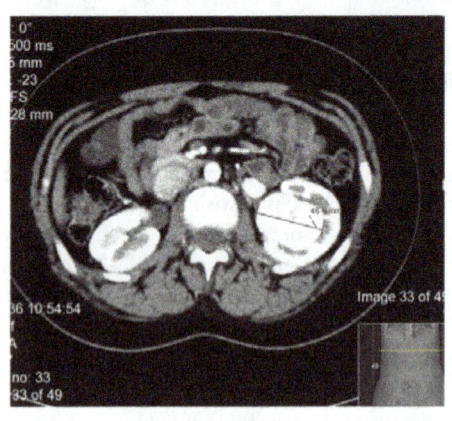

FIGURE 3: CT study.

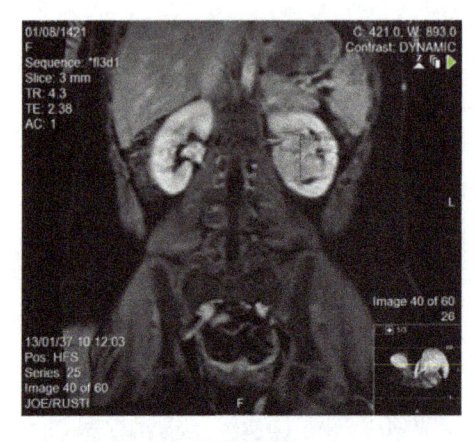

FIGURE 4: MRI study.

oncocytoma is known to have excellent long-term outcomes [11], the diagnosis is made after surgical removal of the tumor because of lack of specific clinical features and imaging findings [12]. Patients with renal oncocytomas need to be monitored closely for any evidence of coexisting renal cell carcinoma or rapid growth in size [10].

In renal oncocytoma patients, CT scans reveal a homogenous well-circumscribed solid mass with a central stellate scar [13]. However, this is only found in 33% of cases [14]. In our case; no central scar was visible by CT.

Furthermore, MRI of renal oncocytoma typically produces homogenous images with low density in T1 weighted sequences, which becomes hyperintense in T2 weighted images [15].

There have been some genetic abnormalities associated with renal oncocytomas, such as loss of chromosome Y or translocations in the 11q13 and loss of heterozygosity on chromosome 14q [10, 12]. However, genetic testing was not performed in this study.

Rarely, oncocytoma can occur as a part of hybrid oncocytic chromophobe tumors (HOCT), which are a subtype of chromophobe renal cell carcinoma (chRCC) that consist of chRCC and renal oncocytoma. This unique presentation has only been reported in two pediatric cases [16, 17]. Furthermore, researchers have shown that primary clear cell carcinoma can coexist with oncocytoma in the same or contralateral kidney [18].

Renal oncocytoma is more prevalent in adults than in children. A literature review revealed that, among the five documented pediatric cases, the youngest age was 10 years, and the eldest was 17 years; most pediatric patients complained of flank pain as a presenting symptom, which is similar to our case. Male to female predominance was 1 : 1 and no cases had any genetic association evident at the time of publication (Table 1) [19].

4. Conclusion

In this case, we present the rare occurrence of renal oncocytoma in a pediatric patient and the importance of considering it as part of the differential diagnosis of a renal mass.

References

[1] L. Zippel, *Zur Kenntnis der oncocytem. Virchow Arch Pathol Anat*, 308, 360, 1942.

[2] M. J. Klein and Q. J. Valensi, "Proximal tubular adenomas of kidney with so-called oncocytic features. A clinicopathologic study of 13 cases of a rarely reported neoplasm," *Cancer*, vol. 38, no. 2, pp. 906–914, 1976.

[3] A. B. Rosenkrantz, N. Hindman, E. F. Fitzgerald, B. E. Niver, J. Melamed, and J. S. Babb, "MRI features of renal oncocytoma and chromophobe renal cell carcinoma," *American Journal of Roentgenology*, vol. 195, no. 6, pp. W421–W427, 2010.

[4] O. N. Kryvenko, M. Jorda, P. Argani, and J. I. Epstein, "Diagnostic Approach to Eosinophilic Renal Neoplasms," *Archives of Pathology & Laboratory Medicine*, vol. 138, no. 11, pp. 1531–1541, 2014.

[5] S. K. Tickoo and M. B. Amin, "Discriminant nuclear features of renal oncocytoma and chromophobe renal cell carcinoma: Analysis of their potential utility in the differential diagnosis," *American Journal of Clinical Pathology*, vol. 110, no. 6, pp. 782–787, 1998.

[6] J. Liu and C. V. Fanning, "Can renal oncocytomas be distinguished from renal cell carcinoma on fine-needle aspiration specimens? A study of conventional smears in conjunction with ancillary studies," *Cancer*, vol. 93, no. 6, pp. 390–397, 2001.

[7] L. Romis, L. Cindolo, J. J. Patard et al., "Frequency, Clinical Presentation and Evolution of Renal Oncocytomas: Multicentric Experience from a European Database," *European Urology*, vol. 45, no. 1, pp. 53–57, 2004.

[8] S. Ahmad, R. Manecksha, B. D. Hayes, and R. Grainger, "Case report of a symptomatic giant renal oncocytoma," *International Journal of Surgery Case Reports*, vol. 2, no. 6, pp. 83–85, 2011.

[9] C. Alamara, E. M. Karapanagiotou, I. Tourkantonis et al., "Renal oncocytoma: A case report and short review of the literature," *European Journal of Internal Medicine*, vol. 19, no. 7, pp. e67–e69, 2008.

[10] D. H. Chao, A. Zisman, A. J. Pantuck, S. J. Freedland, J. W. Said, and A. S. Belldegrun, "Changing concepts in the management of renal oncocytoma," *Urology*, vol. 59, no. 5, pp. 635–642, 2002.

[11] M. A. Benatiya, G. Rais, M. Tahri et al., "Renal oncocytoma: Experience of clinical urology a, urology department, chu ibn sina, rabat, morocco and literature review," *Pan African Medical Journal*, vol. 12, no. 1, 2012.

[12] Y. H. Fan, Y. H. Chang, W. J. S. Huang, H. J. Chung, and K. K. Chen, "Renal oncocytoma: Clinical experience of Taipei Veterans General Hospital," *Journal of the Chinese Medical Association*, vol. 71, no. 5, pp. 254–258, 2008.

[13] L. K. Shin, R. L. Badler, F. M. Bruno, M. Gupta, and D. S. Katz, "Radiology—Pathology Conference," *Clinical Imaging*, vol. 28, no. 5, pp. 344–348.

[14] B. Perez-Ordonez, G. Hamed, S. Campbell et al., "Renal Oncocytoma: A Clinicopathologic Study of 70 Cases," *The American Journal of Surgical Pathology*, vol. 21, no. 8, pp. 871–883, 1997.

[15] P. De Carli, A. Vidiri, L. Lamanna, and R. Cantiani, "Renal oncocytoma: image diagnostics and therapeutic aspects," *Journal of Experimental & Clinical Cancer Research*, vol. 19, no. 3, pp. 287–290, http://www.ncbi.nlm.nih.gov/pubmed/11144520.

[16] A. Gibson and A. Ray, "Rare Case of Hybrid Oncocytoma and Chromophobe Renal Cell Carcinoma in a Pediatric Patient," *Pediatric Blood & Cancer*, vol. 63, no. 6, p. 1127, 2016.

[17] V. Kesik, B. Yalçin, Z. Akçören, M. E. Senocak, B. Talim, and M. Büyükpamukçu, "A rare type of renal cell carcinoma in a girl: hybrid renal cell carcinoma.," *Pediatric Hematology and Oncology*, vol. 27, no. 3, pp. 228–232, 2010.

[18] M. R. Licht, A. C. Novick, R. R. Tubbs, E. A. Klein, H. S. Levin, and S. B. Streem, "Renal Oncocytoma: Clinical and Biological Correlates," *The Journal of Urology*, vol. 150, no. 5, pp. 1380–1383, 1993.

[19] S. Speer, D. Wiseman, M. Moussa, and A. Bütter, "Renal oncocytosis in a pediatric patient: Case report and review of the literature," *Journal of Pediatric Surgery Case Reports*, vol. 3, no. 11, pp. 481–484, 2015.

A Rare Case of Transient Proximal Renal Tubular Acidosis in Pregnancy

Dennis Narcisse,[1] Manyoo Agarwal,[2] and Aneel Kumar[2]

[1] University of Tennessee College of Medicine, Memphis, TN, USA
[2] Department of Internal Medicine, University of Tennessee Health Science Center, Memphis, TN, USA

Correspondence should be addressed to Manyoo Agarwal; manyooagarwal@gmail.com

Academic Editor: Ze'ev Korzets

Renal tubular acidosis (RTA) is a disorder that has improper function of renal acid-base regulation and is rarely encountered during pregnancy. Currently, there is no clear evidence on management and outcomes in patients with this condition. We report a case of a previously healthy 23-year-old female at 30 weeks of gestation who presented with proximal RTA and had spontaneous resolution of the condition shortly after delivery.

1. Introduction

Renal tubular acidosis (RTA) is a group of disorders that are defined by defective renal acid-base regulation. The disease can be inherited, acquired, or idiopathic. RTA is classified into three major forms, which include distal (type 1), proximal (type 2), and hyperkalemic (type 4) forms. Distal RTA is characterized by decreased urinary acid secretion, proximal RTA has an impaired bicarbonate reabsorption, and hyperkalemic RTA is either an aldosterone deficiency or resistance [1].

RTA is rarely encountered during pregnancy and commonly has been reported with maternal substance abuse, such as toluene [2]. Less commonly, it is associated with other maternal diseases such as systemic lupus erythematous, chronic hepatitis, or diabetes [3]. RTA may also have an unclear etiology and sometimes can have a transient course with complete resolution after delivery [2].

We report a case of transient proximal RTA in a previously healthy 23-year-old patient at 30 weeks of gestation that spontaneously resolved after delivery.

2. Case

A 23-year-old previously healthy African American female, gravida 5 para 4, with no significant past medical history presented at 30 weeks of gestation with complaints of generalized weakness and fatigue for the previous two weeks. Review of systems was only significant for polyuria and polydipsia. Physical examination revealed normotensive blood pressure (122/66 mmHg), normal heart rate (72 beats per minute), and a fundus height that was consistent with 30 weeks of gestation. She had no other notable physical exam findings.

Labs revealed WBC 6.5 cells/uL, hemoglobin 13 g/dL, platelets 350, sodium 135 mmol/L, potassium 1.6 mmol/L, chloride 115 mmol/L, bicarbonate 14 mmol/l, BUN 2 mg/dL, creatinine 0.7 mg/dL, glucose 74 mg/dL, albumin 2.5 gm/dL, calcium 8.7 mg/dL, magnesium 2.1 mEq/L, and corrected serum anion gap of 10.55. Arterial blood gas revealed pH of 7.33, PCO_2 25 mmHg, PO_2 110 mmHg, and bicarbonate 13.2 moll/L. Urine studies were significant for urine pH of 5, urine anion gap of −1 (urine sodium 80 mmol/L, urine potassium 40 mmol/L, and urine chloride 121 mmol/L), and transtubular potassium gradient of 18 (serum osmolality 275 mosm/dL/L, urine osmolality 380 mosm/dL, urine potassium 40 mmol/L, and serum potassium 1.6 mmol/l), and both urine protein and glucose were negative.

The patient was subsequently diagnosed with type 2 (proximal) RTA based on the laboratory data ordered above. ANA, anti-SSA, anti-SSB, anti-dsDNA, anti-Smith, HIV, TSH, and hepatitis panel were all normal/nonreactive. During the hospital stay, she initially received a sodium bicarbonate drip totaling 300 mEq. This was eventually transitioned

TABLE 1: Reported cases and outcomes of renal tubular acidosis (RTA) that presented during pregnancy [2, 3, 7–9].

Case	Year	Type of RTA	Outcome
Srisuttayasathien	2015	Distal RTA	Rhabdomyolysis induced by hypokalemia from distal RTA; successful delivery and being healthy on follow-up.
Mallett et al.	2011	Distal RTA (ibuprofen related)	Distal RTA induced by ibuprofen and codeine abuse that resolved after delivery of healthy baby at 37 weeks. Some renal dysfunction persisted on follow-up.
Muthukrishnan et al.	2010	Distal RTA	Persistent hypokalemia leading to rhabdomyolysis; successful delivery and complete resolution of symptoms.
Firmin et al.	2007	Proximal RTA	Delivery of a healthy infant; mild persistence of hypokalemia at 1-year follow-up.
Seoud et al.	2000	Transient RTA	Delivery of a healthy infant; complete resolution of symptoms at follow-up.

to potassium citrate 20 mEq orally three times per day. After one week, she underwent a spontaneous vaginal delivery of a premature fetus; however the baby died shortly after delivery secondary to respiratory failure. The patient was seen at a two-week follow-up visit in the outpatient clinic where serum potassium was 4.3 and serum bicarbonate was 27 mmol/L. Our patient did not require any further potassium or bicarbonate supplementation after pregnancy and her supplementation was then discontinued.

3. Discussion

The kidney has an important role in maintaining normal systemic acid base by controlling bicarbonate reabsorption and acid secretion. Loss of some tubular function can prevent the kidney from maintaining this balance [4]. The group of diseases characterized as renal tubular acidosis (RTA) refers to a condition in which there is normal serum anion gap or hyperchloremic metabolic acidosis in the presence of well-preserved glomerular function. This is caused by the inability of the renal tubule to reabsorb bicarbonate or to secrete hydrogen ions [5]. In most sources, primary RTA is divided into a proximal (type II), distal (type I), and a hyperkalemic form associated with hyperaldosteronism or aldosterone resistance (Type IV).

Distal RTA (type 1) is the most common form of primary RTA in most Western countries. Distal RTA occurs due to the inability of the renal tubules to decrease urine pH and increase urinary ammonium excretion during sustained hyperchloremic metabolic acidosis and hypokalemia [5]. This is caused by a failure to reabsorb bicarbonate by the intercalated cells in the collecting duct [6]. The disease can be inherited or more commonly it can be a complication of other systemic diseases. Distal RTA can also lead to increased loss of urinary calcium resulting in osteopenia, osteomalacia, nephrocalcinosis, and even secondary hyperparathyroidism [2]. Patients with distal RTA typically present with signs and symptoms related to severe hypokalemia such as proximal muscle weakness, polydipsia, and polyuria. Treatment of these patients typically include supplementing with sodium or potassium bicarbonate [6].

Proximal RTA (type 2) is associated with a decreased ability of the proximal nephron to reabsorb bicarbonate. Patients with proximal RTA can be asymptomatic or as in our case present with weakness and paralysis secondary to severe hypokalemia. The hyperchloremic metabolic acidosis in proximal RTA is usually less severe because the tubular system is still capable of retaining bicarbonate distally [6]. This type of RTA is most commonly an inherited condition associated with Fanconi's syndrome, in which there is also a tubular loss of glucose, calcium, phosphate, and amino acids [2].

There is a further subdivision of proximal RTA, which is a rare condition called isolated proximal RTA. This form can either be classified as an autosomal dominant, autosomal recessive, or sporadic isolated proximal RTA. In either the autosomal dominant or recessive form, the RTA usually is a lifelong condition after presentation. However, the sporadic isolated proximal RTA is typically a sporadic event that resolves sometime after treatment [2]. Our case is very likely a presentation of the sporadic isolated proximal RTA because of the spontaneous resolution shortly after treatment and delivery of the fetus.

Pregnancy is reported to worsen either type of RTA. In pregnancy, there is an understood mild physiological respiratory alkalosis and a hyperfiltration in the kidneys secondary to increased blood volume. This hyperfiltration results in an increased loss of some electrolytes leading to a higher requirement of potassium and bicarbonate [3]. Some forms of RTA can cause extreme hypokalemia due to these factors. Both distal and proximal RTA can cause hypokalemia which usually is a result of the renal system attempting to compensate for the metabolic acidosis by excreting potassium [2]. Rhabdomyolysis, commonly caused by severe hypokalemia, is a potentially life threating syndrome that results from the breakdown of muscle fibers that leak into circulation. In pregnancy, there is an increased incidence of hypokalemia induced rhabdomyolysis as seen in a case report by two of the cases in Table 1. In both cases of rhabdomyolysis, the patients presented with muscle pain and severe cramps. Electrolyte abnormalities, renal function, and liver enzymes all need to be monitored and corrected quickly especially in pregnant patients to prevent adverse outcomes [7, 8].

There are some case reports of RTA presenting for the first time in pregnant patients as seen in Table 1. In the medical literature, RTA in pregnancy could be secondary to a maternal systemic disease or ingestion of medications like Dyazide for hypertension during pregnancy or following toluene abuse. Some systemic disorders that have been reported to cause RTA were diabetic ketoacidosis, thyrotoxicosis, alcoholic liver disease, and sickle cell disease. However, in the five cases that were found, only one had a clear cause of RTA. In a report by Mallett et al., the patient had a history of ibuprofen and codeine abusing for the previous six years. The cause of the distal RTA in this case appears clearly linked to her substance abuse, and her renal function and potassium requirements significantly improved after stopping ibuprofen and codeine [9]. In the case by Firmin et al., the previously healthy patient presented with muscle weakness and body pains and was diagnosed with sporadic isolated proximal RTA. The patient responded well to treatment and delivered a healthy infant. Her RTA persisted in a very mild form at her follow-up visits [2]. In the last case, Seoud et al. reported on a previously healthy patient who presented with no signs or symptoms of hypokalemia, but she was incidentally diagnosed with RTA on labs drawn for possible preterm labor. After treatment and delivery of a healthy infant, she gradually had complete resolution of her acidosis and electrolyte abnormalities over the course of six months [3]. In all of the cases found in Table 1, the acidosis did not have any major effect on the fetus.

Previous reports of RTA in pregnancy, however, have offered little discussion on the effects of RTA on fetal development [10]. Severe acute metabolic acidosis in pregnancy has been suggested to cause decreased fetal circulation leading to possible fetal distress or demise [8]. In our case, the patient went into spontaneous premature delivery of the fetus that did not survive. The effects of RTA on fetal outcome are unclear. RTA in pregnancy and the negative effects can be corrected, as seen in Firmin et al. work, whenever the condition is diagnosed early and permanent damage has not yet occurred [2]. However, there have been cases, such as that of Jain et al., where RTA was found to be a cause of multiple loss of pregnancies in a 30-year-old patient [11].

Also, in our case, the patient had no previous past medical history and spontaneously began having hypokalemia symptoms from her sporadic RTA. The patient did not have any evident causes of her disease and did not report any family history or prior complications with previous pregnancies. Seoud et al. reported their patient with proximal RTA initially presented with preterm labor. Their case also resulted in resolution of electrolyte abnormalities in less than a year after delivery [3]. On our patient's labs, there was a very evident hypokalemic hyperchloremic metabolic acidosis, urine studies were consistent with poor compensation by the tubular system, and urinary pH was less than 5.3 with a low serum bicarbonate. The patient had significantly low albumin levels which can cause a reduction in unmeasured anions. For this reason, a corrected anion gap was still collected and it was found to be normal gap of 10.55. These factors are diagnostic for proximal RTA [6]. Treatment goal for proximal RTA is to increase the serum concentration of bicarbonate to as close to normal as possible.

The patient had no systemic disorders and her electrolyte abnormalities quickly resolved after delivery of the preterm fetus. This leads us to believe that our case was isolated sporadic proximal RTA induced during pregnancy. Unfortunately, our patient presented several weeks after being symptomatic, which led to delayed acidosis correction and a preterm delivery. The newborn had respiratory failure and died shortly after birth. It is unclear if earlier treatment would have prevented this outcome.

4. Conclusion

In conclusion, we presented a very rare case of isolated sporadic proximal RTA (type 2) in a previously healthy pregnant patient. She has no past medical history and no clear inciting causes of her presenting condition. She responded well to treatment and one week later delivered a preterm infant who did not survive. Shortly after her delivery, she spontaneously and completely resolved her condition no longer needing any treatment for RTA.

References

[1] J. Yaxley and C. Pirrone, "Review of the diagnostic evaluation of renal tubular acidosis," *The Ochsner Journal*, vol. 16, no. 4, pp. 525–530, 2016.

[2] C. J. Firmin, T. F. Kruger, and R. Davids, "Proximal renal tubular acidosis in pregnancy: a case report and literature review," *Gynecologic and Obstetric Investigation*, vol. 63, no. 1, pp. 39–44, 2007.

[3] M. Seoud, A. Adra, A. Khalil, R. Skaff, I. Usta, and I. Salti, "Transient renal tubular acidosis in pregnancy," *American Journal of Perinatology*, vol. 17, no. 5, pp. 249–252, 2000.

[4] Y. M. Smulders, P. H. J. Frissen, E. H. Slaats, and J. Silberbusch, "Renal tubular acidosis: Pathophysiology and diagnosis," *JAMA Internal Medicine*, vol. 156, no. 15, pp. 1629–1636, 1996.

[5] F. Santos, H. Gil-Peña, and S. Alvarez-Alvarez, "Renal tubular acidosis," *Current Opinion in Pediatrics*, vol. 29, no. 2, pp. 206–210, 2017.

[6] M. Soleimani and A. Rastegar, "Pathophysiology of renal tubular acidosis: Core curriculum 2016," *American Journal of Kidney Diseases*, vol. 68, no. 3, pp. 488–498, 2016.

[7] J. Muthukrishnan, K. Harikumar, R. Jha, and K. Modi, "Pregnancy predisposes to rhabdomyolysis due to hypokalemia," *Saudi Journal of Kidney Diseases and Transplantation*, vol. 21, no. 6, pp. 1127-1128, 2010.

[8] M. Srisuttayasathien, "Hypokalemia-Induced Rhabdomyolysis as a result of Distal Renal Tubular Acidosis in a Pregnant Woman: A Case Report and Literature Review," *Case Reports in Obstetrics and Gynecology*, vol. 2015, pp. 1–3, 2015.

[9] A. Mallett, M. Lynch, G. T. John, H. Healy, and K. Lust, "Ibuprofen-related renal tubular acidosis in pregnancy," *Obstetric Medicine: The Medicine of Pregnancy*, vol. 4, no. 3, pp. 122–124, 2011.

Atypical Haemolytic Uraemic Syndrome Associated with *Clostridium difficile* Infection Successfully Treated with Eculizumab

Joshua M. Inglis,[1] Jeffrey A. Barbara,[2,3] Rajiv Juneja,[2,3] Caroline Milton,[2,3] George Passaris,[2] and Jordan Y. Z. Li[2,3]

[1]*Department of General Medicine, Royal Adelaide Hospital, Adelaide, SA, Australia*
[2]*Department of Renal Medicine, Flinders Medical Centre, Adelaide, SA, Australia*
[3]*School of Medicine, Flinders University, Adelaide, SA, Australia*

Correspondence should be addressed to Jordan Y. Z. Li; Jordan.Li@sa.gov.au

Academic Editor: Yoshihide Fujigaki

Clostridium difficile infection is a rare precipitant of atypical haemolytic uraemic syndrome (aHUS). A 46-year-old man presented with watery diarrhoea following an ileocaecal resection. He developed an acute kidney injury with anaemia, thrombocytopaenia, raised lactate dehydrogenase, low haptoglobin, and red cell fragments. Stool sample was positive for *C. difficile* toxin B. He became dialysis-dependent as his renal function continued to worsen despite treatment with empiric antibiotics and plasma exchange. The ADAMTS13 level was normal consistent with a diagnosis of aHUS. The commencement of eculizumab led to the resolution of haemolysis and stabilisation of haemoglobin and platelets with an improvement in renal function.

1. Background

Atypical haemolytic uraemic syndrome (aHUS) is a rare disorder characterised by thrombocytopaenia and evidence of microangiopathic haemolysis. ADAMTS13 levels are normal and STEC (Shiga toxin-producing *E. coli*) is not present in the stool. The pathogenesis involves activation of complement via the alternative pathway leading to a thrombotic microangiopathy with end-organ involvement predominantly affecting the renal and neurological systems [1]. The precipitants for aHUS include complement regulation deficits, infections, drugs, and pregnancy [2]. *Clostridium difficile* infection has been identified as a rare precipitant [3–7].

2. Case Report

A 46-year-old man with no past medical history and no regular medications presented to a rural hospital with an acute abdomen. An explorative laparotomy revealed a small bowel obstruction secondary to a congenital band with an associated strangulated segment that required an ileocaecal resection. The patient received antibiotic cover with cephazolin, gentamicin, and metronidazole in addition to opioid analgesia. On the tenth postoperative day he had watery diarrhoea. On the following day the patient became anuric with moderate hypertension (BP 160/80).

Blood tests revealed an acute kidney injury with a sudden rise in creatinine from 71 to 307 μmol/L (reference range RR 50–120 μmol/L). The blood film showed red cell fragments (18–24 per HPF) together with an acute anaemia, nadir haemoglobin 68 g/L (RR 110–150 g/L), and thrombocytopaenia, nadir platelet count 87 × 10^9/L (RR 150–450 × 10^9/L). Further blood tests revealed a lactate dehydrogenase (LDH) of 1657 (RR 110–230 U/L), a haptoglobin of 0.09 (RR 0.50–2.50), a bilirubin of 86 (RR 2–24), and a negative direct antibody test (DAT). Complement components were low with C3 of 0.75 (RR 0.85–1.60) and C4 of 0.09 (RR 0.12–0.36). There was a coinciding derangement in the liver function tests with gamma-glutamyl transferase (GGT) 589 IU/L (RR < 60 IU/L), alkaline phosphatase (ALP) 112 IU/L (RR < 55 IU/L), aspartate transaminase (AST) 60 IU/L (RR < 55 IU/L), and alanine transaminase (ALT) 209 IU/l (RR <

TABLE 1: Published reports of C. *difficile*-associated aHUS.

Reference	Age/sex	Kidney	Clinical features	Treatment	Dialysis	Outcome
[3]	51/female	Native	Watery diarrhoea, confusion	Vancomycin	No	Recovery
[4]	46/female	Native	Bloody diarrhoea, vomiting	Metronidazole, plasmapheresis	Yes	Recovery
[5]	62/female	Native	Watery diarrhoea	Metronidazole, plasmapheresis, steroids	Yes	Recovery
[6]	73/female	Native	Watery diarrhoea, respiratory distress, chills, anuria	Metronidazole, steroids	Yes	Recovery
[7]	29/female	Transplant	Diarrhoea, decreased urine output	Vancomycin	Yes	Complete recovery
[7]	52/female	Transplant	Fever, diarrhoea, nausea, vomiting	Metronidazole, plasmapheresis	Yes	Allograft failure and transplant nephrectomy
[7]	63/female	Native	Bloody diarrhoea, fever, confusion	Metronidazole, vancomycin, plasmapheresis	Yes	Partial recovery
Current case	46/male	Native	Watery diarrhoea, anuria	Plasmapheresis, metronidazole, vancomycin and eculizumab	Yes	Recovery

45 IU/L) which was attributed to critical illness. There was an associated coagulopathy with INR 4.9 (range 0.9–1.2), APTT 67 (range 24–38), fibrinogen 3.0 (range 1.5–4), and D-dimer 3.2 that had likely resulted from the hepatic dysfunction.

The stool sample was positive for *Clostridium difficile* toxin B and negative for Shiga toxin on two occasions. Stool culture was negative for other enteric pathogens. ADAMTS13 activity was 69% which is within the normal reference range. Autoimmune screen for ANA, dsDNA, and ANCA was negative. Renal tract ultrasound revealed normal sized kidneys with no hydronephrosis. Liver ultrasound showed hepatomegaly (18 cm) with no evidence of biliary obstruction. Complement factor H *(CFH)* gene analysis did not reveal a mutation.

The patient received daily plasma exchange and haemodialysis in the Intensive Care Unit. Intravenous metronidazole and oral vancomycin were given as antibiotic therapy for *C. difficile*. Multiple blood transfusions were required to maintain the haemoglobin. The patient required intubation and ventilation for hypoxic respiratory failure for a period of 18 days.

Eculizumab infusions were commenced with the cessation of plasma exchange. The protocol involved infusions of 900 mg weekly for four weeks followed by a single infusion of 1200 mg in the fifth week. During the maintenance phase the patient received fortnightly infusions of 1200 mg for one year.

Eculizumab treatment led to a normalisation in haemoglobin, platelet count, LDH, and haptoglobin over the following fortnight. The patient then became dialysis-independent and serum creatinine stabilised at 200 μmol/L prior to discharge.

He continued to receive eculizumab as an outpatient for one year. There was no relapse of disease on eculizumab cessation. He continues to be monitored with regular blood tests. His renal function remains stable at a new baseline creatinine of 130 μmol/L and there is no evidence of haemolysis.

3. Discussion

Atypical haemolytic uraemic syndrome is a clinical diagnosis based on microangiopathic haemolytic anaemia, thrombocytopaenia, and acute kidney injury in the absence of STEC with normal ADAMTS13 activity. Episodes may be precipitated by infection in patients with a genetic susceptibility to complement dysregulation. However, specific complement gene pathway mutations are found in only 50–60% of cases of true aHUS [8].

This case provides further evidence for *C. difficile* infection as a rare precipitant of aHUS. There are seven reported adult cases of *C. difficile*-associated aHUS with this being the first to occur in an adult male and following abdominal surgery [3–7]. The characteristics of these cases are listed in Table 1. While all cases have shared similar clinical presentations of anaemia, thrombocytopaenia and acute kidney injury, the nature of diarrhoea has varied with both watery and bloody stools being reported. Confusion has been reported in four of eight reported cases suggesting that neurological involvement may occur. However, confusion was not present in our case.

Various treatments have been used in the reported cases of *C. difficile*-associated aHUS including antibiotics, steroids, and plasma exchange with generally favourable outcomes in all but one patient who developed allograft failure and required graft nephrectomy [7]. There have been no documented recurrences of *C. difficile*-associated aHUS.

Terminal complement inhibitors have emerged as an effective therapy for aHUS. Eculizumab has been shown to control haemolysis and lead to improvements in renal function [9]. This is the first reported case of *C. difficile*-associated aHUS to be treated with eculizumab in addition to conventional therapies. The patient responded favourably with resolution of haemolysis, normalisation of haemoglobin and platelets, and an improvement in renal function. There has been no recurrence of disease two years after ceasing eculizumab. Eculizumab may be an effective agent for achieving resolution of haemolysis and stabilising renal function in patients with *C. difficile*-associated aHUS.

Disclosure

The authors confirm that this case report has not been published previously except in abstract format.

References

[1] D. Kavanagh, S. Raman, and N. S. Sheerin, "Management of hemolytic uremic syndrome," *F1000Prime Reports*, vol. 6, article no. A119, 2014.

[2] D. Kavanagh, T. H. J. Goodship, and A. Richards, "Atypical haemolytic uraemic syndrome," *British Medical Bulletin*, vol. 77-78, no. 1, pp. 5–22, 2006.

[3] A. Mogyorosi and M. D. Carley, "Hemolytic-uremic syndrome associated with pseudomembranous colitis caused by clostridium difficile," *Nephron*, vol. 76, no. 4, p. 491, 1997.

[4] C. C. Mbonu, D. L. Davison, K. M. El-Jazzar, and G. L. Simon, "Clostridium difficile Colitis Associated With Hemolytic-Uremic Syndrome," *American Journal of Kidney Diseases*, vol. 41, no. 5, pp. e14.1–e14.5, 2003.

[5] M. Keshtkar-Jahromi and M. Mohebtash, " Hemolytic uremic syndrome and ," *Journal of Community Hospital Internal Medicine Perspectives (JCHIMP)*, vol. 2, no. 3, p. 19064, 2012.

[6] E. Kalmanovich, O. Kriger-Sharabi, E. Shiloah, N. Donin, Z. Fishelson, and M. J. Rapoport, "Atypical hemolytic uremic syndrome associated with Clostridium difficile infection and partial membrane cofactor protein (CD46) deficiency," *Israel Medical Association Journal*, vol. 14, no. 9, pp. 586-587, 2012.

[7] A. S. Alvarado, S. V. Brodsky, T. Nadasdy, and N. Singh, "Hemolytic uremic syndrome associated with clostridium difficile infection," *Clinical Nephrology*, vol. 81, no. 4, pp. 302–306, 2014.

[8] M. Noris and G. Remuzzi, "Atypical hemolytic-uremic syndrome," *The New England Journal of Medicine*, vol. 361, no. 17, pp. 1676–1687, 2009.

[9] C. M. Legendre, C. Licht, P. Muus et al., "Terminal complement inhibitor eculizumab in atypical hemolytic-uremic syndrome," *The New England Journal of Medicine*, vol. 368, no. 23, pp. 2169–2181, 2013.

Therapeutic Approach to the Management of Severe Asymptomatic Hyponatremia

Thaofiq Ijaiya, Sandhya Manohar, and Kameswari Lakshmi

Department of Medicine, Montefiore New Rochelle Hospital, Albert Einstein College of Medicine, New Rochelle, NY, USA

Correspondence should be addressed to Thaofiq Ijaiya; tundeijaiya@gmail.com

Academic Editor: Phuong Chi Pham

Hyponatremia is an electrolyte imbalance encountered commonly in the hospital and ambulatory settings. It can be seen in isolation or present as a complication of other medical conditions. It is therefore a challenge to determine the appropriate therapeutic intervention. An understanding of the etiology is key in instituting the right treatment. Clinicians must not be too hasty to correct a random laboratory value without first understanding the physiologic principle. We present such a case of a patient who presented with sodium of 98 mmol/L, the lowest recorded in the current literature, and yet was asymptomatic. Following appropriate management driven by an understanding of the underlying pathophysiologic mechanism, the patient was managed to full recovery without any clinically significant neurological sequelae.

1. Introduction

Hyponatremia is the most commonly identified electrolyte abnormality in hospitalized adults [1, 2] and known to have an association with mortality. Symptoms can range from nausea and malaise, with mild reduction in the serum sodium, to lethargy, decreased level of consciousness, and, in severe cases, seizures and coma [3, 4]. Overt neurologic symptoms are due to very low serum sodium levels (usually less than 115 mEq/L), resulting in intracerebral osmotic fluid shifts and brain edema. Cases of severe hyponatremia presenting with no neurologic symptoms are rare [5]. We report a case of severe, asymptomatic hyponatremia with a sodium level of 98 mmol/L, which to the best of our knowledge is the lowest recorded level in the current literature.

2. Case Report

A 48-year-old female presented to our emergency room (ER) with facial injuries following a mechanical fall. She denied any dizziness, chest pain, palpitations, or unsteadiness of her gait prior to this.

Her history was remarkable for alcoholic liver disease with prior episodes of nonvariceal gastrointestinal bleeding. She continues to consume alcohol on a regular basis, usually 2 bottles of beer per day and her last drink was a day prior to her fall. She also smokes up to a pack of cigarettes a day. Her home medications were potassium supplement and multivitamins.

On physical examination, she had a pulse rate of 78/min and a blood pressure of 154/59 mmHg with no orthostatic changes. She appeared comfortable and well oriented to time, place, and person. She had moist mucous membrane and no JVD. She had multiple lacerations on her face that were sutured in the ER, along with multiple bilateral ecchymotic patches on her legs. Her neurological exam showed mild impairment in her balance and coordination. Rest of the physical examination was unremarkable.

Blood work showed serum sodium concentration was 98 mmol/L, and other laboratory data are listed in Table 1. Her baseline serum sodium from a year ago was consistently between 125 and 129 mmol/L with no symptoms reported and there was no intervention at that time. Her stools were positive for occult blood. A chest X-ray and a CT head were normal.

A decision was made to admit the patient to the Intensive Care Unit for closer monitoring of her sodium levels. Her volume status was considered to be low initially due to presumed gastrointestinal bleed as well as the low urine sodium and

TABLE 1: Laboratory data at the time of admission.

Sodium 98 mmol/L
Potassium 2.6 mmol/L
Magnesium 1.1 mmol/L
Blood urea nitrogen 19 mg/dL
Creatinine 0.71 mg/dL
Creatine kinase 2366 IU/L
Measured osmolality 235 mOsm/kg
Calculated osmolarity 208 mOsm/kg
Glucose 97 mg/dL
Cortisol 43mcg/dL
TSH 1.55 mIU/L
Total bilirubin 1.8 mg/dL
INR 1.5
Hemoglobin 6.0 mg/dL
Mean corpuscular vol. 93
White blood cell 8,000/mcL
Platelet 67,000/mcL
Folate 9.1 ng/mL
Vitamin B12 1500 pg/mL
Blood alcohol level 82 mg/dL
Urine osmolality 317 mOsm/kg
Urine sodium 17 mmol/L
Urine potassium 31 mmol/L
Urine chloride 25 mmol/L
Direct bilirubin 0.6 mg/dL
AST/ALT 404/113 IU/L

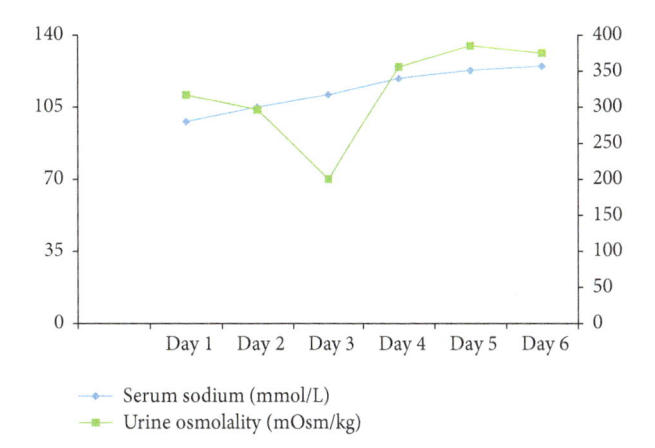

FIGURE 1: Daily trend of serum sodium plotted on left y-axis and urine osmolality plotted on right y-axis.

high urine osmolality. A volume challenge with one litre of 0.9% saline was initially given. A repeat serum sodium level obtained 2 hours later was 100 mmol/L. She was subsequently transfused with 2 units of packed red cells. However, urine osmolality remained elevated (337 mOsm/kg) following this with no significant change in serum sodium levels suggesting an underlying persistent high ADH state. Absence of typical symptoms of severe hyponatremia suggested a chronic etiology as did her moderate hyponatremia from a year earlier.

She was placed on fluid restriction of up to 800 ml/day. Her hypokalemia and hypomagnesemia were corrected with infusions of potassium chloride and magnesium sulphate. With this approach, her serum sodium increased by 7 mmol in the first 24 hours (Figure 1). She had a gradual improvement in her sodium concentration with her levels reaching 125 mmol/L over a six-day period. She had a CT of the chest, abdomen, and pelvis and it did not reveal any significant findings. Her liver dysfunction was managed supportively during her hospital course. The patient was subsequently discharged without any neurological sequelae and follow-up planned with nephrology as well as hepatology.

3. Discussion

Hyponatremia is the clinical manifestation of a wide variety of diseases and identifying the underlying mechanism is crucial in instituting the right treatment [6, 7]. An inappropriate treatment may cause more harm than the initial presenting condition; thus, clinicians need to be familiar with the diagnosis and management of various forms of hyponatremia. The determination of the underlying pathophysiologic mechanism requires a detailed history with emphasis on medications and social habits, a thorough physical exam to assess the volume status, and the valuable input of laboratory and radiological data.

Serum sodium is one of the main determinants of serum osmolality. A fall in serum sodium concentration results in the development of cerebral edema from the sudden changes in osmolality. The brain's adaptation to the process begins immediately after the initial fall in serum osmolality and is completed in 2-3 days [8]. The brain adapts by losing its organic solutes with a resultant osmotic movement of water out of the cell, thus reducing brain swelling [9]. The hyponatremia in such a patient where the brain has acclimatized to a new homeostasis is considered to be chronic hyponatremia [8]. When the hyponatremia is corrected, this process of adaptation in the brain reverses. An aggressive reversal of chronic hyponatremia does not give the brain sufficient time for reuptake of the organic solutes and water resulting in cell shrinkage and demyelination. This is known as osmotic demyelination [10]. It can lead to irreversible neurologic dysfunction, seizures, coma, and, in severe cases, death.

The determination of chronicity is a challenging clinical scenario. It is suggested to consider the patient's history, prior baseline laboratory data as well as the neurological clinical picture to determine chronicity. It is important for the clinician to be aware of this challenge as impulsive decisions can lead to deleterious effects during treatment [11]. Our patient presented with profoundly low serum sodium concentration which appears to have been chronic in nature considering her lack of neurological symptomatology. When in doubt, it is safer to presume the condition to be chronic and be cautious in the management.

Although the existence of truly asymptomatic hyponatremia has been questioned [12, 13], our patient did not manifest with any clinically significant neurological symptoms like seizures or confusion. It could be argued that her mild gait imbalance was related to her hyponatremia although our patient did not provide a history to make that association. The gait abnormality described in this case may be due to other neurological dysfunctions (e.g., cortical atrophy, cerebellar dysfunction) stemming from her chronic alcohol use. Her neurological exam also did not change despite the correction of her sodium. Renneboog et al. have described in their study an association between mild chronic hyponatremia with an increasing incidence of gait and attention impairments [13]. But the general consensus supports the evidence that clinical presentation of severe hyponatremia is influenced more by the rate of decline of the sodium level as against the absolute value [14, 15].

The hyponatremia in our patient was determined to be multifactorial and attributable to a combination of hypovolemic hyponatremia superimposed on chronic hyponatremia related to syndrome of inappropriate antidiuretic hormone secretion (SIADH). The low potassium store, which was attributed to her poor nutrition status from alcoholism, was also likely a propagating factor. Potassium is an osmotically active solute like sodium and the repletion of low potassium levels will increase the serum osmolality and result in the shifting of sodium from intracellular to extracellular space [16]. Monitoring and provision of other osmotically active substrates such as serum phosphate and magnesium are also necessary in the correction of hyponatremia by reducing osmolality differences between compartments [17]. Our patient was managed with the guiding principle that the serum sodium concentration should be corrected at a rate of no more than 10 meq/L in the first 24 hours, 18 meq/L in the first 48 hours, and 20 meq/L in the first 72 hours to prevent iatrogenic brain injury and central pontine myelinolysis [18, 19]. It is recommended that, in high-risk patient groups (severe malnutrition, alcoholism, or advanced liver disease), therapeutic target range should be below the limits that have been established for patients without these conditions as they are at higher risk of osmotic demyelination [19]. Hypertonic saline is not recommended in the management of asymptomatic hyponatremia [18].

Our patient humbled us with a perilously low serum sodium level of 98 mmol/L which to the best of our knowledge is one of the lowest serum sodium concentration reported in the current literature. Joseph et al. discuss a patient with serum sodium of 99 mmol/L who improved on fluid restriction without any neurological sequelae [20]. Accurate diagnosis of the etiology by understanding the underlying mechanism at play is key to a successful correction. Severe hyponatremia, even with such critically low sodium concentration, with appropriate management and diligent monitoring can be managed to the extent of full recovery without any clinically significant neurological sequelae.

References

[1] G. Gill, "Hyponatraemia: biochemical and clinical perspectives," *Postgraduate Medical Journal*, vol. 74, no. 875, pp. 516–523, 1998.

[2] J. A. Owen and D. G. Campbell, "A comparison of plasma electrolyte and urea values in healthy persons and in hospital patients," *Clinica Chimica Acta*, vol. 22, no. 4, pp. 611–618, 1968.

[3] A. I. Arieff, F. Llach, S. G. Massry, and A. Kerian, "Neurological manifestations and morbidity of hyponatremia: Correlation with brain water and electrolytes," *Medicine*, vol. 55, no. 2, pp. 121–129, 1976.

[4] S. J. Ellis, "Severe hyponatraemia: complications and treatment," *QJM*, vol. 88, no. 12, pp. 905–909, 1995.

[5] R. H. Sterns, J. E. Riggs, and S. S. Schochet Jr., "Osmotic demyelination syndrome following correction of hyponatremia," *New England Journal of Medicine*, vol. 314, no. 24, pp. 1535–1542, 1986.

[6] J. A. Clayton, I. R. Le Jeune, and I. P. Hall, "Severe hyponatraemia in medical in-patients: aetiology, assessment and outcome," *Quarterly Journal of Medicine*, vol. 99, no. 8, pp. 505–511, 2006.

[7] D. S. Shapiro, M. Sonnenblick, I. Galperin, L. Melkonyan, and G. Munter, "Severe hyponatraemia in elderly hospitalized patients: prevalence, aetiology and outcome," *Internal Medicine Journal*, vol. 40, no. 8, pp. 574–580, 2010.

[8] I. Douglas, "Hyponatremia: why it matters, how it presents, how we can manage it," *Cleveland Clinic Journal of Medicine*, vol. 73, no. 3, pp. 4–12, 2006.

[9] R. H. Sterns and S. M. Silver, "Brain volume regulation in response to hypo-osmolality and its correction," *The American Journal of Medicine*, vol. 119, no. 7, supplement 1, pp. S12–S16, 2006.

[10] B. O. Saeed, D. Beaumont, G. H. Handley, and J. U. Weaver, "Severe hyponatraemia: Investigation and management in a district general hospital," *Journal of Clinical Pathology*, vol. 55, no. 12, pp. 893–896, 2002.

[11] A. H. Tzamaloukas, D. Malhotra, B. H. Rosen, D. S. C. Raj, G. H. Murata, and J. I. Shapiro, "Principles of management of severe hyponatremia," *Journal of the American Heart Association*, vol. 2, no. 1, Article ID e005199, 2013.

[12] G. Decaux, "Is asymptomatic hyponatremia really asymptomatic?" *American Journal of Medicine*, vol. 119, no. 7, pp. S79–S82, 2006.

[13] B. Renneboog, W. Musch, X. Vandemergel, M. U. Manto, and G. Decaux, "Mild chronic hyponatremia is associated with falls, unsteadiness, and attention deficits," *The American Journal of Medicine*, vol. 119, no. 1, pp. e1–e8, 2006.

[14] J. C. Ayus and A. I. Arieff, "Pathogenesis and prevention of hyponatremic encephalopathy," *EndocrinolMetabClin North Am*, vol. 22, no. 2, pp. 425–446, 1993.

[15] C. L. Fraser and A. I. Arieff, "Epidemiology, pathophysiology, and management of hyponatremic encephalopathy," *American Journal of Medicine*, vol. 102, no. 1, pp. 67–77, 1997.

[16] M. K. Nguyen and I. Kurtz, "Role of potassium in hypokalemia-induced hyponatremia: lessons learned from the edelman equation," *Journal of Clinical and Experimental Nephrology*, vol. 8, no. 2, pp. 98–102, 2004.

[17] P.-M. T. Pham, P.-A. T. Pham, S. V. Pham, P.-T. T. Pham, P.-T. T. Pham, and P.-C. T. Pham, "Correction of hyponatremia and osmotic demyelinating syndrome: have we neglected to think intracellularly?" *Clinical and Experimental Nephrology*, vol. 19, no. 3, pp. 489–495, 2015.

[18] R. H. Sterns, S. U. Nigwekar, and J. K. Hix, "The treatment of hyponatremia," *Seminars in Nephrology*, vol. 29, no. 3, pp. 175–318, 2009.

[19] J. G. Verbalis, S. R. Goldsmith, A. Greenberg, R. W. Schrier, and R. H. Sterns, "Hyponatremia treatment guidelines 2007: expert panel recommendations," *The American Journal of Medicine*, vol. 120, no. 11, supplement 1, pp. S1–S21, 2007.

[20] F. Joseph, M. Kaliyaperumal, N. Moss, F. Qedwai, C. Hill, and A. A. Khan, "Severe hyponatremia - how low can you go?" *Endocrine Abstracts*, vol. 13, p. P43, 2007.

Severe Symptomatic Hyponatremia Secondary to Escitalopram-Induced SIADH: A Case Report

Rishi Raj,[1] Aasems Jacob,[1] Ajay Venkatanarayan,[2] Mohankumar Doraiswamy,[2] and Manjula Ashok[2]

[1]University of Kentucky, Lexington, KY 40536, USA
[2]Monmouth Medical Center, Long Branch, NJ 07740, USA

Correspondence should be addressed to Rishi Raj; rishiraj91215@gmail.com

Academic Editor: Yoshihide Fujigaki

Hyponatremia is a well-known medication related side effect of selective serotonin reuptake inhibitors; despite its association with escitalopram, the newest SSRI is very rare. We did a review of literature and came across only 14 reported case of this rare association of SIADH with escitalopram. We hereby report a case of a 93-year-old female who presented with generalized tonic-clonic seizure and was diagnosed with severe hyponatremia due to escitalopram-induced syndrome of inappropriate antidiuretic hormone secretion (SIADH). With this article, we want to emphasize clinicians about this rare side effect of escitalopram use and look for the risk factors leading to SIADH.

1. Background

The syndrome of inappropriate antidiuretic hormone secretion (SIADH) is a well-known cause of hyponatremia. It is a diagnosis of exclusion and can be secondary to pulmonary disorders, infections, malignant diseases, central nervous system disorders, or drugs [1]. Selective serotonin reuptake inhibitors (SSRIs) are a well-known cause of SIADH with a threefold increased risk compared to other antidepressants [2]. Hyponatremia from escitalopram, one of the newest SSRI is rare with only few reported cases in literature. Here, we report a case of severe hyponatremia which was associated with escitalopram. The importance of the report lies in the fact that SSRIs are one of the most widely used antidepressants and it is imperative for the clinicians to be more widely aware of the life-threatening nature of the side effect of this seemingly benign medication.

2. Case Presentation

A 93-year-old Caucasian female was brought to emergency room for gradual decline in mental status over a course of one week. Her past medical history was significant for coronary artery disease, hypertension, diabetes mellitus, hyperlipidemia, and mild cognitive dysfunction. Her medications included aspirin 81 mg daily, metoprolol 25 mg daily, amlodipine 10 mg daily, and atorvastatin 20 mg daily. Four days prior to the onset of symptoms, she was started on escitalopram 10 mg daily by her primary care physician for newly diagnosed depression. She had a routine blood work immediately prior to the outpatient visit and on retrospective review was found to have a serum sodium level of 136 mEq/L. Patient developed drowsiness and inability to maintain conversation after four days of starting escitalopram. Her mental status continued to gradually decline over the course of next few days and on the day of presentation, which was seven days from the onset of symptoms, she was noted to have intermittent severe agitation. She did not have fever, chills, neck rigidity, myalgia, recent trauma, or fall. There was no reported seizure activity or loss of consciousness. At the time of admission, patient was afebrile, blood pressure was 134/57 mm Hg, pulse rate was 75 beats/min, and respiratory rate of 18 and saturating was 99% on room air. Her BMI was 27.1. She was noted to be lethargic and was only responsive to painful

Table 1: Laboratory results at admission.

Laboratory Test	Levels	Reference Range
Serum Sodium	105 mEq/L	135–145 mEq/L
Serum Chloride	74 mEq/L	99-109 mEq/L
Serum Osmolality	234 mosm/kg	275–295 mosm/kg
Serum Creatinine	0.69 mg/dL	0.40-1.10 mg/dL
Blood Urea Nitrogen (BUN)	10 mg/dL	5-21 mg/dL
Urine Sodium	68 mEq/L	25-150 mEq/L
Urine Chloride	75 mEq/L	75-170 mEq/L
Urine Osmolality	468 mosm/kg	50-1400 mosm/kg
Morning Cortisol	49.2 mcg/dL	1.0-75.0 mcg/dL
Thyroid Stimulating Hormone (TSH)	0.86 mcIU/mL	0.5- 5.0 mcIU/mL

Table 2: Diagnostic criteria for the syndrome of inappropriate antidiuretic hormone secretion (SIADH).

Essential criteria
1. True plasma hypoosmolality (<275 mOsm/kg H2O)
2. Inappropriate urinary response to hypoosmolality (urine osmolality >100 mOsm/kg H2O)
3. Euvolemia; no edema, ascites, or signs of hypovolemia
4. Elevated urine sodium (>30 mEq/L) during normal sodium and water intake
5. No other causes of euvolemic hyponatremia
Supplemental criteria
1. No significant increase in serum sodium after volume expansion, but improvement with fluid restriction.
2. Unable to excrete >80% of a water load (20 cc/kg) in 4 hours and/or failure to achieve urine osmolality <1mOsm/kg H2O

stimuli. Mucous membranes were moist, and the skin turgor was intact. Her GCS score was 7 (E2V1M4). Neurological examination was negative for any gross focal neurological deficits. The rest of the physical examination was unremarkable. While, in the emergency room, patient was noted to have generalized tonic-clonic seizure which was controlled with a single dose of intravenous lorazepam 1 mg. Initial laboratory investigation results are presented in Table 1, along with reference range values. Notably, patient's serum osmolality was 234 mosm/kg (normal range: 275–295 mosm/kg), urine osmolality was 468 mosm/kg, serum sodium was 105 mEq/L (normal range: 135–145 mEq/L), and urinary sodium was 68 mEq/L (normal range 25-150 mEq/L). Her thyroid-stimulating hormone (TSH) and early morning free cortisol were 0.8 μIU/mL (normal range 0.5-5.0 μIU/mL) and 49.2 μg/dL (normal range 1-75 μg/dL), respectively. Chest X-ray as well as CT Head without contrast were unremarkable.

3. Diagnosis

Based on her clinical findings of witnessed seizure, laboratory findings of severe hyponatremia, hypoosmolality, elevated urine osmolality, and elevated urinary sodium in the presence of normal adrenal and thyroid function, a diagnosis of acute severe symptomatic hypotonic hyponatremia or SIADH was made based on the diagnostic criteria (Table 2). The current symptoms were attributed to initiation of escitalopram due to the temporal relation.

4. Treatment

Escitalopram was discontinued on the day of admission. She was started on 3% hypertonic saline at 20 ml/hr with frequent monitoring of her sodium levels with a goal sodium correction of less than 10 mEq/L in 24 hrs. Patient was put on water restriction to less than one liter per day. She was also given 2 doses of Tolvaptan 15 mg on Day 3 and Day 5 of hospitalization. Patient did not have any further episodes of seizures. Her sodium levels started to trend up and her sodium levels became normal on the 6th day of hospitalization (Figure 1). The patient was finally discharged home on Day 6. Sodium levels on discharge were 135 mEq/L. She was discharged without any SSRI. Repeat sodium levels on 1 week and 2 weeks were 138 mEq/L and 142 mEq/L, respectively. She was eventually started on Mirtazapine 15 mg at bedtime on outpatient follow-up and her sodium levels remained within normal range at 3 and 6 months.

5. Discussion & Review of Literature

SIADH is defined as euvolemic hypotonic hyponatremia (serum sodium level of less than 135mmol/L), inappropriately elevated urine osmolality (usually more than 200 mmol/kg) relative to plasma osmolality, and an elevated urine sodium level (typically greater than 20 mmol/L) with normal renal, adrenal, and thyroid functions. Since Schwartz et al. first described it about 6 decades ago in 1957 in two patients, SIADH now has a long list of potential causes including malignant neoplasms, nonmalignant pulmonary diseases, central nervous system disorders, and drugs. In a single center retrospective study, Shepshelovich et al. compared different drug classes and showed a higher incidence of SIADH with antidepressants mainly SSRIs compared to other drug classes [3]. SSRIs are becoming increasingly leading because of SIADH with a reported incidence of 1 out of 200 patients per year [4]. SSRIs are first-line drugs for the treatment of geriatric depression owing to their safety, easy dose titration, and low rates of anticholinergic and cardiovascular adverse events [5]. Among SSRIs, escitalopram is the newest SSRI and was FDA approved in 2002. It is composed of only (S)-enantiomer of citalopram and inhibits the binding of serotonin (5-HT) to serotonin transporter (SERT), resulting in increased 5-HT concentration in synaptic cleft, which leads to increased binding of 5-HT to postsynaptic receptors causing improvement in the depression symptoms [6]. Experimental studies have revealed that enhanced serotonergic tone result in stimulation of antidiuretic hormone (ADH) secretion resulting in hyponatremia, provided water intake is sufficient [7]. As a matter of fact, since the publication of the above literature, there has been increasingly higher

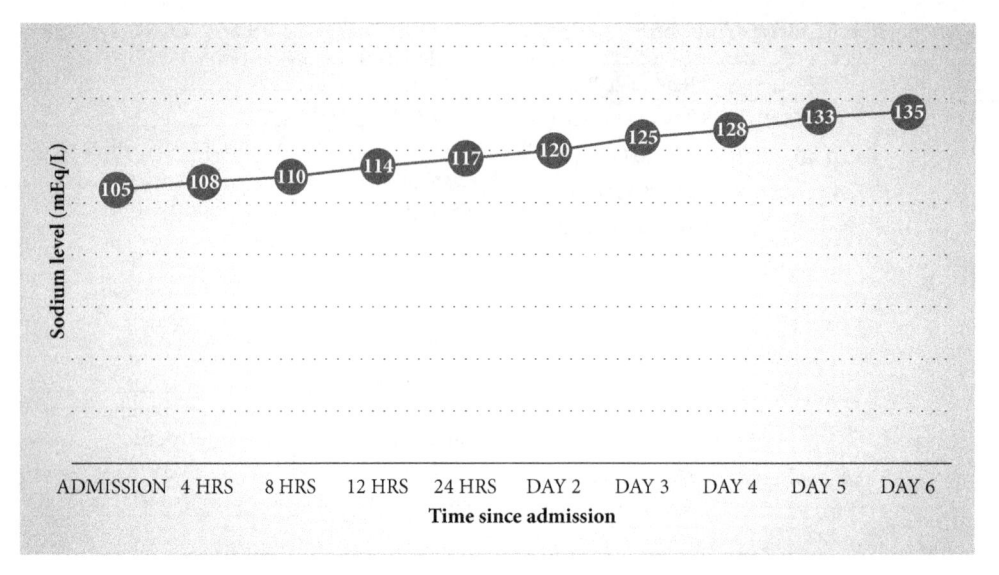

Figure 1: Sodium levels of the patient during the course of treatment.

number of reports on escitalopram-induced SIADH. We aimed to identify these cases with detailed characteristics and present an extensive review of SIADH associated with escitalopram use which has not been included in the previous reviews. We reviewed literature published between January 1, 2002, and March 31, 2018, through search on Medline and found fourteen reported cases of SIADH associated with escitalopram use (Table 3). We also went through reference sections of each of these reports to identify other missing articles.

Nashoni et al. reported the first case of hyponatremia associated with escitalopram in 2004 in a 62-year-old female which occurred 3 weeks following initiation of escitalopram [8]. Majority of these reported escitalopram-induced SIADH were in females (64.28%). While age more than 65 years was found to be risk factor for SSRI-induced SIADH [2], this association was not seen with escitalopram, although the number of cases were limited to draw a definitive statistical conclusion. 50% of reported cases were in patients below 65 years of age. The youngest reported case was in a 47-year-old male who presented with seizures within 4 days of initiation of the drug while the oldest patient was a 97-year-old female [9, 10]. The mean serum sodium levels on presentation were 115 mEq/L.

The most common symptoms at presentation included confusion, seizures, and weakness. None of the reported cases had asymptomatic presentation which signifies underreporting of the association between escitalopram and SIADH. Similar to other SSRIs, the risk of hyponatremia is the highest during the first weeks with the earliest onset being within 2 days of starting escitalopram but can also occur even after 2 months of medication initiation [10, 11]. The median time of onset of symptoms was 7 days. Many of the patients reported in the literature were on multiple medications known to cause hyponatremia especially thiazide, proton pump inhibitor, and other psychiatric medications; however, a temporal association was drawn to escitalopram in all the cases [8, 9, 12–15]. Diken et al. reported a case of a 59-year-old male who underwent coronary artery bypass graft and developed hyponatremia with sodium levels of 107 mEq/L about 1 week following concomitant use of escitalopram 10 mg once daily and hydrochlorothiazide 50 mg once daily. Interestingly, this particular patient had prior history of use of escitalopram without any side effects [15].

The main modality of management in SIADH is water restriction, although in severe symptomatic cases hypertonic saline (3%) and drugs such as loop diuretics (furosemide), demeclocycline, and vaptans should be used [16]. Water restriction is the most important treatment modality in patients with SIADH. Those who do not respond fully or respond only partially can be treated with salt tablets and diuretics. Demeclocycline has been used previously which lead to acute kidney injury and hence its use has been limited. Vaptans, a selective V2 receptor antagonist (Tolvaptan and Conivaptan) can be safely used for treatment of SIADH in carefully monitored patients [17, 18]. High cost and overcorrection remain a potential risk for vaptans [18]. In all 14 cases, hyponatremia improved after discontinuation of the drug and active treatment for SIADH with fluid restriction and administration of hypertonic saline. However, in our case Tolvaptan was used for correction of hyponatremia. Rapid correction of hyponatremia leads to serious neurologic problems with the most severe including osmotic demyelination syndrome and hence close monitoring of sodium during the treatment of SIADH is of paramount importance [16, 19]. One patient had complication secondary to treatment of hyponatremia resulting in central pontine myelinolysis [20].

In 2012, Tsai et al. reported a case of 73-year-old female with history of dementia with Lewy bodies who developed delirium after being on escitalopram for 2 months. She was found to have serum sodium of 124 mEq/L on presentation. She recovered to baseline within 2 weeks following discontinuation of medication. Her delirium and hyponatremia (122 mEq/L), however, recurred after escitalopram

TABLE 3: Summary of all reported cases of SIADH associated with escitalopram.

Case Report	Age	Sex	Escitalopram Dose	Onset (Days)	Sodium Levels (mEq/L)	Presenting Symptoms	Treatment given	Resolution (Weeks)	Comorbid conditions	Medications	Remarks
Nashoni et al, 2004 [8]	62	F	10 mg	21	110	Syncope	Medication discontinuation	1 week	Hypertension, Hyperlipidemia, Atrial fibrillation, Protein C deficiency, Osteoporosis	Losartan, Simvastatin, Sotalol, Warfarin, Calcium, Vitamin D	Patient was later treated with Mirtazapine for depression
Nirmalani et al, 2006 [22]	50	M	20 mg	28	121	Weakness, Dizziness	Medication discontinuation, Fluid Restriction	5 days	Depression with Psychotic features, Hypertension, COPD, Osteoarthritis, GERD	Risperidone	
Adiga et al, 2006 [12]	81	F	10 mg	21	120	Generalized weakness & Recurrent Falls	Medication discontinuation, Hypertonic saline	1 week	Alzheimer's disease, Hypertension, Osteoporosis	Ramipril, Alendronic acid, Donepezil, Mirtazapine, HCTZ	Patient noted to have Renal tubular defect
Grover et al, 2007 [14]	67	F	10 mg	28	127	Delirium	Medication discontinuation	4 weeks	Bipolar affective disorder, Hypertension, Diabetes mellitus	Sodium valproate, HCTZ, Gliclazide, Aspirin, Losartan	Patient was later treated with Mirtazapine & Valproate for Moderate depression
Grover et al, 2007 [14]	75	M	10 mg	10	126	Seizures	Medication discontinuation	2 weeks	Hypertension, Generalized anxiety disorder	Atenolol, Amlodipine	Patient was later treated with Mirtazapine for Generalized Anxiety disorder
Covyeou et al, 2007 [13]	75	F	Unknown	5	116	Unknown	Medication discontinuation	5 days	Hypertension	Amlodipine, HCTZ, Aspirin, Omeprazole, Alprazolam	
Koski et al, 2009 [9]	97	F	5 mg	7	113	Recurrent Falls & Confusion	Medication discontinuation, Fluid restriction, Hypertonic saline	Unknown	Hypertension, Anxiety, UTI (diagnosed 1 day prior to hospitalization)	Tolterodine, Atenolol, Furosemide, Lisinopril, Docusate, Ciprofloxacin (started 1 day prior to hospitalization)	
Tsai et al 2012 [11]	73	F	10 mg	>60	124, 122	Delirium	Medication discontinuation, Fluid restriction	2 weeks, 1 week	Lewy body dementia	Trihexyphenidyl, Bethanechol, Tamsulosin	Failed rechallenge of escitalopram as patient developed Hyponatremia

TABLE 3: Continued.

Case Report	Age	Sex	Escitalopram Dose	Onset (Days)	Sodium Levels (mEq/L)	Presenting Symptoms	Treatment given	Resolution (Weeks)	Comorbid conditions	Medications	Remarks
Pae et al, 2013 [10]	47	M	5 mg	2	110	Seizure	Medication discontinuation	4 days	Quadriplegia with Spinal A-V Malformation Depression	No other medication	
Soysal et al, 2014 [23]	76	F	10 mg	28	113	Confusion Lethargy Incontinence	Medication discontinuation Hypertonic saline	Unknown	Hypertension Diabetes mellitus, Alzheimer's disease Sleep disorder	Losartan Sitagliptin Rivastigmine Memantine Trazodone	
Diken et al, 2016 [15]	59	M	10 mg	7	107	Confusion, Hallucination, Drowsiness	Medication discontinuation Fluid restriction Hypertonic saline	4 days	COPD Diabetes mellitus	Aspirin, metoprolol perindopril amiodarone Spironolactone Hydrochlorothiazide	Recent introduction of hydrochlorothiazide
Parmar et al, 2016 [20]	50	M	10 mg	3	94	Seizure	Medication discontinuation	5 days	Hypertension Panic disorder	Telmisartan Aspirin	Developed central pontine myelinolysis from rapid correction of sodium
Rawal et al, 2017 [24]	54	F	Unknown	4	116	Seizure	Medication discontinuation Fluid restriction	Unknown	Hypertension Depression	Telmisartan Salt restriction	
Vidyasagar et al, 2017 [25]	58	F	Unknown	14	107	Severe Constipation	Medication discontinuation High salt diet Fluid restriction	Unknown	Seronegative spondyloarthropathy Diabetes mellitus Dysthymia	Prednisolone, Hydroxychloroquine Methotrexate Insulin	

was rechallenged. During the rechallenge phase, she had an early onset of symptomatic hyponatremia at 4 days [11]. This case signifies that rechallenge of escitalopram leads to SIADH with early initiation of the medication. The mean time for normalization of serum sodium levels after discontinuation of escitalopram and active treatment was found to be 5.8 days among the ten reported cases with data on resolution time. Mirtazapine was noted to be a good choice of antidepressant for those patients who developed escitalopram associated SIADH on review of literature [8, 14].

6. Conclusion

Our case highlights the clear association of escitalopram use with SIADH in the absence of any significant medical comorbidity or concomitant drug use. With our literature review of all the published case reports, we could infer that female gender and use of concomitant medication may be the risk factors for SIADH in patients taking escitalopram. However, more data is needed for obtaining meaningful conclusion regarding the risk factors and associations. Hyponatremia in most cases started within first week of treatment and resolved within 2 weeks after discontinuation of the medication. Patients being started on escitalopram and other SSRIs should be informed about this life-threatening adverse effect and the warning signs. Factors leading to overhydration like water intake for urinary tract infections and ingestion of excess water during exercise can lead to precipitation of SIADH [21]. We suggest regular serum electrolyte monitoring in patients receiving escitalopram and always evaluate patients for hyponatremia when presenting with symptoms of weakness, confusion, or seizures. Patient who once developed SIADH on escitalopram should not be ideally rechallenged with the same medication due to risk of causing more severe SIADH and may be started on alternative antidepressants like Mirtazapine.

References

[1] M. Sahay and R. Sahay, "Hyponatremia: A practical approach," *Indian Journal of Endocrinology and Metabolism*, vol. 18, no. 6, p. 760, 2014.

[2] K. L. Movig, H. G. Leufkens, A. W. Lenderink et al., "Association between antidepressant drug use and hyponatraemia: a case-control study," *British Journal of Clinical Pharmacology*, vol. 53, no. 4, pp. 363–369, 2002.

[3] D. Shepshelovich, A. Schechter, B. Calvarysky, T. Diker-Cohen, B. Rozen-Zvi, and A. Gafter-Gvili, "Medication-induced SIADH: distribution and characterization according to medication class," *British Journal of Clinical Pharmacology*, vol. 83, no. 8, pp. 1801–1807, 2017.

[4] C. Fonzo-Christe and N. Vogt, "Susceptibility of the elderly patient to hyponatremia induced by selective serotonin reuptake inhibitors," *Therapie*, vol. 55, no. 5, pp. 597–604, 2000, http://www.ncbi.nlm.nih.gov/pubmed/Available from.

[5] P. D. Bowen, "Use of Selective Serotonin Reuptake Inhibitors in the Treatment of Depression in Older Adults: Identifying and Managing Potential Risk for Hyponatremia," *Geriatric Nursing*, vol. 30, no. 2, pp. 85–89, 2009.

[6] S. M. Stahl, "Mechanism of action of serotonin selective reuptake inhibitors. Serotonin receptors and pathways mediate therapeutic effects and side effects," *Journal of Affective Disorders*, vol. 51, no. 3, pp. 215–235, 1998.

[7] L. Kovacs and G. L. Robertson, "Syndrome of Inappropriate Antidiuresis," *Endocrinology and Metabolism Clinics of North America*, vol. 21, no. 4, pp. 859–875, 1992.

[8] E. Nahshoni, A. Weizman, D. Shefet, and N. Pik, "A Case of Hyponatremia Associated With Escitalopram," *Journal of Clinical Psychiatry*, vol. 65, no. 12, p. 1722, 2004.

[9] R. R. Koski, J. A. Covyeou, and M. Morissette, "Case Report of SIADH Associated With Escitalopram Use," *Journal of Pharmacy Practice*, vol. 22, no. 6, pp. 594–599, 2009.

[10] C.-U. Pae, G.-Y. Park, S. Im, S. B. Ko, and S.-J. Lee, "Low-dose escitalopram-associated hyponatremia," *Asia-Pacific Psychiatry*, vol. 5, no. 2, pp. E90–E90, 2013.

[11] P. Tsai, H. Chen, S. Liao, M. M. Tseng, and M. Lee, "Recurrent escitalopram-induced hyponatremia in an elderly woman with dementia with Lewy bodies," *General Hospital Psychiatry*, vol. 34, no. 1, pp. 101.e5–101.e7, 2012.

[12] GU. Adiga and TS. Dharmarajan, "Renal tubular defects from antidepressant use in an older adult: an uncommon but reversible adverse drug effect," *Clin Drug Investi*, vol. 26, no. 10, pp. 607–611, 2006, http://go.galegroup.com.ezproxy2.library.drexel.edu/ps/i.do?p=AONE&u=drexel_main&id=GALE%7CA199858434&v=2.1&it=r&sid=summon.

[13] J. A. Covyeou and C. W. Jackson, "Hyponatremia Associated with Escitalopram," *The New England Journal of Medicine*, vol. 356, no. 1, pp. 94-95, 2007.

[14] S. Grover, P. Biswas, G. Bhateja, and P. Kulhara, "Escitalopram-associated hyponatremia [4]," *Psychiatry and Clinical Neurosciences*, vol. 61, no. 1, pp. 132-133, 2007.

[15] A. I. Diken, A. Yalçinkaya, Ö. Erçen Diken et al., "Hyponatremia due to escitalopram and thiazide use after cardiac surgery," *Journal of Cardiac Surgery*, vol. 31, no. 2, pp. 96-97, 2016.

[16] P. Gross, "Clinical management of SIADH," *Therapeutic Advances in Endocrinology and Metabolism*, vol. 3, no. 2, pp. 61–73, 2012.

[17] H. D. Zmily, S. Daifallah, and J. K. Ghali, "Tolvaptan, hyponatremia, and heart failure," *International Journal of Nephrology and Renovascular Disease*, vol. 4, pp. 57–71, 2011.

[18] M. A. Humayun and I. C. Cranston, "In-patient Tolvaptan use in SIADH: care audit, therapy observation and outcome analysis," *BMC Endocrine Disorders*, vol. 17, no. 1, 2017.

[19] R. H. Sterns, "Treatment of Severe Hyponatremia," *Clinical Journal of the American Society of Nephrology*, vol. 13, no. 4, pp. 641–649, 2018.

[20] P. Arpit, M. Piyali, T. Manjari, and S. Rajesh, "Escitalopram Induced Hyponatremia," *Escitalopram Induc Hyponatremia ASEAN J Psychiatry*, vol. 17, no. 2, 2016.

[21] T. Hew-Butler, M. H. Rosner, S. Fowkes-Godek et al., "Statement of the 3rd International Exercise-Associated Hyponatremia Consensus Development Conference, Carlsbad, California, 2015," *British Journal of Sports Medicine*, vol. 49, no. 22, pp. 1432–1446, 2015.

[22] A. Nirmalani, S. L. Stock, and G. Catalano, "Syndrome of Inappropriate Antidiuretic Hormone Associated with Escitalopram Therapy," *CNS Spectrums*, vol. 11, no. 06, pp. 429–432, 2006.

[23] P. Soysal and A. T. Isik, "Severe Hyponatremia Due to Escitalopram Treatment in an Elderly Adult with Alzheimer's Disease," *Journal of the American Geriatrics Society*, vol. 62, no. 12, pp. 2462-2463, 2014.

[24] G. Rawal, R. Kumar, and S. Yadav, "Severe hyponatremia associated with escitalopram," *Journal of Family Medicine and Primary Care*, vol. 6, no. 2, p. 453, 2017.

[25] S. Vidyasagar, K. Rao, M. Verma, AD. Tripuraneni, N. Patil, and D. Bhattacharjee, "Escitalopram induced SIADH in an elderly female: A case study," *Psychopharmacol Bull*, vol. 47, pp. 64–67, 2017, http://www.ncbi.nlm.nih.gov/pubmed/2893601.

Cisplatin-Induced Renal Salt Wasting Requiring over 12 Liters of 3% Saline Replacement

Phuong-Chi Pham,[1] Pavani Reddy,[1] Shaker Qaqish,[1] Ashvin Kamath,[1] Johana Rodriguez,[2] David Bolos,[2] Martina Zalom,[2] and Phuong-Thu Pham[3]

[1]*Olive View-UCLA Medical Center, Division of Nephrology and Hypertension, Sylmar, CA 91342, USA*
[2]*Olive View-UCLA Medical Center, Division of Hematology and Oncology, Sylmar, CA 91342, USA*
[3]*Ronald Reagan UCLA Medical Center, Kidney Transplant, Los Angeles, CA 90095, USA*

Correspondence should be addressed to Phuong-Chi Pham; pctp@ucla.edu

Academic Editor: Yoshihide Fujigaki

Cisplatin is known to induce Fanconi syndrome and renal salt wasting (RSW). RSW typically only requires transient normal saline (NS) support. We report a severe RSW case that required 12 liters of 3% saline. A 57-year-old woman with limited stage small cell cancer was admitted for cisplatin (80 mg/m^2) and etoposide (100 mg/m^2) therapy. Patient's serum sodium (SNa) decreased from 138 to 133 and 125 mEq/L within 24 and 48 hours of cisplatin therapy, respectively. A diagnosis of syndrome of inappropriate antidiuretic hormone secretion (SIADH) was initially made. Despite free water restriction, patient's SNa continued to decrease in association with acute onset of headaches, nausea, and dizziness. Three percent saline (3%S) infusion with rates up to 1400 mL/day was required to correct and maintain SNa at 135 mEq/L. Studies to evaluate Fanconi syndrome revealed hypophosphatemia and glucosuria in the absence of serum hyperglycemia. The natriuresis slowed down by 2.5 weeks, but 3%S support was continued for a total volume of 12 liters over 3.5 weeks. Attempts of questionable benefits to slow down glomerular filtration included the administration of ibuprofen and benazepril. To our knowledge, this is the most severe case of RSW ever reported with cisplatin.

1. Introduction

Cis-diamminedichloroplatinum (CDDP), commonly known as cisplatin, is a chemotherapeutic agent used in the treatment of various cancers including carcinomas, germ cell tumors, lymphomas, and sarcomas. Its antitumor effect is thought to reflect its ability to cross-link with purine bases on DNA, thus interfering with DNA repair mechanisms and leading to DNA damage and tumor cell apoptosis [1]. However, cisplatin is also known to be associated with many adverse effects including gastrointestinal disturbances, hearing loss, allergic reactions, and a multitude of renal problems including electrolyte disturbances, renal tubular acidosis, acute kidney injury with reduced glomerular filtration, Fanconi syndrome, nephrogenic diabetes insipidus, and renal salt wasting (RSW). The pathogenesis of cisplatin-induced renal injuries is thought to be due to renal vasoconstriction and cellular apoptosis and necrosis mediated by altered cell cycle regulation, death receptor signaling, and increased oxidative stress and inflammatory state [1–3].

In a recent literature review, Hamdi et al. analyzed 18 patients who were reported with cisplatin-induced RSW. Patients developed RSW as soon as 12 hours and up to 4 months following cisplatin therapy. Cisplatin dosage used ranged from 80 to 600 mg/m^2. Renal salt wasting typically only requires transient normal saline (NS) support. With the exception of one patient who required approximately 2.6 L of 3% saline infusion over 2 days, all 17 others only required normal saline support with or without supplemental oral sodium chloride tablets [4, 5]. We herein report a severe RSW case that required 12 liters of 3% saline (6156 mEq Na) over a 3.5-week course, followed by oral sodium chloride supplement for an additional 2 weeks. Preventive and therapeutic considerations for cisplatin-induced RSW will also be discussed.

2. Case Presentation

A 57-year-old woman presented with 4 weeks of shortness of breath, dyspnea on exertion, and nonproductive cough. Imaging studies revealed a lung mass extending into the mediastinum with narrowing of the left pulmonary artery and total left upper lobe collapse. Patient was diagnosed with limited stage small cell carcinoma of the lung (SCCL). Initial therapy included cisplatin 80 mg/m^2 on day 1 and etoposide 100 mg/m^2 on days 1 to 3 with plan to include radiation at cycle 2. Prior to the administration of cisplatin, patient's serum sodium (SNa) was 134–137 mEq/L. Following the first cisplatin dose, her SNa decreased to 133 mEq/L and 125 mEq/L by 24 and 48 hours, respectively. The acute hyponatremia was initially attributed to the continuous infusion of 5% dextrose half-normal saline in association with presumed lung cancer induced SIADH. However, despite empirical free water restriction, her SNa decreased to 119 mEq/L within 72 hours. Patient developed acute headache, nausea, and fatigue. Renal service was consulted.

Medications included fluticasone nasal spray twice daily, amoxicillin-clavulanic acid 875 mg twice daily, omeprazole 20 mg daily, and empirical intravenous stress dose of hydrocortisone 100 mg q 8 h. As needed medications included metoclopramide 10 mg q 6 h and albuterol 2.5 mg nebulizer treatment q 4 h.

Physical exam revealed blood pressure 123/76 mmHg, heart rate 70 beats per minute, and respiratory rate 18 per minute. Patient was uncomfortable with generalized headaches and nausea but alert and oriented to situation, person, place, and time. Oral mucosa was dry. Heart, lungs, abdomen, and extremities were unremarkable. Neurological exam was nonfocal.

3. Results

Laboratory Findings. Urine studies revealed osmolality (Uosm) 693 mosm/kg, UNa 205 mEq/L, and potassium (UK) 40 mEq/L in association with increasingly high urine output (average 100–150 mL/h, up to 600 mL/h of urine with UNa + UK up to 265 + 73 mEq/L, resp.). Cisplatin-induced proximal tubular injury with sodium wasting was suspected. Additional laboratory testing revealed glucosuria in the absence of significant serum hyperglycemia (urine glucose 1000 mg/dL, concurrent serum glucose ranged from 117 mg/dL to 141 mg/dL), low-molecular weight proteinuria (0.3 g protein/g creatinine, concurrent albumin/creatinine ratio of 27.7 mcg/mg creatinine), and hypophosphatemia (2.4 mg/dL from baseline of 4.2 mg/dL 1 week previously), all consistent with proximal tubular injury. Serum calcium was also noted to trend downwards from a baseline of 8.78 ± 0.46 mg/dL two days before to 8.25 ± 0.39 mg/dL two days following cisplatin therapy. There was no change noted in serum magnesium. Other routine evaluations for hyponatremia including thyroid stimulating hormone and morning serum cortisol levels were within normal limits.

Patient was started on 3% saline infusion. Her daily effective electrolyte loss (urine sodium and potassium) averaged at 634 ± 183 mEq/d, with a maximum of 1050 mEq.

Patient required approximately 12 L of 3% saline infusion over a 3.5-week period to correct the initial hyponatremia and maintain salt equilibrium prior to gaining sufficient renal recovery for switching to oral sodium supplements. During the worst phase of renal salt wasting, patient required up to 47 g of NaCl or 18.5 g of sodium supplement daily. During the natriuretic phase, attempts to slow her glomerular filtration, thus filtered sodium and potassium load, included ibuprofen 200 mg thrice daily and benazepril 10 mg twice daily (Table 1). It is unclear if our medical therapy ameliorated any renal salt wasting. Addition of fludrocortisone 0.1 mg bid empirically prior to resulting of cortisol did not appear to ameliorate the massive natriuresis. Patient also received intermittent K-phosphate and magnesium supplement during the hospital course. Full clinical renal recovery occurred by 5.5 weeks.

4. Discussion

In the setting of malignancy, hyponatremia commonly arises from excess free water intake in association with SIADH, poor solute intake, or, less commonly, adrenal insufficiency due to metastatic disease. Since current patient was initially euvolemic and had no problem with oral intake or known adrenal insufficiency, the diagnosis of SIADH was entertained. Despite empirical free water restriction of one liter a day, patient developed rapid worsening hyponatremia (SNa dropped from 125 mEq/L to 119 mEq/L within eight hours) and acute onset headaches, nausea without vomiting, and clinical evidence of hypovolemia (dizziness and dry oral mucosa) in association with polyuria (up to 4 L a day) of high urine sodium plus potassium content (Table 1). The worsening hyponatremia despite free water restriction and inappropriate and incessant polyuria of high urinary electrolyte content despite volume depletion ruled out SIADH while raising concerns for either cisplatin-induced RSW or undiagnosed adrenal insufficiency. Both SIADH and adrenal insufficiency were eventually definitively ruled out with low vasopressin level (2.4 pg/mL normal range [1.0 to 13.3 pg/mL]) and normal morning cortisol level and lack of response to empirical fludrocortisone therapy, respectively. The diagnosis of cisplatin-induced RSW was thus made.

Cisplatin-induced kidney injury is rare but may lead to acute tubulointerstitial nephritis, tubular necrosis, proximal S3 tubular damage with salt wasting (K^+, Mg^{2+}, Ca^{2+}, PO_4^{2-}), Fanconi syndrome, and even nephrogenic diabetes insipidus. Given significant natriuresis and hypophosphatemia, mild tubular proteinuria, and glucosuria in the absence of hyperglycemia, patient was felt to have developed Fanconi syndrome and RSW. Of interest, patient's daily urinary sodium loss was up to 8.9-fold the sodium content of her daily hospital-prepared meals (average sodium content of 2.0 ± 0.2 gm daily), assuming she ate all of her meals. To our knowledge, this is the most severe case of cisplatin-induced RSW ever reported. The reason for severe salt wasting in current case is not known. Patient has no underlying kidney disease and was not receiving any diuretic or nephrotoxic agent that could have potentiated the natriuresis. While we successfully supported patient with high volume 3% saline followed by salt tablets, preventive measures are vital.

TABLE 1: Hospital course of patient with cisplatin-induced renal salt wasting.

Hospital day	Laboratory findings						Total (Na + K) urinary loss (mEq/L)	Management	
	SNa (mEq/L)	U(Na + K) (mEq/L)	Uosm (mosm/Kg)	Sosm (mosm/Kg)	SPhos (mg/dL)	Urine volume (mL)		Medications	3% NS (mL)
1	138							Cisplatin	
2	133								
3	125, 122, 119, 124, 123	205 + 40	693	262	3.1				300
4	125, 122	212 + 21	907		2.8	3800	885		800
5	124, 127, 126	190 + 38	806		2.7	4050	923		875
6	129, 133, 128, 132	242 + 42	847		2.8	3100	880		750
7	130, 136	270 + 46	832		3	2450	774		500
8	133, 128, 134	250 + 34	903		2.9	2445	694		670
9	132, 122, 124	250 + 32	760		2.8	2460	693		1400
10	132, 131, 130, 135	245 + 15	636		2.7	2485	646		850
11	134, 133	235 + 56	827		2.9	1630	474	Benazepril	650
12	136, 133	212 + 23	810		2.8	2425	569		500
13	133, 129	265 + 42	768		2.7	1950	598		600
14	134, 131	258 + 41	731		3.1	2500	747	Ibuprofen	0
15	132, 130	246 + 73			3.1	1820	580		1000
16	130, 129	246 + 22	637		3.2	1925	515		500
17	129, 138, 126, 130, 131	199 + 87	734		4.1	2375	679		500
18	131, 131	189 + 39			4.5	2850	649		1000
19	138, 138, 135	255 + 54	783		3.1	2200	679		500
20	135	162 + 44	787			3600	741		0
21	135	232 + 54	540			3670	1049		0
22	130, 129, 131					2650	0		0
23	126, 127	225 + 43	660			1750	469		250
24	131, 131, 127	250 + 46	774			1600	473		250
25	130, 127, 131, 134	147 + 69	625			1750	378		250
26	135, 135	197 + 21	528			1800	392		
27	139	145 + 19	404			1700	278		
28	137, 130, 134	218 + 26	675			2225	542		
29	131, 135	209 + 47				2100	537		
30	132					1020			
31	138								
Total									12145

SNa: serum sodium; U(Na + K): urine sodium plus potassium; Uosm: urine osmolality; Sosm: serum osmolality; SPhos: serum phosphorus; NS: normal saline.

Normal saline support during cisplatin therapy is likely the key preventive therapy. The protective effects of NS are thought to involve the ability of the chloride ion concentration to stabilize the CDDP molecule, suppress the formation of CDDP metabolites, and reduce the conversion of CDDP to its aquated products. The latter have higher protein binding capacity and thus greater tissue accumulation and damage [6].

Despite the lack of clinical data, concurrent use of commonly used antioxidants including N-acetylcysteine, vitamin C, and vitamin E has been suggested due to their reported efficacy in animal studies and low toxicity profile. Other clinically available agents considered for renoprotection against cisplatin include salicylates for anti-inflammation, allopurinol for the reduction of reactive oxygen species generation, fibrates for the reduction of free fatty acid accumulation and suppression of apoptosis, and resveratrol for antioxidative, anti-inflammatory, and cytoprotective properties [2].

Alternatively, replacement of cisplatin with carboplatin may be considered in cases with either known contraindication with cisplatin or documented severe cisplatin-induced nephrotoxicity. Nonetheless, it must be recognized that cisplatin has unequivocal superiority over carboplatin in terms of antitumor effect on various malignancies [7]. Subsequent continuation of cisplatin administration can become a difficult clinical decision and must be carefully discussed among the healthcare team and affected patients.

5. Conclusions

Clinicians must exert great caution when administering cisplatin due to its severe and potentially life-threatening salt wasting complication. Preventive measures, particularly early normal saline infusion with or without concurrent use of antioxidants, anti-inflammatory agents, or both, must be considered to prevent adverse outcomes. In patients with established severe cisplatin-induced RSW, considerations for an alternative agent may be advisable.

References

[1] S. Dasari and P. Bernard Tchounwou, "Cisplatin in cancer therapy: Molecular mechanisms of action," *European Journal of Pharmacology*, vol. 740, pp. 364–378, 2014.

[2] G.-S. Oh, H.-J. Kim, A. Shen et al., "Cisplatin-induced kidney dysfunction and perspectives on improving treatment strategies," *Electrolyte and Blood Pressure*, vol. 12, no. 2, pp. 55–65, 2014.

[3] A.-M. Florea and D. Büsselberg, "Cisplatin as an anti-tumor drug: Cellular mechanisms of activity, drug resistance and induced side effects," *Cancers*, vol. 3, no. 1, pp. 1351–1371, 2011.

[4] T. Hamdi, S. Latta, B. Jallad, F. Kheir, M. N. Alhosaini, and A. Patel, "Cisplatin-induced renal salt wasting syndrome," *Southern Medical Journal*, vol. 103, no. 8, pp. 793–799, 2010.

[5] P. J. Lammers, L. White, and L. J. Ettinger, "Cis-platinum-induced renal sodium wasting," *Medical and Pediatric Oncology*, vol. 12, no. 5, pp. 343–346, 1984.

[6] The FDA Recommended Sodium Intake. SFGate, http://healthyeating.sfgate.com/fda-recommended-sodium-intake-1873.html.

[7] R. A. Fulco, M. Vannozzi, P. Collecchi et al., "Effect of normal saline on cisplatin pharmacokinetics and antitumor activity in mice bearing P388 leukemia," *Anticancer Research*, vol. 10, no. 6, pp. 1603–1610, 1990.

Scleroderma Renal Crisis Debute with Thrombotic Microangiopathy: A Successful Case Treated with Eculizumab

Maite Hurtado Uriarte,[1] Carolina Larrarte,[2] and Laura Bravo Rey[3]

[1]Nephrologist, University Hospital San Rafael, RTS Baxter, Bogota, Colombia
[2]Nephrologist, University Hospital Militar, RTS Baxter, Bogota, Colombia
[3]Medical student, Javeriana University, Bogota, Colombia

Correspondence should be addressed to Laura Bravo Rey; laurabravor@hotmail.com

Academic Editor: Władysław Sułowicz

We had the challenged to treat a 40-year-old female with Systemic Scleroderma who was showing unspecific symptoms. During her time at the hospital she rapidly develops renal dysfunction, associated with hypertension. She required renal replacement therapy initiation and we observed a decline in hemoglobin and platelets numbers. We confirm a microangiopathic hemolytic anemia and rule out other immune diseases or thrombotic thrombocytopenic purpura. Systemic Sclerosis is a chronic immune disorder of unknown origin that it is not completely understood. It is believed that environmental factors may contribute and also altered genes may be implicated in the immune system's function. Microangiopathic hemolytic anemia occurs in 43% of patients who develop scleroderma renal crisis and an activation of the complement system through the classical pathway may be involved. Given that context we decided to treat the patients with C5 blocker Eculizumab and obtain an extraordinary positive response.

1. Introduction

Systemic sclerosis (SSc) is a chronic and complex autoimmune disorder that it is not fully understood. It is characterized by microvascular endothelial cell apoptosis, excessive extracellular matrix protein deposition and perivascular infiltration of mononuclear cells, producing damage and progressive fibrosis of the skin and visceral organs (lungs, heart, and kidney). It has been divided into two categories; (i) limited and (ii) diffuse [1–3]. The first affects only the skin of distal extremities and face, usually characterized by a very slow clinical course. On the other hand, the diffuse type affects wide areas of skin and internal organs. Neither category has completely effective treatment available, mainly as a result of the lack of knowledge of its pathogenesis, which is an obstacle for the prescription of the right treatment or at least for taking the appropriate measures to slow down its adverse effects [4].

It has been seen that environmental factors may contribute [5]; immune genes are also involved in the abnormal regulation of T and B cells and the activation of the complement system through the classical pathway, which targets the vascular and connective tissue [6–8].

Scleroderma renal crisis is defined by: first, severe or worsening arterial hypertension, and second a quick and progressive kidney failure, in both cases in the absence of any other case [9].

The most recent data shows that renal crisis is found in 1% of cases with limited scleroderma; on the other hand, in the diffuse type it was found between 4 to 11% [10] and in some reports up to 25% [9].

Abnormalities found on real biopsy are "onion bulbs" in the arteries (Figures 1-2) caused by endothelial injury, in which intimal proliferation and vascular remodeling lead to the obstruction of the vascular lumen and the reduction of glomerular filtration rate [10].

2. Case Presentation

We present the case of a 40-year-old woman with a history of systemic sclerosis, diagnosed 3 years ago. She arrived

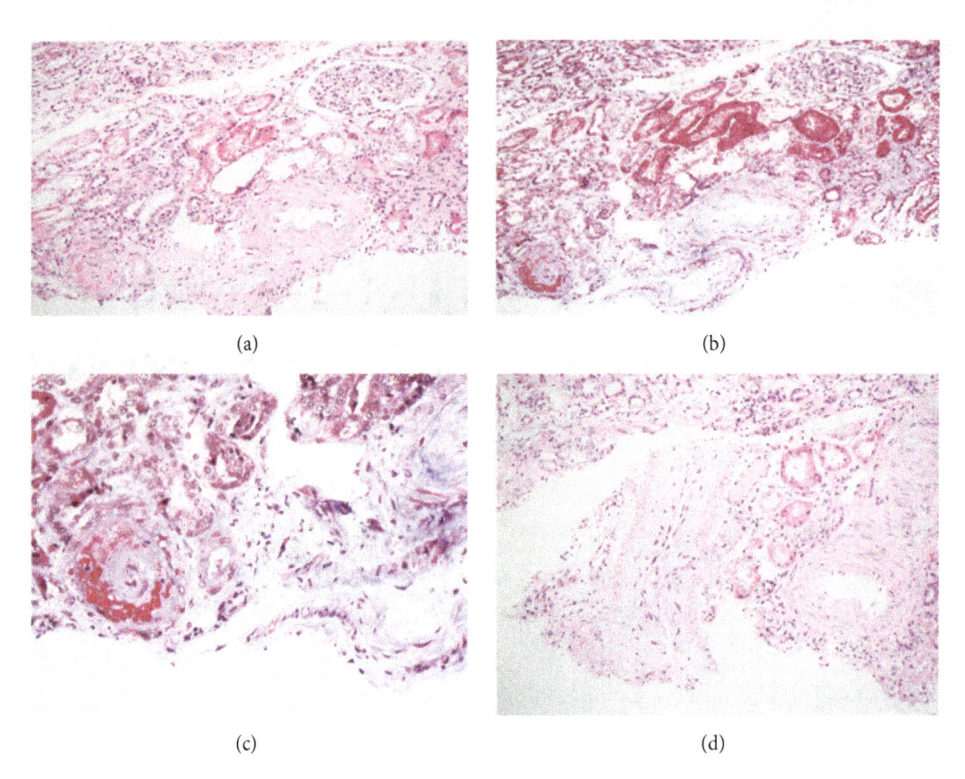

FIGURE 1: Renal parenchyma with glomerular ischemia. ((a) Hematoxylin y Eosin 10X, (b) Trichrome 10X), associated with vascular changes in interlobular arteries: fibrinoid necrosis of the intima with fragmentation of erythrocytes, ((c) Tricromico 20X) and mucoid expansion of the intima with luminal obliteration, and ((d) haematoxylin and eosin 10X).

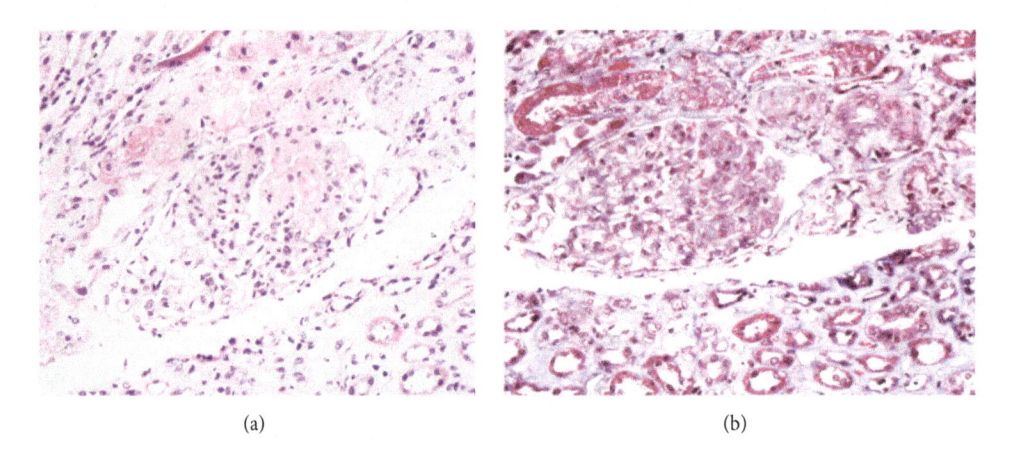

FIGURE 2: Glomerulus with subendothelial edema towards the vascular pole and arterioles with luminal obliteration due to endothelial edema and fibrinoid necrosis. ((a) Hematoxylin and 40X eosin and (b) Trichrome 40X).

without treatment, due to a poor toleration of the medication metrotexate. She requested medical help in different opportunities for unspecific symptoms for 3 months including; nausea, vomiting, dizziness, asthenia and loss of weight. She didn't demonstrate any improvement and arrived with an uncertain diagnosis. Our institution observed symptoms, showing a decline in her renal function (creatinine 1,6 mg/dl and Uremic nitrogen blood BUN 41,3), with a urine test showing hematuria 28 xc, associated with hypertension 214/140 mmHg. Initially she was treated for an infection, showing rapid renal deterioration to creatinine 6,67 mg/dl and BUN 96,77 mg/dl with oliguria and overload. We started conventional treatment with IECA and calcium channel blockers, the patient showed no response, on the contrary her renal functiondeclined to the point that RRT was needed (Figure 3). At the same time, the patient developed a deep thrombocytopenia and anemia, showing smear schistocytes in the blood, elevated Lactate Dehydrogenase (LDH), and consumption of haptoglobin (Figures 4-5.) We ruled out Thrombotic Thrombocytopenic Purpura (TTP) because ADAMST 13 was normal; we also dismissed different immunologic disease. Kidney histopathology showed

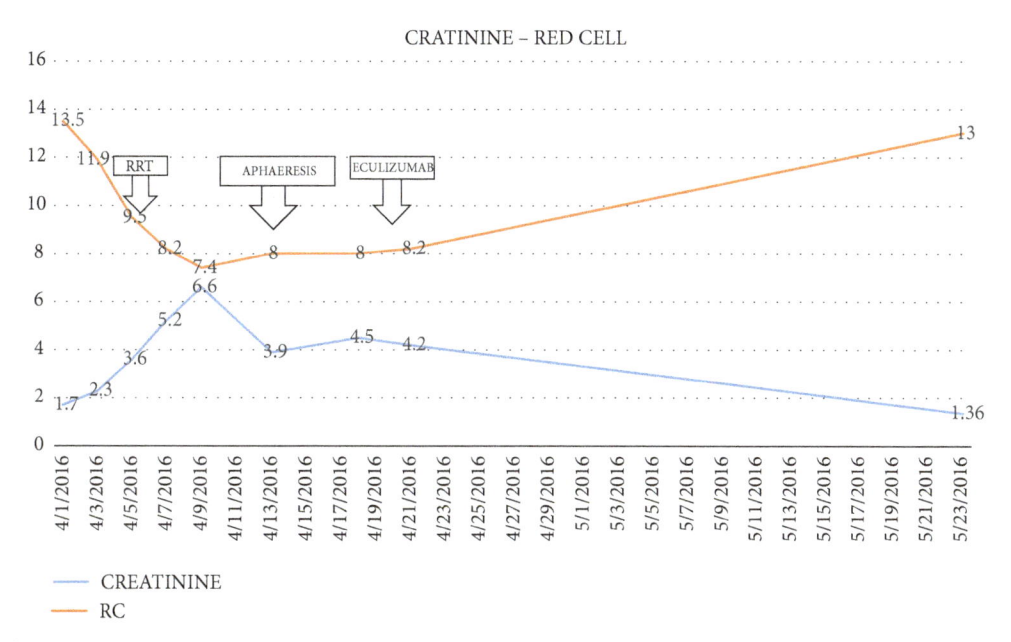

FIGURE 3: Initial increase of creatinine levels showing decrease of renal function and decrease of red blood cells, hemolytic anemia, the breaking point on day 9, after 10 days after trying with RRT and aphaeresis Eculizumab therapy was started with a subsequently recovery of red cell line and creatinine level.

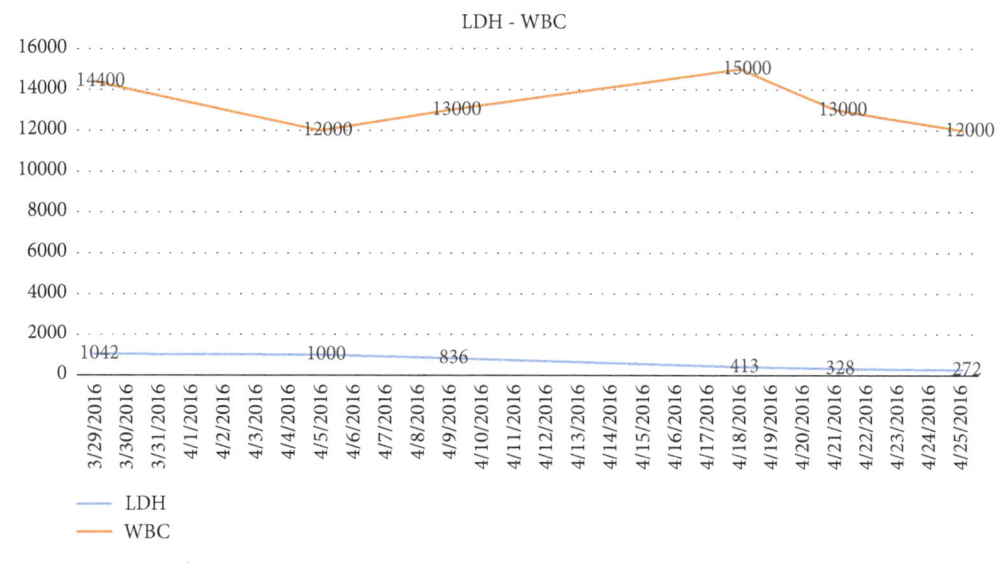

FIGURE 4: We keep track of white blood cells and LDH showing the impact on all blood lines and hemolytic anemia.

Thrombotic Microangiopathy (TMA), therefore we started plasma exchange getting slight improvement. Our patient showed a dramatic decline in renal, hematologic, and cardiac functions, therefore we decided to initiate treatment using C5 blocker with previous vaccination against encapsulated bacteria, resulting in an improvement in platelet count and red cells within the first week. 6 months later the patient showed full renal recovery and as a result RRT treatment was no longer needed.

Given the dramatic morbidity and mortality of this disease, in particular in the context of our incomplete understanding of its roots, we believe that to present this case may be relevant as it shows a successful outcome that may lead to new ways to approach the research needed to develop more suitable methods and treatments.

3. Discussion–Conclusions

Our understanding of the pathogenesis of renal damage in systemic sclerosis remains incomplete; however it seems to result from a series of factors affecting the kidney. The primary process is the injury of the endothelial cells, which results in intimal proliferation of renal arteries (Figures 1-2). We do not know with certainty the physiopathology, but recent findings suggest that an activation of the complement

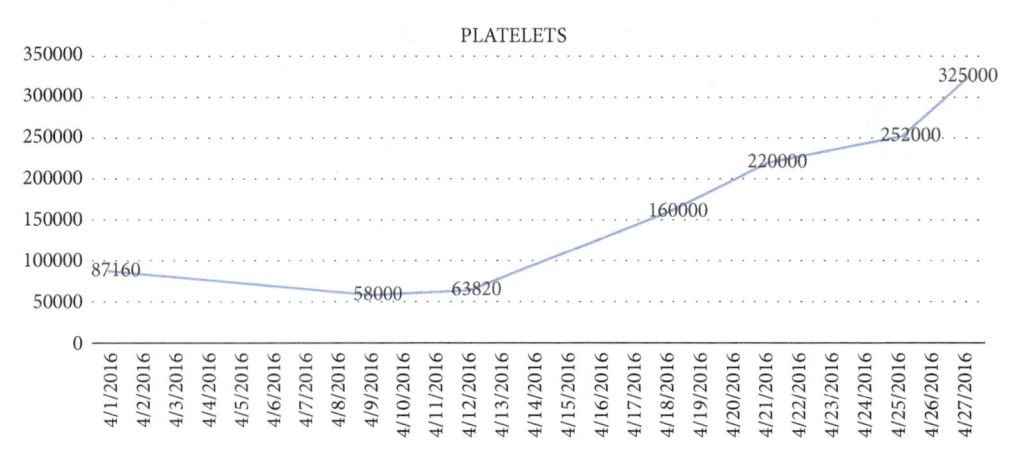

FIGURE 5: This graphic shows the platelet count decrease at the beginning of the disease; that is the reason of suspect Thrombotic thrombocytopenic purpurea; we can see the ascending curve after day 19 with the start of Eculizumab therapy.

system through the classical pathway may be are involved. It is believed that certain proteins are involved in either promoting or maintaining an inflammatory state, such as a variation on factor H as associated with endothelial cells damage [11, 12].

The renin Angiotensin System plays an important role in this complication. That is why ACE inhibitors alter survival substantially. Before the use of this, less than 10% of patients survived the first year; after the use of this drug, 5-year survival increased to 65%. Nevertheless, almost 40% of the patients are still going to require dialysis, and 25% will die within one year [9].

As microangiopathic hemolytic anemia occurs in 43% of patients who have scleroderma renal crisis, it has been suggested that an activation of the complement system through the classical pathway may be involved.

As a result of the dramatic clinical and histological severity and the lack of responses to the conventional treatment; IECA, calcium channel blockers, and plasma exchange, recently the use C5 blocker eculizumab has been proposed.

Eculizumab is a humanized recombinant immunoglobulin G2/4 monoclonal antibody directed against the complement component C5; by binding to complement component C5, the drug inhibits the generation of C5a and C5b-9, and thus subsequently inhibits the lysis and endothelial damage.

Disclosure

This manuscript was presented as a poster at the World Congress of Nephrology, Mexico, 2017, and published as a poster at the International Society of Nephrology academy page.

References

[1] F. Ingegnoli, L. Carmona, and I. Castrejon, "Systematic review of systemic sclerosis- specific instruments for the EULAR Outcome Measures Library: An evolutional database model of validated patient-reported outcomes," *Seminars in Arthritis and Rheumatism*, vol. 46, no. 5, pp. 609–614, 2017.

[2] R. E. Pellar and J. E. Pope, "Evidence-based management of systemic sclerosis: Navigating recommendations and guidelines," *Seminars in Arthritis and Rheumatism*, vol. 46, no. 6, pp. 767–774, 2017.

[3] T. Tay, N. Ferdowsi, M. Baron et al., "Measures of disease status in systemic sclerosis: A systematic review," *Seminars in Arthritis and Rheumatism*, vol. 46, no. 4, pp. 473–487, 2017.

[4] M. Baron, "Special issue on rheumatology targeted therapy in systemic sclerosis," *Rambam Maimonides Medical Journal*, vol. 7, no. 4, pp. 1–6, 2016.

[5] P. Chairta, P. Nicolaou, and K. Christodoulou, "Genomic and genetic studies of systemic sclerosis: A systematic review," *Human Immunology*, vol. 78, no. 2, pp. 153–165, 2017.

[6] G. Murdaca, M. Contatore, R. Gulli, P. Mandich, and F. Puppo, "Genetic factors and systemic sclerosis," *Autoimmunity Reviews*, vol. 15, no. 5, pp. 427–432, 2016.

[7] L. I. Sakkas and D. P. Bogdanos, "Systemic sclerosis: New evidence re-enforces the role of B cells," *Autoimmunity Reviews*, vol. 15, no. 2, pp. 155–161, 2016.

[8] J. Esposito, Z. Brown, W. Stevens et al., "The association of low complement with disease activity in systemic sclerosis: a prospective cohort study," *Arthritis Research & Therapy*, vol. 18, no. 1, 2016.

[9] L. Mouthon, G. Bussone, A. Berezné, L.-H. Noël, and L. Guillevin, "Scleroderma renal crisis," *The Journal of Rheumatology*, vol. 41, no. 6, pp. 1040–1048, 2014.

[10] S. Simin and M. Aliakbarian, "Scleroderma and renal crisis," *Journal of Medical Sciences*, vol. 7, no. 4, pp. 707–709, 2007.

[11] A. Devresse, S. Aydin, M. Le Quintrec et al., "Complement activation and effect of eculizumab in scleroderma renal crisis," *Medicine*, vol. 95, no. 30, p. e4459, 2016.

[12] "._FACTOR H.pdf".

Acute Hypocalcemia and Metabolic Alkalosis in Children on Cation-Exchange Resin Therapy

Aadil Kakajiwala,[1,2] Kevin T. Barton,[1] Elisha Rampolla,[2] Christine Breen,[2] and Madhura Pradhan[2,3]

[1]Division of Pediatric Nephrology, Washington University in St. Louis School of Medicine, St. Louis, MO, USA
[2]Divisions of Nephrology, The Children's Hospital of Philadelphia, Philadelphia, PA, USA
[3]Perelman School of Medicine, The University of Pennsylvania, Philadelphia, PA, USA

Correspondence should be addressed to Aadil Kakajiwala; akakajiwala@wustl.edu

Academic Editor: Salih Kavukcu

Background. Sodium polystyrene sulfonate (SPS) is a chelating agent used for the treatment of hyperkalemia. SPS has a wide range of exchange capacity requiring close monitoring of serum electrolytes. We observed two patients who developed acute hypocalcemia and increased metabolic alkalosis after initiating SPS therapy. We report these cases to draw attention to the potential risk of this medication in pediatric patients. *Case Diagnosis/Treatment.* Two children with chronic kidney disease on dialysis were started on SPS for hyperkalemia. Within a week after initiation of the medication, both patients developed hypocalcemia on routine labs without overt clinical manifestations. The hypocalcemia was rapidly corrected with oral supplementation and discontinuation of SPS. *Conclusions.* Severe hypocalcemia can develop after SPS therapy. The metabolic alkalosis in these patients associated with the hypocalcemia put them at increased risk for complications. Hence, careful attention must be paid to the state of calcium metabolism in all patients receiving SPS. Often calcium supplementation is required to maintain normal calcium levels.

1. Introduction

Sodium polystyrene sulfonate (SPS) is a cross-linked polymer, used in the treatment of hyperkalemia. It contains sulfonic groups bound to sodium ions that are easily exchanged for other cations in solution. When taken orally or rectally, the resin exchanges sodium ions for potassium ions in the intestine before being excreted. SPS may also be added to formula as a chelating agent to decrease potassium load.

SPS has such a wide range of exchange capacity that close monitoring of serum electrolytes is necessary. Its principle side effect has been excessive sodium load, but hypokalemia, hypocalcemia, and even tetany have been described after SPS therapy [1, 2]. We report two patients who developed acute hypocalcemia and increased metabolic alkalosis after initiating SPS therapy. These cases draw attention to the potential risk of this medication in pediatric patients.

2. Case Presentation

2.1. Case 1. An 18-month-old male child with steroid resistant nephrotic syndrome due to diffuse mesangial sclerosis rapidly progressed to end stage renal disease. He was initially started on hemodialysis followed by chronic peritoneal dialysis (PD). His chronic medications included lansoprazole, hydrocortisone, sevelamer, levothyroxine, amlodipine, epogen, ferrous sulfate, multivitamin, erythromycin, and albuterol. His main source of nutrition was a peptide-based formula that provided 1008 mg of calcium, 540 IU of vitamin D, and 30.4 mEq of potassium per day. The dialysate contained 2.5 mEq/l of calcium.

A year after being on PD, he developed persistent hyperkalemia (serum potassium 5.2 to 5.9 mEq/L) with increased doses of enalapril and was started on 0.5 g/kg of SPS. A month later, routine blood work noted improved serum potassium at 3.9 mEq/l, metabolic alkalosis (serum bicarbonate of

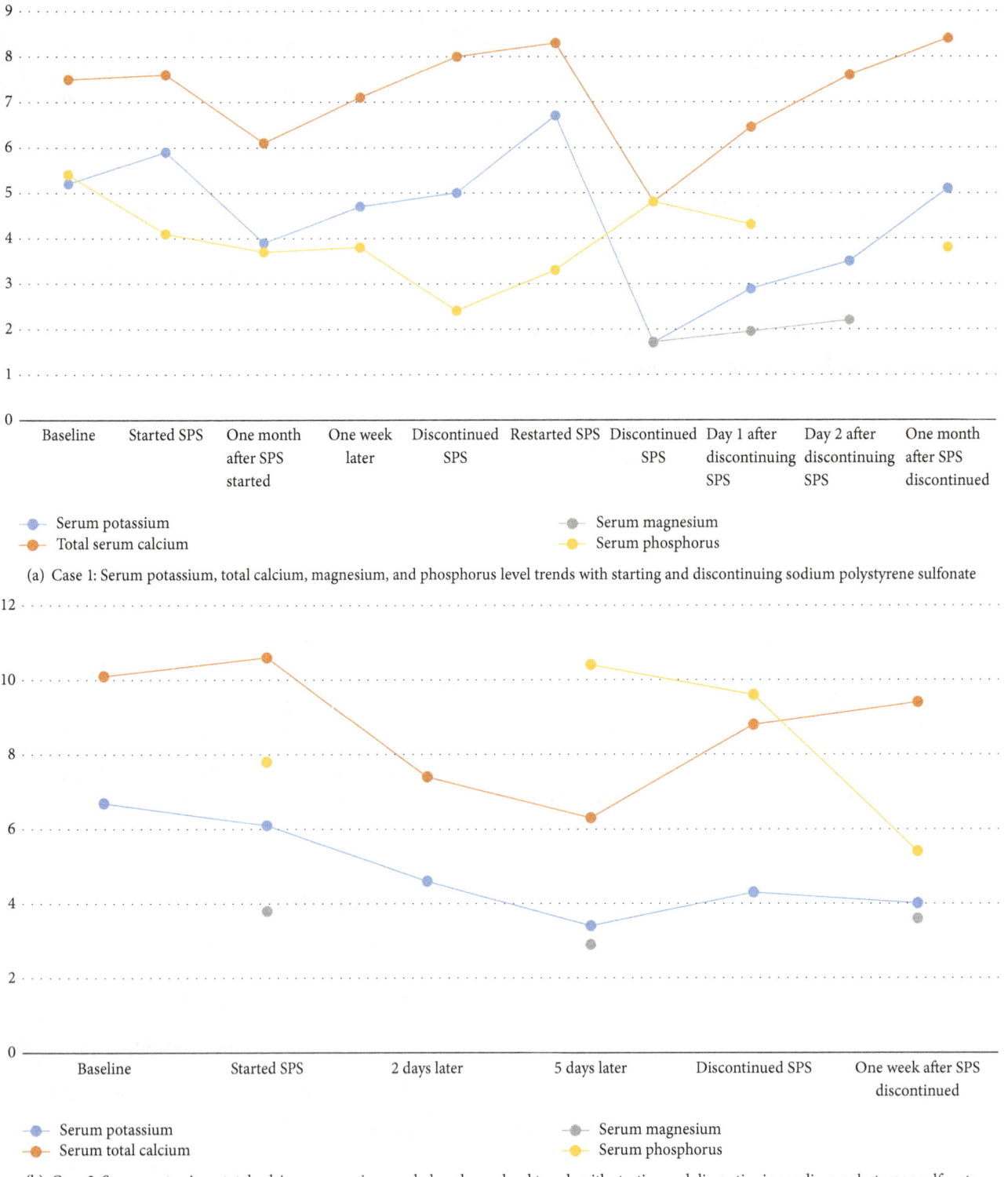

(a) Case 1: Serum potassium, total calcium, magnesium, and phosphorus level trends with starting and discontinuing sodium polystyrene sulfonate

(b) Case 2: Serum potassium, total calcium, magnesium, and phosphorus level trends with starting and discontinuing sodium polystyrene sulfonate

FIGURE 1

35 mEq/l), hypocalcemia (calcium of 6.1 mg/dl, serum albumin of 3.3 g/dl), and phosphorus of 3.7 mg/dL (Figure 1(a)). Intact PTH level had increased in the last month from 118.4 pg/ml to 180.4 pg/ml and 25(OH)-Vitamin D checked 6 months earlier was 33 ng/dL. On examination, heart rate was about 130/min and blood pressure was 102/58 mmHg. He had no tetany, normal deep tendon reflexes, a negative Chvostek sign, and no electrocardiogram (EKG) changes.

He was started on 0.1 mcg of calcitriol weekly and 350 mg of calcium carbonate supplement three times a day (administered in between feeds). In a week his potassium was 4.7 mEq/L and calcium improved to 7.1 mg/dL. The following month, he had a potassium of 5 mEq/L, serum bicarbonate of 36 mEq/L, serum calcium concentration of 8 mg/dl (albumin of 3.7 g/dL), phosphorus of 2.4 mg/dl, and intact PTH level of 190 pg/ml. He had blood pressure of about 90/60 mmHg and enalapril was stopped. Sevelamer was decreased from 4.8 g to 3.2 g and SPS was discontinued.

A week later, he was noted to have a serum potassium concentration of 6.7 mEq/L, serum bicarbonate of 30 mEq/L, calcium of 8.3 mg/dl, and phosphorus of 3.3 mg/dL. He was started on 30 g of SPS (0.8 g of SPS per mEq of potassium in the formula) added to his formula for decanting. He was continued on calcium carbonate three times a day (administered with bolus feeds) and sevelamer was discontinued. Repeat serum potassium concentration was 5 mEq/L.

He had episodes of vomiting and diarrhea while being on SPS. About one week later, he had routine blood work done which was again notable for hypokalemia (serum potassium concentration of 1.7 mEq/L), persistent metabolic alkalosis (serum bicarbonate 35 mEq/L), and severe hypocalcemia (serum calcium of 4.8 mg/dL, albumin level of 3.3 g/dL). The serum phosphorus level was 4.8 mg/dL and magnesium 1.72 mg/dL. In the ED, he had a transient breath holding spell, heart rate of about 120/min and blood pressure of 114/55 mmHg, no tetany, normal deep tendon reflexes, and a normal EKG. He was treated with intravenous calcium and potassium. SPS was discontinued, calcium supplements were increased to 810 mg/day, and he was dialyzed on high calcium (3.5 mEq/L) dialysate fluid with 1 mEq/L of potassium. At the time of discharge his serum potassium concentration was 4.3 mEq/L, calcium concentration was 7.9 mg/dL, serum phosphorus level was 4 mg/dL, and magnesium level was 2.2 mg/dL. Most recently, he has maintained a stable calcium of about 9.4 mg/dL while off of SPS.

2.2. Case 2. Second case is male with chronic kidney disease (CKD) secondary to posterior urethral valves who was maintained on chronic PD since 8 months of age.

At 17 months of age, while on PD, his serum potassium and phosphorus were low at 3.0 mEq/L and 2.9 mg/dL, respectively, for which he was started on 15 mEq of potassium phosphate supplements per day. He was not receiving SPS at that time. Two weeks later, he developed stridor with agitation and was diagnosed with croup. He improved after treatment with racemic epinephrine and dexamethasone. The following week, his symptoms returned and he again was diagnosed with croup. His laboratory tests were significant for severe hypocalcemia (serum calcium of 4.2 mg/dL and ionized calcium < 0.25 mmol/L). This episode was attributed to recent initiation of potassium phosphate. Hypocalcemia resolved with intravenous and enteral calcium supplementation and discontinuation of potassium phosphate.

At 28 months of age, his chronic medications included cholecalciferol (400 IU daily), lansoprazole, 2.5 mEq daily potassium chloride, somatotropin, metoclopramide, Nephronex, ferrous sulfate, and epogen. He was on formula feeds with Suplena (given by mouth and G-tube) that contained 570 mg of calcium, 45 IU of vitamin D daily, and 15.5 mEq of potassium. The dialysate contained 2.5 mEq/L of calcium. His serum bicarbonate level was 26 mEq/l, serum calcium was 10.1 mg/dl (albumin concentration of 3.9 g/dl), phosphorus was 7.3 mg/dl, intact PTH concentration was 801 pg/ml, and 25(OH)-Vitamin D concentration was 67.2 ng/ml. The cholecalciferol was discontinued. Sevelamer (1600 mg added to the formula for decanting) was started at this visit. About one week later he underwent lysis of intra-abdominal adhesions due to pain and abdominal distention with PD. Due to recurrence of symptoms and leakage of PD fluid, he was admitted for initiation of hemodialysis (HD) due to ultrafiltration failure.

At the time of initiation of HD he had a serum bicarbonate concentration of 31 mEq/l and calcium of 8.6 mg/dl. His was dialyzed on a 2.5 mEq/l calcium bath. He was started on 0.25 mcg of intravenous calcitriol; intravenous epogen and potassium supplements were discontinued. His Sevelamer was changed to 400 mg four times a day with feeds.

Five days after discharge, he developed a hemoglobin level of 6.9 g/dl requiring a 20 ml/kg red blood cell transfusion and was started on maintenance intravenous iron. He was continued on a 2 mEq/L potassium and 2.5 mEq/L calcium dialysate bath. Two days later, during his outpatient HD treatment, he was noted to have hyperkalemia (potassium of 6.6 mEq/L) and was switched to a 1 mEq/L potassium dialysate bath. He had persistent hyperkalemia at his next dialysis visit (potassium level of 6.1 mEq/L) and was started on 10 g of SPS daily. At this time his serum bicarbonate was 28 mEq/L, calcium was 10.6 mg/dL, phosphorus was 7.8 mg/dL, magnesium was 3.8 mg/dL, and intact PTH was 1539 pg/ml (Figure 1(b)). He also had persistent diarrhea. Two days after starting SPS, he had potassium of 4.6 mEq/L and calcium of 7.4 mg/dL. Three days later the patient was noted to be hypokalemic (potassium of 3.4 mEq/L) and he had metabolic alkalosis (serum bicarbonate of 32 mEq/L), hypocalcemia (calcium of 6.3 mg/dL), phosphorus of 10.4 mg/dL, and magnesium 2.9 mg/dL. His heart rate was about 90/min and blood pressure about 110/60 mmHg and he had no tetany, normal deep tendon reflexes, and a negative Chvostek sign. He was admitted and started on calcium carbonate dosed at 200 mg of elemental calcium three times a day (later increased to 270 mg of elemental calcium) and SPS was discontinued. An EKG showed nonspecific ST-T wave abnormalities and normal QT. Telemetry showed appropriate sinus bradycardia overnight without evidence of heart block. His new dialysate contained 1 mEq/L potassium and 4 mEq/L calcium. Calcium levels improved to 8.1 mg/dL, serum bicarbonate of 27 mEq/L, and phosphorus (postdialysis) of 4.4 mg/dL prior to discharge home. Most recently, he has maintained a stable calcium of about 8.8 mg/dL and potassium of 3.7 mEq/L off SPS.

3. Discussion

Both the children with CKD and on dialysis were started on SPS for hyperkalemia. Within a week after initiation of the medication, both developed hypocalcemia on routine labs without overt clinical manifestations. The hypocalcemia was

TABLE 1: Potassium sparing agents for management of hyperkalemia [3].

	Sodium polystyrene sulfonate (SPS)	Sodium zirconium cyclosilicate	Patiromer
FDA approval	Approved	Still pending	Approved in adults
Mechanism of action	Nonspecific sodium-cation exchange resin	Selective potassium cation binding agent	Calcium based cation exchange resin
Adverse effects	Colon necrosis, GI disturbances, hypokalemia, hypomagnesemia, hypocalcemia, metabolic alkalosis	GI disturbances, hypokalemia	GI disturbances, hypokalemia, hypercalcemia, hypomagnesemia

rapidly corrected with oral supplementation and discontinuation of SPS.

Potassium exchange resins are used to treat hyperkalemia in CKD frequently. It removes potassium by exchanging sodium ions for potassium ions in the intestine before the resin is excreted. Hypokalemia, hypocalcemia, and even tetany have been described after SPS therapy [1, 2]. A study done by Greenman et al. on patients with congestive heart failure and edema treated with exchange resin therapy showed that four of the twelve patients had abnormally low calcium values after prolonged treatment and three others had only slight decrease in their serum calcium levels [4]. The affinity of ion-exchangers for cations of bivalent elements such as calcium is greater than that for univalent ions such as potassium. Among the univalent ions, the affinity for hydrogen ions exceeds most others [5]. There is a steady loss of calcium in the gut which leads to a risk of gradual demineralization of bone when patients are maintained on cation exchangers for months to years. These studies noted that when patients developed hypocalcemia, the serum calcium levels increased only temporarily with supplementation. The rapid removal of calcium is likely due to deposition in the bones [2, 5]. Our patients however, were noted to have an acute drop in their serum calcium levels within a week of initiation of SPS therapy. Their hypocalcemia responded rapidly to calcium supplementation.

Multiple studies have been done measuring the calcium and potassium content in formulas pretreated with SPS. A retrospective study in Seattle done in 2013 showed, within 72 hours, there was an average 24% decrease in serum potassium after pretreatment of formula or breastmilk with SPS [6]. In 1972, Starbuck showed a decrease in potassium and calcium ion content and an increase in sodium content of milk treated with SPS [7]. A more recent study by Bunchman et al. showed an average drop in calcium levels by 66% in formula pretreated with 1 gm SPS per milliequivalent of potassium in the formula. Human testing in five patients did not show any clinical symptoms of hypocalcemia [8]. Hobbs et al. suggested the use of adult renal formulas that are low in minerals to manage nutrition of hyperkalemic infants with CKD without complications [9].

There are case reports of metabolic alkalosis occurring in patients receiving alkali therapy along with SPS [1, 10]. This occurs because, in the presence of an ion exchange resin, the salt formed by interaction of the antacid with hydrochloric acid in the stomach does not neutralize the bicarbonate in the small bowel. The bicarbonate that is reabsorbed by the gut cannot be excreted in the presence of poor renal function, leading to metabolic alkalosis.

Newer agents, including sodium zirconium cyclosilicate and patiromer have been studied for the use management of chronic hyperkalemia in patients with CKD [3, 11, 12]. Details comparing currently available drugs used for hyperkalemia are shown in Table 1.

Metabolic acidosis of chronic renal failure usually protects patients from overt symptoms of hypocalcemia. Tetany or seizures may occur when acidosis is corrected rapidly without correcting hypocalcemia at the same time.

Severe hypocalcemia can develop after SPS therapy. The metabolic alkalosis in these patients associated with the hypocalcemia put them at increased risk for complications. This report illustrates the necessity of very close monitoring of electrolytes, calcium, and phosphorus balance in pediatric patients on dialysis. Often calcium supplementation is required to maintain normal calcium levels. Newer agents including patiromer and sodium zirconium cyclosilicate are potentially safer medications for management of hyperkalemia in patients with CKD.

References

[1] H. A. Ziessman, "Alkalosis and seizure due to a cation-exchange resin and magnesium hydroxide," *Southern Medical Journal*, vol. 69, no. 4, pp. 497–499, 1976.

[2] D. Macaulay and G. Watson, "Tetany following cation-exchange resin therapy," *The Lancet*, vol. 264, no. 6828, pp. 70-71, 1954.

[3] M. Chaitman, D. Dixit, and M. B. Bridgeman, "Potassium-binding agents for the clinical management of Hyperkalemia," *Pharmacy and Therapeutics*, vol. 41, no. 1, p. 43, 2016.

[4] L. Greenman, J. B. Shaler, and T. S. Danowski, "Biochemical disturbances and clinical symptoms during prolonged exchange resin therapy in congestive heart failure," *The American Journal of Medicine*, vol. 14, no. 4, pp. 391–403, 1953.

[5] W. Dock and N. R. Frank, "Cation exchangers: Their use and hazards as AIDS in managing edema," *American Heart Journal*, vol. 40, no. 4, pp. 638–645, 1950.

[6] K. Thompson, J. Flynn, D. Okamura, and L. Zhou, "Pretreatment of formula or expressed breast milk with sodium polystyrene sulfonate (Kayexalate®) as a treatment for hyperkalemia in infants with acute or chronic renal insufficiency," *Journal of Renal Nutrition*, vol. 23, no. 5, pp. 333–339, 2013.

[7] W. C. Starbuck, "Reduction of potassium and calcium in milk by sodium sulfonated polystyrene resins," *Kidney International*, vol. 2, no. 3, pp. 175–177, 1972.

[8] T. E. Bunchman, E. G. Wood, M. H. Schenck, K. A. Weaver, B. L. Klein, and R. E. Lynch, "Pretreatment of formula with sodium polystyrene sulfonate to reduce dietary potassium intake," *Pediatric Nephrology*, vol. 5, no. 1, pp. 29–32, 1991.

[9] D. J. Hobbs, T. R. Gast, K. B. Ferguson, T. E. Bunchman, and G.-M. Barletta, "Nutritional management of hyperkalemic infants with chronic kidney disease, using adult renal formulas," *Journal of Renal Nutrition*, vol. 20, no. 2, pp. 121–126, 2010.

[10] H. J. Baluarte, J. Prebis, M. Goldberg, and A. B. Gruskin, "Metabolic alkalosis in an anephric child caused by the combined use of Kayexalate and Basaljel," *The Journal of Pediatrics*, vol. 92, no. 2, pp. 237–239, 1978.

[11] M. R. Weir, G. L. Bakris, D. A. Bushinsky et al., "Patiromer in patients with kidney disease and hyperkalemia receiving RAAS inhibitors," *The New England Journal of Medicine*, vol. 372, no. 3, pp. 211–221, 2015.

[12] D. K. Packham, H. S. Rasmussen, P. T. Lavin et al., "Sodium zirconium cyclosilicate in hyperkalemia," *The New England Journal of Medicine*, vol. 372, no. 3, pp. 222–231, 2015.

Denosumab-Induced Severe Hypocalcaemia in Chronic Kidney Disease

Ryan Jalleh,[1] Gopal Basu,[1,2] Richard Le Leu,[1] and Shilpanjali Jesudason[1,2]

[1]Central and Northern Adelaide Renal and Transplantation Service, Royal Adelaide Hospital, Adelaide, South Australia, Australia
[2]Department of Medicine, University of Adelaide, South Australia, Australia

Correspondence should be addressed to Ryan Jalleh; ryan.jalleh@sa.gov.au

Academic Editor: Yoshihide Fujigaki

Background. Hypocalcaemia is increasingly recognized as a complication of denosumab use in Chronic Kidney Disease (CKD) patients with osteoporosis. Despite Therapeutic Goods Administration (TGA) notifications in 2013, we have subsequently encountered several cases of denosumab-induced hypocalcaemia, raising concern about lack of widespread awareness among prescribing practitioners. *Aims.* We reviewed the morbidity and healthcare intervention needs of CKD patients with hypocalcaemia attributed to denosumab. *Methods.* A retrospective case series of CKD patients with clinically significant hypocalcaemia after exposure to denosumab, encountered at the tertiary care referral hospital from December 2013 to February 2017, was undertaken. *Results.* Eight patients (52-85 years of age) with stage 4-5 CKD developed clinically significant hypocalcaemia (corrected calcium 1.45±0.21mmol/L) following denosumab therapy for osteoporosis. Seven of the eight patients required inpatient management with three patients requiring intravenous calcium replacement and cardiac monitoring in a high dependency unit. Our study also identified additional factors that could potentially contribute to hypocalcaemia such as lack of calcium supplementation, use of noncalcium based phosphate binders, absence of or use of lower doses of calcitriol supplementation, low vitamin D levels, concomitant treatment with loop diuretics, history of parathyroidectomy, or presence of acute medical illness. *Conclusion.* Multiple cases of severe hypocalcaemia in CKD patients following denosumab exposure were encountered after TGA warnings, resulting in considerable morbidity and intensive healthcare interventions in CKD patients. We advocate greater awareness amongst the medical profession, careful consideration before using denosumab in CKD patients, and close follow-up after administration to prevent morbidity.

1. Introduction

Denosumab is a fully humanised monoclonal antibody used for treatment of osteoporosis. Denosumab binds to the ligand to the receptor activator of nuclear factor kappa B (RANK-L)[1], the osteoclast differentiating factor, thereby preventing RANK-L from binding to RANK, consequently inhibiting downstream pathways of osteoclast formation, activity, and survival. Thus, it decreases bone resorption, increases bone mineral density (BMD), and reduces the risk of fragility fractures. It is a useful alternative to bisphosphonates in management of osteoporosis especially in patients who are intolerant or unresponsive to bisphosphonates. Unlike bisphosphonates, denosumab is not renally cleared, and hence its dosing is simplified in chronic kidney disease (CKD) patients in whom bisphosphonates are considered contraindicated [2]. In addition, its ease of administration as a subcutaneous injection has rapidly raised its popularity among clinicians.

However, the use of denosumab in CKD patients is not without risk. Hypocalcaemia is a known adverse event with incidence 14-15% reported among CKD patients [3, 4]. The Therapeutic Goods Administration (TGA) has issued medication safety updates of hypocalcaemia in 2013 and additionally of prolonged QT interval due to hypocalcaemia in 2016 [5, 6]. However, there is limited information for the safety in patients with CKD and consequently several cases of patients with hypocalcaemia after denosumab were encountered in the recent years [3, 7]. This case series was conducted to highlight the morbidity and healthcare interventions needed

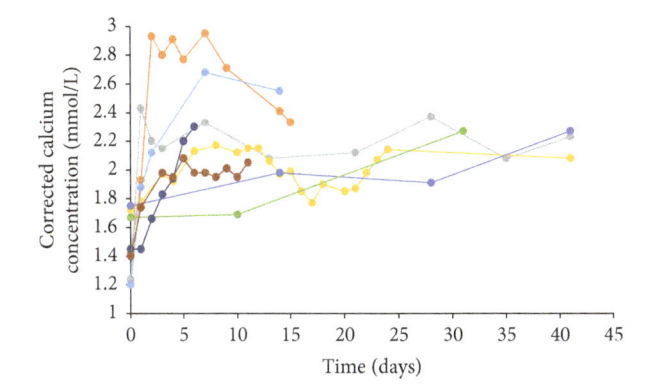

FIGURE 1: Corrected calcium levels on admission day (time 0) and subsequently (n=8 cases).

to manage this complication and thereby raise awareness of the risk of hypocalcaemia in CKD patients receiving denosumab.

2. Materials and Methods

We performed a retrospective case series of patients with CKD stage 4 or 5, who developed clinically significant hypocalcaemia following denosumab therapy and presented to a tertiary hospital between December 2013 and February 2017. Cases were referred by nephrologists at the institution who had patients with CKD stage 4 or 5, had at least one dose of subcutaneous denosumab 60mg, and had hypocalcaemia (corrected calcium <2.10) identified at any time following the dose of denosumab. The clinical data, collected by review of medical records and in liaison with the primary care general practitioners, included stage of chronic kidney disease, profile of corrected calcium, phosphate levels, parathyroid hormone levels, alkaline phosphatase (ALP), vitamin D levels, T-score from the most recent dual-energy X-ray absorptiometry (DEXA) scan preceding the denosumab, dosing history, and time of onset of hypocalcaemia. This study was approved by our institution's Human Research Ethics Committee.

The calcium level was corrected for low serum albumin using the following formula [9]:

$$\text{Corrected calcium (mmol/L)} = \text{total serum calcium (mmol/L)} + 0.02 \left(40 - \text{serum albumin [g/L]}\right) \quad (1)$$

3. Results

A total of eight CKD patients with symptomatic hypocalcaemia were identified from Dec 2013 to Feb 2017 aged between 52 and 85 years. A summary of the biochemical parameters and the patient's current calcium/vitamin D therapy are described in Tables 1 and 2.

The number of doses of denosumab before developing hypocalcaemia varied from a single dose in most patients up to 6 doses. The onset of hypocalcaemia from the last dose of denosumab ranged from 2 to 12 weeks with a mean of 6.6 weeks (median 8 weeks).

Seven of the eight patients required hospital admission. Calcium levels at and after admission are shown in Figure 1. Three patients required intravenous calcium replacement with cardiac monitoring in an intensive care/high dependency unit. Four patients were managed in the ward and one patient was managed as an outpatient.

Four of the eight patients were not receiving regular calcium supplementation, which is associated with an increased risk of severe hypocalcaemia [7]. All three cases that required high dependency support were not on concurrent calcium supplements when commenced on denosumab. Two of the three patients admitted to a high dependency unit were on regular furosemide for management of congestive cardiac failure. The increased calcium loss via diuresis may have increased their risk of hypocalcaemia. Five out of eight cases were on a less than daily dosing of calcitriol and four out of eight cases had low levels of vitamin D. None of the patients were receiving cinacalcet.

Seven out of 8 patients had additional factors that could potentially contribute or worsen denosumab-related hypocalcaemia including use of noncalcium based phosphate binders (1 case), absence of or use of low doses of calcitriol (less than daily doses) supplementation (5 cases), low levels of vitamin D (4 cases), concomitant treatment with loop diuretics (2 cases), history of parathyroidectomy (1 case), and presence of an acute medical illness with reduced oral intake (1 case).

There was no significant correlation between time from denosumab dose to hypocalcaemia and the severity of hypocalcaemia (Pearson correlation coefficient $r = 0.19$, $r^2 = 0.036$ ($p = 0.65$)). There was no correlation between calcium level at presentation and length of stay. All patients required close outpatient monitoring of calcium levels on discharge with frequent medical follow-up encounters. In all cases, following the presentation of hypocalcaemia, the use of denosumab was discouraged.

4. Discussion

Chronic kidney disease, mineral and bone disorder (CKD-MBD), is frequently present in stage 4 to 5 CKD and can cause fragility fractures as well as a low bone mineral density.[10] In CKD stage 4-5 patients, a history of fragility fractures and DEXA results is unable to differentiate osteoporosis from CKD-MBD. However, the treatment of CKD-MBD is different from that of osteoporosis. This distinction is difficult but important as denosumab and other antiresorptive agents may not be beneficial in the setting of CKD-MBD. The gold standard of discriminating between the various forms of renal bone disease is transiliac bone biopsy performed with prior double tetracycline labelling.[10] However, due to cost and invasiveness, this procedure is not frequently done in clinical practice and none of the cases reported above underwent this form of testing.

As CKD progresses, there is decreased phosphate clearance and this is thought to be the driving mechanism that

TABLE 1: Baseline clinical data for 8 patients with CKD stages 4 to 5 who were on denosumab treatment.

Case	Sex	CKD stage	Serum Creatinine (μmol/L)	eGFR (ml/min/1.73m²)	Ca2+ prior to denosumab	Corr Ca²⁺ (Ref: 2.10 – 2.55 mmol/L) at presentation	PO₄³⁻ (Ref: 0.65 – 1.45 mmol/L)	PTH (Ref: 0.8 – 5.5 pmol/L)	ALP (Ref: 30 – 110 units/L)	Vitamin D (Ref: 60 – 160 nmol/L)	T-score
1	F	5	394	11	2.21	1.42	1.85	55.4	61	75	-3.0
2	F	4	207	20	2.28	1.24	1.02	83.9	77	27	-
3	M	4	289	18	2.11	1.30	2.63	58.2	399	45	-2.5
4	F	5	645	5	2.20	1.20	2.71	80.1	54	54	-2.5
5	F	5D	601	5	2.44	1.80	1.68	59.6	74	90	-3.0
6	F	4T	221	20	2.18	1.70	1.65	15.5	93	62	-1.3†
7	F	4T	234	18	2.38	1.50	0.69	-	101	88	-4.4
8	M	5	410	11	2.14	1.40	1.40	33.3	76	32	-2.7

5D = stage 5 CKD on dialysis and 4T = stage 4 CKD with a renal transplant. All results (including serum phosphate, PTH, ALP, and vitamin D) were obtained closest to the time of presentation with hypocalcaemia in patients who were symptomatic or nadir of hypocalcaemia in patients who were asymptomatic and being actively monitored. All T-scores were obtained based on bone densitometry of the femur except for case 6† who had forearm bone densitometry due to bilateral hip joint replacements. eGFR was calculated using the CKD-EPI formula [8]; Ref = reference range.

TABLE 2: Baseline clinical data for 8 patients with CKD stages 4 to 5 who were on denosumab treatment.

Case	Number of denosumab doses	Length of hospital stay	Ward/HDU/Outpatient	Time from dose of denosumab to calcium nadir (weeks)	Time to normal calcium level (weeks)	Calcium dose regime prior to admission	Calcitriol dose regime prior to admission	History of fragility fracture
1	1	2	Ward	12	2	1g TDS	250ng twice weekly	No
2	1	4	HDU	4	8	Nil	Nil	Yes
3	1	25	Ward	8	11	1g TDS	250ng daily	No
4	3	11	HDU	8	7	Nil	250ng alternate daily	Yes
5	4	1	Outpatient	9	8	500mg TDS	250ng thrice weekly	No
6	6	7	Ward	8	2	Nil	250ng daily	No
7	1	8	Ward	2	1	500mg TDS	250ng daily	No
8	1	10	HDU	2	1	Nil	Nil	No

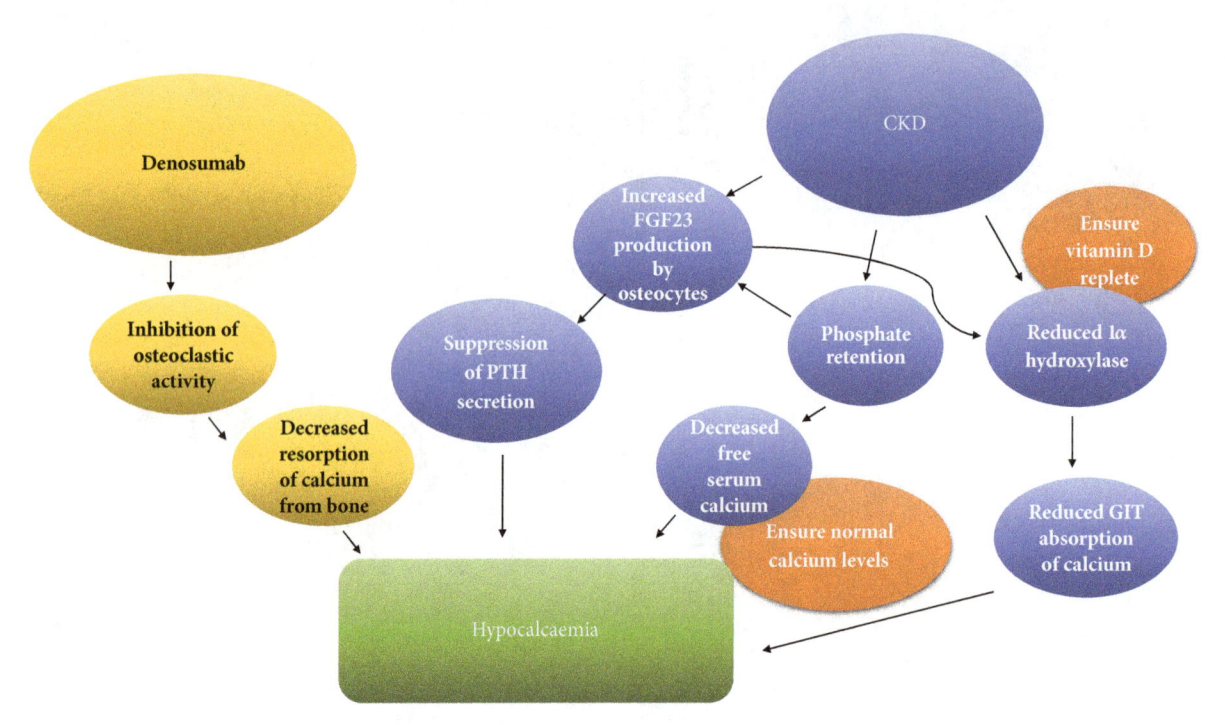

FIGURE 2: A summary of mechanisms for increased risk of hypocalcaemia with denosumab in patients with CKD.

results in increased production of fibroblast growth factor-23 (FGF-23) mainly by osteocytes.[11–13] In addition to reduced production of 1α hydroxylase in CKD due to decreased functional renal tissue, there is also inhibition of the enzyme due to FGF-23 accumulation.[11] Ultimately, this results in reduced absorption of calcium from the gastrointestinal tract potentially exacerbating hypocalcaemia. In addition, FGF-23 suppresses PTH secretion which may impair the ability of the kidneys to maintain calcium homeostasis [14]. There are multiple mechanisms that predispose CKD patients to hypocalcaemia (Figure 2).

Denosumab downregulates osteoclast activity in CKD patients, increasing their predisposition to hypocalcaemia. Many patients with CKD could already be suffering from low bone turnover and denosumab could potentially worsen this and possibly increase the risk of fractures. There is a paucity of evidence for the use of denosumab in CKD stage 4 to 5 and it is currently unclear if denosumab provides benefit. Significantly, in the original denosumab trial, the FREEDOM study [1, 15], only 73 of 7808 patients recruited had CKD stage 4 and none of the patients had CKD stage 5. Patients with secondary hyperparathyroidism, associated with the CKD stage 4 to 5 population, were also excluded from the study. Thus, the results from FREEDOM study are clearly not widely applicable for patients with advanced CKD and those with secondary hyperparathyroidism.

Despite the lack of robust evidence of benefit, and warnings of possible harm, denosumab continues to be used in patients with advanced CKD and cases of hypocalcaemia secondary to denosumab use continue to be reported, as demonstrated by this case series. The cases described outline the potentially life-threatening severity of morbidity that may occur. Most of our patients required hospitalisation, with half requiring intensive care unit admissions for intravenous calcium replacement and cardiac monitoring. Importantly, significant hypocalcaemia often occurred some weeks after denosumab administration. These cases highlight the unpredictability of hypocalcaemia and the need for heightened awareness and closer biochemical monitoring for CKD patients receiving denosumab. A critical review of the patients' comorbidities and other medications that regulate calcium and parathyroid hormone to identify risk factors for hypocalcaemia (or impaired response to hypocalcaemia) is important before considering denosumab use in patients with CKD.

The denosumab product information [16] includes a special warning regarding hypocalcaemia and states that this must be corrected prior to initiating therapy. Consistent with the findings in this case series, it warns that patients with the following may have a predisposition to hypocalcaemia: severe renal impairment, history of hypoparathyroidism, thyroid or parathyroid surgery, malabsorption syndromes, and excision of small intestine. It recommends monitoring of calcium in these cases especially within the first two weeks of initiating therapy and prior to each dose. Similar to our recommendations, it also advises that all patients should be instructed on the symptoms of hypocalcaemia and the importance of maintaining calcium levels with adequate calcium and vitamin D supplementation. In addition to following the recommendations on the product information, based on our experience, we have developed further clinical practice points for clinicians considering denosumab therapy in patients with advanced CKD, which may prevent serious hypocalcaemia. (Box 1). This approach is supported by a

> Practice points for clinicians:
> *Prior to denosumab administration*:
> (1) Consult with the patient's primary nephrologist prior to commencement of denosumab in patients with Stage 4–5 CKD. Review the indication for denosumab.
> (2) Check baseline calcium level prior to each dose of denosumab.
> (3) Correct hypocalcaemia prior to initiating therapy. Review calcium-based phosphate binders and calcitriol supplementation dosing, or initiate this therapy if hypocalcaemic.
> (4) Identify other medications that may predispose to hypocalcaemia such as loop diuretics (frusemide), calcimimetics (cinacalcet), steroids, bisphosphonates, calcitonin, barbiturates and ketoconazole.
> *After denosumab administration*:
> (1) Clearly notify denosumab administration to all clinicians involved to raise awareness of potential hypocalcaemia.
> (2) Calcium levels should be monitored at least weekly following denosumab administration, for up to 12 weeks.
> (3) Identify declining calcium levels early. Optimize calcium and calcitriol therapy early to prevent severe hypocalcaemia.
> *Information for patients*:
> (1) Patients with Stage 4–5 CKD should be counselled about the increased risk of hypocalcaemia with denosumab.
> (2) Patients should understand the importance of blood tests for detecting hypocalcaemia early.
> (3) Patients should be advised about the signs and symptoms of hypocalcaemia.
> (4) Patients should be advised to seek immediate medical attention should the following occur: unusual fatigue, paraesthesia, muscle spasm, twitching, stiffness, confusion and/or seizures.

Box 1: Based on the authors' experience, our recommended practice points while considering denosumab in CKD patients to address potential hypocalcaemia.

pilot study by Chen et al. [17]. In this study, 12 patients on renal replacement therapy received denosumab for treatment of secondary hyperparathyroidism. Consistent with our findings, = a high risk of hypocalcaemia in patients with CKD is noted; however with aggressive calcium and calcitriol supplementation, use of high calcium dialysate, and weekly blood tests monitoring calcium in the first month of initiating denosumab, none of the patients needed inpatient admission for management of hypocalcaemia.

A limitation of this study is that it is a retrospective, observational study with a small number of reported patients. The total incidence of hypocalcaemia among all CKD patients receiving denosumab was not known and there was a lack of information for why denosumab was administered to the patients. Furthermore, patients with asymptomatic hypocalcaemia where biochemical monitoring was not undertaken could not be identified. Further research is required to determine the optimal regime for early identification and prevention of hypocalcaemia in patients with chronic kidney disease receiving denosumab.

5. Conclusions

Denosumab can cause hypocalcaemia in patients with CKD. Given the number of cases that we have observed, there may be a lack of awareness of the risk of hypocalcaemia, the need for close monitoring of calcium levels, and the paucity of evidence of the effectiveness of denosumab in CKD stages 4-5. We urge clinicians to exercise caution when using denosumab in patients with advanced CKD, to consult with the patient's nephrologist when initiating treatment, and to arrange biochemical monitoring after administration.

Disclosure

The authors confirm that the results presented in this paper have not been published previously in whole or part, except in abstract format. The abstract was presented as a poster at 2017 Annual Scientific Meeting of the Australian and New Zealand Society of Nephrology.

References

[1] S. R. Cummings, J. S. Martin, M. R. McClung et al., "Denosumab for prevention of fractures in postmenopausal women with osteoporosis," *The New England Journal of Medicine*, vol. 361, no. 8, pp. 756–765, 2009.

[2] F. Festuccia, M. T. Jafari, A. Moioli et al., "Safety and efficacy of denosumab in osteoporotic hemodialysed patients," *Journal of Nephrology*, vol. 30, no. 2, pp. 271–279, 2017.

[3] A. L. H. Huynh, S. T. Baker, A. J. Stewardson, and D. F. Johnson, "Denosumab-associated hypocalcaemia: incidence, severity and patient characteristics in a tertiary hospital setting," *Pharmacoepidemiology and Drug Safety*, vol. 25, no. 11, pp. 1274–1278, 2016.

[4] G. A. Block, H. G. Bone, L. Fang, E. Lee, and D. Padhi, "A single-dose study of denosumab in patients with various degrees of renal impairment," *Journal of Bone and Mineral Research*, vol. 27, no. 7, pp. 1471–1479, 2012.

[5] Therapeutic Goods Administration, "Denosumab and severe hypocalcaemia," *Australian Prescriber*, vol. 32, no. 2, 2013.

[6] Therapeutic Goods Administration, "Denosumab and QT prolongation," *Australian Prescriber*, vol. 7, no. 4, 2016.

[7] V. Dave, C. Y. Chiang, J. Booth, and P. F. Mount, "Hypocalcemia post denosumab in patients with chronic kidney disease stage 4-5," *American Journal of Nephrology*, vol. 41, no. 2, pp. 129–137, 2015.

[8] A. S. Levey and L. A. Stevens, "Estimating GFR using the CKD epidemiology collaboration (CKD-EPI) creatinine equation: More accurate GFR estimates, lower CKD prevalence estimates, and better risk predictions," *American Journal of Kidney Diseases*, vol. 55, no. 4, pp. 622–627, 2010.

[9] R. B. Payne, A. J. Little, R. B. Williams, and J. R. Milner, "Interpretation of serum calcium in patients with abnormal serum proteins," *British Medical Journal*, vol. 4, no. 5893, pp. 643–646, 1973.

[10] P. D. Miller, "Chronic kidney disease and osteoporosis: evaluation and management," *Bonekey Reports*, vol. 3, 2014.

[11] P. Hu, Q. Xuan, B. Hu, L. Lu, J. Wang, and Y. H. Qin, "Fibroblast growth factor-23 helps explain the biphasic cardiovascular effects of vitamin D in chronic kidney disease," *International Journal of Biological Sciences*, vol. 8, no. 5, pp. 663–671, 2012.

[12] O. Gutierrez, T. Isakova, E. Rhee et al., "Fibroblast growth factor-23 mitigates hyperphosphatemia but accentuates calcitriol deficiency in chronic kidney disease," *Journal of the American Society of Nephrology*, vol. 16, no. 7, pp. 2205–2215, 2005.

[13] H. Komaba and M. Fukagawa, "FGF23: A key player in mineral and bone disorder in CKD," *Nefrología*, vol. 29, no. 5, pp. 392–396, 2009.

[14] I. Z. Ben-Dov, H. Galitzer, V. Lavi-Moshayoff et al., "The parathyroid is a target organ for FGF23 in rats," *The Journal of Clinical Investigation*, vol. 117, no. 12, pp. 4003–4008, 2007.

[15] S. A. Jamal, Ö. Ljunggren, C. Stehman-Breen et al., "Effects of denosumab on fracture and bone mineral density by level of kidney function," *Journal of Bone and Mineral Research*, vol. 26, no. 8, pp. 1829–1835, 2011.

[16] "Denosumab product information," Australia (NSW): Amgen Australia, 2018 [revised 2018 Jul 18].

[17] C.-L. Chen, N.-C. Chen, C.-Y. Hsu et al., "An open-label, prospective pilot clinical study of denosumab for severe hyperparathyroidism in patients with low bone mass undergoing dialysis," *The Journal of Clinical Endocrinology & Metabolism*, vol. 99, no. 7, pp. 2426–2432, 2014.

Porphyria Cutanea Tarda in a Patient with End-Stage Renal Disease: A Case of Successful Treatment with Deferoxamine and Ferric Carboxymaltose

Natacha Rodrigues,[1] Fernando Caeiro,[1] Alice Santana,[1] Teresa Mendes,[1] and Leonor Lopes[2]

[1]Hemodialysis Unit Diaverum Cruz Vermelha Portuguesa, Lisbon, Portugal
[2]Department of Dermatology, Centro Hospitalar Lisboa Norte, Lisbon, Portugal

Correspondence should be addressed to Natacha Rodrigues; rodrigues120@hotmail.com

Academic Editor: David Mudge

Porphyria cutanea tarda (PCT) is a rare disease, with a strong association with hepatitis C virus. PCT is particularly problematic in end-stage renal disease patients as they have no renal excretion of porphyrins and these are poorly dialyzed. Also, conventional treatment of PCT is compromised in these patients as hydroxychloroquine is contraindicated, phlebotomies with the stipulated frequency are poorly tolerated in already anaemia-prone patients, and iron-chelating agents are less efficient in removing iron and contribute to worsening anaemia. The authors report a patient on haemodialysis, with hepatitis C infection, that is diagnosed with PCT. Despite the good clinical results with deferoxamine, she became dependent on blood transfusions because of her ferropenic state. Every time oxide iron was started, the patient developed clinical features of the disease, resolving after the suspension of the drug. A decision was made to start the patient on ferric carboxymaltose, which was well tolerated without disease symptoms and need of further blood transfusions. This case suggests that deferoxamine is efficient in treatment of porphyria cutanea tarda. Also, ferric carboxymaltose may be a valuable option for refractory anaemia in patients with this disease and end-stage renal disease, as it seems to provide iron without clinical relapse of the disease.

1. Introduction

Although dermatological manifestations in patients with end-stage renal disease (ESRD) can be very common, such as pruritus, xerosis, and pigmentation, other cutaneous disorders are quite rare [1]. Sporadic *porphyria cutanea tarda* (PCT) is such a disease, occurring in less than 5% of dialysis patients [2]. Despite the low prevalence, there is a strong association between the sporadic form of PCT and hepatitis C virus (HCV) infection that has been demonstrated in multiple studies [3].

Although rare, PCT has particular issues in ESRD patients. Not only do these patients have no renal excretion of porphyrins and these are poorly dialyzed, but also although the treatment of PCT in the general population is well established, in ESRD patients hydroxychloroquine is contraindicated, frequent phlebotomies tend to be poorly tolerated by these already anaemia-prone patients, and iron-chelating agents are less efficient in removing iron and contribute to worsening anaemia.

2. Case Report

We report the case of a 46-year-old melanodermic woman with end-stage renal disease of unknown aetiology. She started haemodialysis (HD) in 1996 and received a cadaveric kidney transplant in 1997. After transplantation, she had cytomegalovirus infection, colon adenocarcinoma, and chronic renal allograft dysfunction. She restarted haemodialysis in 2003 due to graft dysfunction.

She also had HCV infection (genotype 1a) and she was put on pegylated interferon-alpha-2a 180 mcg/week from July 2010 to July 2011; however, a negative viral load was not attained with this treatment regimen.

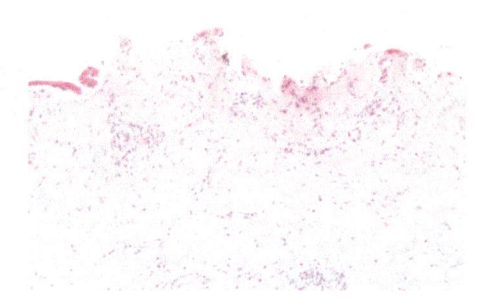

FIGURE 1: Cutaneous biopsy tissue. Skin biopsy specimens showing epidermal detachment with minimal dermal inflammatory infiltrate, festooning of dermal papillae with thickening of basement membrane, and deposits of eosinophilic hyaline material (PAS positive) on the wall of superficial vascular plexus (H&E 100x).

TABLE 1: Laboratory results.

	Result	Reference
Haemoglobin	104 g/L	100–120 g/L
WBC count	6.06×10^9/L	3.8–10.8×10^9/L
Platelet count	138×10^9/L	150–450×10^9/L
C-reactive protein	0.04 mg/L	<0.8 mg/L
Transferrin saturation	43%	>30%
Ferritin	267 µg/L	200–500 µg/L
ALT	53 U/L	<20 U/L
AST	34 U/L	<42 U/L
G-GT	133 U/L	8–65 U/L
Total plasma porphyrin	1052.3 ug/L	<32.5 ug/L
Plasma uroporphyrin	983.3 ug/L	<11.8 ug/L
Plasma heptacarboxylporphyrin	24.3 ug/L	<3.8 ug/L
Plasma hexacarboxylporphyrin	13.4 ug/L	<1.3 ug/L
Plasma pentacarboxylporphyrin	27.3 ug/L	<27.3 ug/L
Plasma coproporphyrin I	2.5 ug/L	<6.4 ug/L
Plasma coproporphyrin II	1.5 ug/L	<8 ug/L
Faecal porphyrins	All normal	
Urinary porphyrins	Anuric	

ALT, alanine aminotransferase; AST, aspartate aminotransferase; G-GT, gamma-glutamate transpeptidase. The reference values for haemoglobin, ferritin, and transferrin saturation are in concordance with KDIGO considering ESRD patients.

In March of 2014, she presented with bullous dermatosis evolving both upper limbs, more exuberant on the dorsal aspect of the hands and forearms, and oral enanthema more prominent in the lower lip, interfering with meals. Despite her skin and mucosal lesions, physical examination was otherwise unremarkable. She did not have any family history of porphyria, photosensitivity, or prior episodes of this dermatosis. She was not on oestrogen replacement therapy or had a history of alcoholism. At this time, she was on epoetin 160 U/kg/week IV, alfacalcidol 1 mcg/HD session, Generis saccharated iron oxide 50 mg/week, and carvedilol 12,5 mg/bid. The lesions were biopsied: epidermal detachment with minimal dermal inflammatory infiltrate, festooning of dermal papillae with thickening of basement membrane, and deposits of eosinophilic hyaline material on the wall of superficial vascular plexus (Figure 1).

The laboratory investigation is presented in Table 1 and showed an appropriate haemoglobin, normal white blood cell count, platelet count, C-reactive protein level, transferrin saturation, ferritin, alanine aminotransferase, aspartate aminotransferase, and slightly increased gamma-glutamate transpeptidase. Serologic tests were negative for HIV and hepatitis B and were positive for hepatitis C. The patient had elevated levels of total plasma porphyrin, uroporphyrin, and heptacarboxylporphyrin and hexacarboxylporphyrin; she had normal levels of pentacarboxylporphyrin, coproporphyrin I, and coproporphyrin II. Faecal porphyrin levels were normal. Urinary porphyrins were not measured because she was anuric.

With these findings, she was diagnosed with porphyria cutanea tarda. Phlebotomy was not an option considering the anaemia secondary to chronic renal disease in a patient already under a significant dose of epoetin. Generis saccharated iron oxide was suspended and she was started on deferoxamine 4 mg/kg/week (intravenous infusion in the end of dialysis session) for 6 weeks. Skin lesions disappeared and laboratorial revaluation showed haemoglobin of 98 g/L, transferrin saturation of 16%, and ferritin of 140 µg/L.

During the subsequent months, a progressive drop in haemoglobin levels was registered, despite augmentation of epoetin dose to 600 U/kg/week. She became symptomatic with fatigue; her haemoglobin was 77 g/L, transferrin saturation was 6%, and ferritin was 16 µg/L. A red blood cell transfusion was administered and despite the transitory response repeated transfusions were needed. After one year, it was decided to restart Generis saccharated oxide iron 50 mg/week; however, skin lesions returned with the previous pattern. Generis saccharated oxide iron was suspended, resulting in skin lesion remission and as her anaemia became symptomatic, the patient maintained the need for regular red blood cell transfusions. This prompted the medical team to search for alternative iron therapies in order to avoid the need for repeated red blood cell transfusions and surpass the recurrent lesions which appeared to be linked to the use of saccharated oxide iron. Ferric carboxymaltose was administered in a dose of 500 mg and the patient tolerated this treatment with no skin lesions, ferritin elevation to 49 µg/L, and increased response to epoetin. No more red blood cell transfusions were required. The administration of ferric carboxymaltose was repeated after two months with good results. The patient is now medicated with 120 U/kg/week epoetin, has haemoglobin of 114 g/L, and has started HCV treatment with direct acting antivirals.

3. Discussion

Deficiency or altered activity of enzymes responsible for heme biosynthetic pathway leads to a group of diseases nominated porphyrias. Clinical manifestations are predominantly visceral or cutaneous, depending on the affected enzyme and what step of the pathway is compromised, resulting in both the accumulation of some certain porphyrins and the deficit of others. The most common of these rare disorders is porphyria cutanea tarda (PCT) caused by an activity deficit of the fifth enzyme in the heme synthetic pathway uroporphyrinogen decarboxylase (UROD) [4]. Genetic factors can contribute to increased susceptibility, namely, heterozygosity for UROD mutation, reducing activity to 50% of normal activity, or hemochromatosis mutations, increasing iron absorption. Acquired factors are well known such as alcohol, smoking, oestrogen, human immunodeficiency virus, hepatitis C virus, and secondary causes of iron overload. The precise mechanism by which HCV infection might cause or act as a trigger for PCT in predisposed subjects is not known but is thought to be related to alterations in iron metabolism [5]. Patients on haemodialysis may be prone to PCT by their occasional exposure to iron overload states through intravenous iron, blood transfusions, and the accumulation of porphyrins not totally removed by the dialytic technique [6].

The diagnosis of PCT implies dermatologic manifestations such as itching and painful skin lesions, chronic photosensitivity with blisters, bullae, scarring, increased skin fragility, and hyper-hypopigmentation, affecting sun-exposed areas, hirsutism, and alopecia. It also implies increased plasma or urine porphyrins formed before the UROD step such as uroporphyrin, heptacarboxylporphyrin, hexacarboxylporphyrin, and pentacarboxylporphyrin (urine analysis not validated for patients with end-stage renal disease (ESRD)) with concomitant normal levels of coproporphyrins [7].

The first-line treatment for PCT is phlebotomy with removal of 450 mL every two weeks and low-dose hydroxychloroquine along with identifying and minimising predisponent factors present in each patient and skin protection from sunlight until porphyrin levels have normalised [8]. Unfortunately, patients with ESRD present specificities that make treatment a true challenge. Not only is hydroxychloroquine contraindicated in ESRD, but also phlebotomies are normally not tolerated in already anaemia-prone patients as well as in patients with poor venous access. Iron-chelating agents are less efficient in removing iron than phlebotomy [9] but have been proposed as an option in ESRD with anaemia.

The administration of iron-chelating agents, namely, deferoxamine, for the treatment of PCT allowed remission in our patient, although our patient did not have a very high ferritin concentration, corroborating the hypothesis of this drug being a good option for patients with ESRD and anaemia.

The consequent ferropenic status after the treatment with deferoxamine contributed to the refractory anaemia developed by the patient afterwards and she became symptomatic. On one hand, red blood cell transfusions contain not only young but also old erythrocytes, meaning that a considerable portion of them will be caught by the spleen in a short time after transfusion and the erythrocytes' catabolism will result in production of porphyrins, which is not obviously desirable in a patient suffering of PCT. On the other hand, in a patient with ESRD, ferropenic status, and symptomatic anaemia under already maximized erythropoiesis-stimulating agent therapy and with known association of trigger of PCT with previous iron administration, we considered red blood cell transfusion as an appropriate therapy on that moment.

In an attempt to end with the dependency of red blood cell transfusions, saccharated oxide iron was reintroduced and resulted in relapse of PCT. The suspension of saccharated oxide iron was sufficient to achieve remission; however, the ferropenic state contributed considerably to dependence on red blood cell transfusions, leading the authors to try a different approach and to administer ferric carboxymaltose with success. Although the rationale for ferric carboxymaltose not precipitating PCT relapse is not fully understood, the answer is certainly related to the fact that different iron carbohydrate complexes have different pharmacokinetic/pharmacodynamic characteristics and specific reactivities. The success of this case may be related to the fact that, compared to saccharated ferric oxide, ferric carboxymaltose is a more stable, large sized complex formulated as a colloidal solution with physiological pH and therefore releases less amounts of iron at a time over a long period of time [10], which might result in less saturation of the heme pathway with less accumulation of porphyrins and is therefore not enough to trigger PCT manifestations. Studies are necessary to validate this hypothesis.

4. Conclusion

Deferoxamine is an efficient treatment for porphyria cutanea tarda in end-stage renal disease patients. Furthermore, ferric carboxymaltose may be a valuable option for refractory anaemia in these patients, as it seems to provide iron without clinical relapse of the disease conversely to other iron formulations. However, studies are necessary to validate this hypothesis.

References

[1] O. Lupi, L. Rezende, M. Zangrando et al., "Cutaneous manifestations in end-stage renal disease," *Anais Brasileiros de Dermatologia*, vol. 86, no. 2, pp. 319–326, 2011.

[2] P. Vasconcelos, H. Luz-Rodrigues, C. Santos, and P. Filipe, "Desferrioxamine treatment of porphyria cutanea tarda in a patient with HIV and chronic renal failure," *Dermatologic Therapy*, vol. 27, no. 1, pp. 16–18, 2014.

[3] J. P. Gisbert, L. García-Buey, J. M. Pajares, and R. Moreno-Otero, "Prevalence of hepatitis C virus infection in porphyria cutanea tarda: systematic review and meta-analysis," *Journal of Hepatology*, vol. 39, no. 4, pp. 620–627, 2003.

[4] C. Badenas, J. To-Figueras, J. D. Phillips, C. A. Warby, C. Muñoz, and C. Herrero, "Identification and characterization of novel uroporphyrinogen decarboxylase gene mutations in a large series of porphyria cutanea tarda patients and relatives," *Clinical Genetics*, vol. 75, no. 4, pp. 346–353, 2009.

[5] K. Miura, K. Taura, Y. Kodama, B. Schnabl, and D. A. Brenner, "Hepatitis C virus-induced oxidative stress suppresses hepcidin

expression through increased histone deacetylase activity," *Hepatology*, vol. 48, no. 5, pp. 1420–1429, 2008.

[6] S. Seubert, A. Seubert, K. W. Rumpf, and H. Kiffe, "A porphyria cutanea tarda-like distribution pattern of porphyrins in plasma, hemodialysate, hemofiltrate, and urine of patients on chronic hemodialysis," *Journal of Investigative Dermatology*, vol. 85, no. 2, pp. 107–109, 1985.

[7] A. C. Deacon and G. H. Elder, "ACP Best Practice No 165: front line tests for the investigation of suspected porphyria," *Journal of Clinical Pathology*, vol. 54, no. 7, pp. 500–507, 2001.

[8] A. K. Singal, C. Kormos-Hallberg, C. Lee et al., "Low-dose hydroxychloroquine is as effective as phlebotomy in treatment of patients with porphyria cutanea tarda," *Clinical Gastroenterology and Hepatology*, vol. 10, no. 12, pp. 1402–1409, 2012.

[9] E. Rocchi, P. Gibertini, M. Cassanelli et al., "Iron removal therapy in porphyria cutanea tarda: phlebotomy versus slow subcutaneous desferrioxamine infusion," *British Journal of Dermatology*, vol. 114, no. 5, pp. 621–629, 1986.

[10] P. Geisser and S. Burckhardt, "The pharmacokinetics and pharmacodynamics of iron preparations," *Pharmaceutics*, vol. 3, no. 1, pp. 12–33, 2011.

Extended Peritoneal Dialysis and Renal Recovery in HIV-Infected Patients with Prolonged AKI: A Report of 2 Cases

Donlawat Saengpanit,[1] Pongpratch Puapatanakul,[1] Piyaporn Towannang,[2] and Talerngsak Kanjanabuch[1,2,3]

[1]Division of Nephrology, Department of Medicine, Faculty of Medicine, Chulalongkorn University, Bangkok, Thailand
[2]CAPD Excellent Center, King Chulalongkorn Memorial Hospital, Bangkok, Thailand
[3]Kidney and Metabolic Research Unit, Department of Medicine, Faculty of Medicine, Chulalongkorn University, Bangkok, Thailand

Correspondence should be addressed to Talerngsak Kanjanabuch; golfnephro@hotmail.com

Academic Editor: Yoshihide Fujigaki

Peritoneal dialysis (PD) has recently been established as a treatment option for renal replacement therapy (RRT) in patients with acute kidney injury (AKI). Its efficacy in providing fluid and small solute removal has also been demonstrated in clinical trials and is equivalent to hemodialysis (HD). However, effect of RRT modality on renal recovery after AKI remains a controversy. Moreover, the setting of human immunodeficiency virus- (HIV-) infected patients with AKI requiring RRT makes the decision on RRT initiation and modality selection more complicated. The authors report here 2 cases of HIV-infected patients presenting with severe AKI requiring protracted course of acute RRT. PD had been performed uneventfully in both cases for 4–9 months before partial renal recovery occurred. Both patients eventually became dialysis independent but were left in chronic kidney disease (CKD) stage 4. These cases highlight the example of renal recovery even after a prolonged course of dialysis dependence. Thus, PD might be a suitable option for HIV patients with protracted AKI.

1. Introduction

Acute kidney injury (AKI) has been increasingly recognized in human immunodeficiency virus- (HIV-) infected patients and associated with poor outcomes [1]. The management of the HIV-infected patients with AKI requires meticulous attention to the control of fluid status, electrolytes, acid-base balance, and uremic toxin removal, in a similar manner as in those without HIV infection. Peritoneal dialysis (PD) is an overlooked modality of renal replacement therapy (RRT) for AKI as it is mainly considered in patients with end-stage renal disease (ESRD) [2]. However, acute PD remains a viable treatment option for selected cases of HIV-infected patients with AKI, especially in those who are hemodynamically unstable, having severe bleeding disorders, or when other modalities are unavailable [3]. PD has several advantages as an RRT in AKI patients including wide availability, ease of performance, nonvascular access placement, ability to remove large amounts of fluid in hemodynamically unstable patients, gradual but effective correction of acid-base and electrolyte imbalance, no need for anticoagulation, and high biocompatibility [3]. Above all, PD provides better preservation of residual kidney function (RKF) compared to hemodialysis (HD) in ESRD patients [4]. In those patients with potentially reversible etiology of AKI, treatment with PD may also have a higher likelihood of recovery of endogenous renal function [5].

We presented 2 cases of HIV-infected patients with severe AKI requiring acute RRT in which PD had been undertaken uneventfully. A few months later, recovery of renal function followed and PD was discontinued safely.

2. Case Report

2.1. Case 1. A 49-year-old Dutch male patient came to King Chulalongkorn Memorial Hospital (KCMH) with a complaint of low-grade fever and profuse sweating at night for 1 week. Three weeks earlier, he was diagnosed HIV infection when antiretroviral medications comprising of tenofovir, emtricitabine, and efavirenz were prescribed. He denied taking any over-the-counter drugs. The physical examination was unremarkable except for a body temperature of 38°C. He also had normotension (blood pressure 125/75 mmHg) without orthostatic hypotension or other signs of volume depletion. The chest X-ray showed miliary pulmonary nodules compatible with miliary tuberculosis which was later confirmed by positive polymerase-chain-reaction for *Mycobacterium tuberculosis* in his sputum. Disseminated tuberculosis was promptly diagnosed, and antituberculosis treatment (isoniazid, rifampicin, pyrazinamide, and ethambutol) was planned. However, he also had severe azotemia at admission (BUN 53.6 mmol/L, Cr 1,230 μmol/L) in contrast to his baseline values from one month earlier (Cr 115 μmol/L). At that time, there were no evidences of uremic symptoms or volume overload, and he still voided 500 mL of urine per day. Urinalysis revealed isosthenuria with bland urinary sediments (specific gravity 1.010, pH 5.0, albuminuria trace, glycose negative, WBC 0–1/hpf, and RBC 0–1/hpf). Renal ultrasonography demonstrated normal size and contour of both kidneys. Urine biomarker for renal tubular injury, neutrophil gelatinase-associated lipocalin (NGAL), was markedly elevated (7,891 ng/mL). Acute kidney injury was diagnosed and likely caused by nephrotoxic acute tubular necrosis (ATN) even though a renal biopsy had not been done. In the absence of other offending drugs or conditions, tenofovir was suspected to be a causal drug for ATN resulting in an adjustment of the antiretroviral regimen (abacavir, lamivudine, and raltegravir).

In the absence of uremic symptom or volume overload, PD was, nevertheless, initiated due to high level of nitrogen catabolites. The flexible double-cuffed PD catheter was inserted on day 4 of admission, and automated PD (Homechoice cycler®; Baxter) using a total dialysate (Dianeal®; Baxter) volume of 10 L (initial fill volume of 700 mL, 14 cycles, 20 hours) was promptly started on the same day of the catheter insertion. PD dose was gradually increased to achieve the total dialysate volume of 20 L per day in the next few days. The delivered dose of PD by total weekly Kt/V and total weekly creatinine clearance (CCr) were 3.23 and 97.84 L/week, respectively. After a week of automated PD, nitrogen catabolites decreased gradually (BUN 27.8 mmol/L, Cr 840 μmol/L). At one month, his urine volume had increased to 1 L per day, but measured renal CCr was still at 4 mL/min/1.73 m^2 which reflected inadequate recovery of renal function. He was discharged on day 31 of admission with continuation of automated PD at a total dialysate volume of 10 L per day. At follow-up visit, the patient showed gradually improvement in renal function and the dose of PD was tapered accordingly. Eventually, PD could be discontinued at 4 months after the onset of AKI. The patient attained stable serum Cr of 124 μmol/L and measured CCr of 29 mL/min/1.73 m^2 afterwards.

2.2. Case 2.
A 58-year-old Thai female patient with hypertension, hyperlipidemia, and type 2 diabetes mellitus was infected with HIV 1.5 years ago. She had been taking antiretroviral drugs including tenofovir, emtricitabine, and boosted darunavir thereafter and achieved virological control after 6 months of therapy. Her CD4-positive T-lymphocyte count was 532/mm^3 (40%). Her other medications were amlodipine 5 mg/day, enalapril 10 mg/day, fenofibrate 300 mg/day, and metformin 500 mg/day. She gradually developed anorexia, nausea, and fatigue over two weeks' duration. She also noticed a decrease in her daily urine volume and new-onset nocturia together with swelling in both of her legs particularly in the evening. She reported no fever, rash, or joint pain. She denied taking over-the-counter medication or nonsteroidal anti-inflammatory drugs. On examination, she was alert and had normal vital signs except for mild hypertension (body temperature 37.0°C, pulse rate 70/min, respiratory rate 16/min, and blood pressure 140/70 mmHg). She also had mildly pale conjunctivae and pitting edema in both of her legs. Laboratory tests showed severe azotemia (BUN 21.4 mmol/L, Cr 1,370 μmol/L) compared to baselines labs 1 month earlier (Cr 124 μmol/L). She also had hyponatremia, hypokalemia, metabolic acidosis, and elevated muscle enzyme (sodium 127 mEq/L, potassium 5.5 mEq/L, chloride 94 mEq/L, bicarbonate 10 mEq/L, and creatine phosphokinase 1,904 U/L; normal value 22–165 U/L). Urinalysis revealed isosthenuria, albuminuria, leukocyturia, and microhematuria without dysmorphic RBC (specific gravity 1.010, proteinuria 2+, glucose negative, WBC 3–5/hpf, and RBC 20–30/hpf). Renal ultrasonography demonstrated normal size but mildly increased parenchymal echogenicity of both kidneys without hydroureter or hydronephrosis. AKI was diagnosed. Differential diagnoses of AKI included tenofovir-induced ATN, HIV-associated nephropathy/immune complex glomerulonephritis, and rhabdomyolysis.

RRT was initiated soon after admission due to uremia and volume overload. After successful insertion of flexible double-cuff PD catheter, automated PD (Homechoice cycler; Baxter) using total dialysate (Dianeal; Baxter) volume of 10 L was started (fill volume of 2 L, five cycles, therapy time 12 hours) on the first day of admission resulting in adequate control of fluid, electrolytes, and acid-base balance. The doses of PD by total weekly Kt/V and total weekly CCr were 3.63 and 91.94 L/week, respectively. Renal biopsy was later performed revealing evidence of acute granulomatous interstitial nephritis (AIN) and ATN without evidence of glomerular or vascular injury. Antiretroviral drugs-induced ATN/AIN was diagnosed. The attending physician then switched antiretroviral regimen to stavudine/lamivudine/boosted darunavir regimen. During fourth week of admission, her urine volume had increased to 0.8–1.0 L per day but the measured renal CCr was still low (6.62 mL/min/1.73 m^2). She was discharged from the hospital anyway and was prescribed to continue automated PD during night time at home (night intermittent PD; NIPD) at a similar dose (fill volume of 2 L, five cycles, therapy time 12 hours). Eventually, PD was successfully discontinued 9 months after the onset of AKI in August 2014. At that time, her serum Cr was 159 μmol/L, and measured renal CCr was stable at 17.3 mL/min/1.73 m^2 with daily urine volume of 2,480 mL. Afterwards, she remained in chronic kidney disease (CKD) stage 4 with stable renal function for another whole year.

3. Discussion

AKI has been demonstrated to occur at a 2 to 3 times higher incidence in hospitalized HIV-infected patients compared to those without HIV infection and is associated with poor long-term outcomes, including increased risk of cardiovascular events, ESRD, and mortality [1]. The common causes of AKI in HIV-infected patients are volume depletion, septicemia, and nephrotoxic medications [6]. In cases where RRT is warranted, acute PD has been established as a viable option for selected patients, particularly those who are hemodynamically unstable and have severe coagulation defects, or when other modalities are not readily available [2]. Moreover, performing PD in HIV-infected patients reduces exposure of healthcare workers to contaminated blood and needle, putting them at a lower risk of acquiring the infection. As for patients' outcomes, PD has been shown to provide better preservation of residual kidney function (RKF) in long-term dialysis patients compared to HD [4]. In AKI setting, the outcomes of patients including survival and metabolic control were comparable between daily intermittent HD and PD using high volume prescription (36–44 L of dialysate per day) [5].

Renal recovery after AKI in HIV-infected patients has not been well-described. In a large cohort of 489 hospitalized HIV-infected patients, in which 18% developed AKI, renal recovery occurred in 67.2%, and rate of recovery decreased with increasing severity of AKI according to "Risk Injury Failure Loss of kidney function End-stage kidney disease" (RIFLE) criteria (Risk, 85.2%; Injury 61.9%; Failure, 43.8%) [7]. Time to renal recovery of AKI in HIV-infected is also rarely described. Generally, renal recovery in AKI, especially in cases of ATN, usually occurs within an average of 1–3 weeks. However, on a rare occasion, it may take up to several months for kidney to recover, mostly dependent on severity and duration of the insulting causes of ATN [8]. There is conflicting evidence whether PD helps renal recovery in a patient with AKI. One randomised controlled trial in Brazil comparing high volume PD and daily intermittent HD in AKI patients showed similar rate of recovery in both groups (28% versus 26%; $p = 0.84$) but patients undergoing PD had shorter time to renal recovery (7.2 ± 2.6 days versus 10.6 ± 4.7 days; $p = 0.04$) [5]. On the other hand, in another randomised controlled trial comparing high volume PD and extended HD (duration 6–8 hours per session, 6 times per week) in 143 critically ill patients with ATN, rate of renal recovery and time to recovery were similar in two groups [9]. Whether PD has better effect on renal recovery compared to HD remained controversial.

Many possible mechanisms may account for the better preservation of RKF in PD and may involve in renal recovery after an episode of AKI. For example, abrupt fluctuation in volume and osmotic load are fewer in PD patients, so their hemodynamic status during dialysis is more stable than HD. This may be associated with more stable glomerular capillary pressure and more constant glomerular filtration. An episode of renal ischemia caused by rapid fluctuation of osmolality and contraction of the circulatory volume is more frequent during HD than PD. Mild overhydration of some patients on PD may contribute to better RKF preservation. The membrane used in hemodialysers is less biocompatible than the peritoneal membrane, leading to rapid loss of RKF caused by repeated exposure to inflammatory mediators such as IL-1 that generated by the extracorporeal circulation [10].

Our patients presented with severe nonoliguric AKI caused by ATN/AIN both of which underwent PD as an RRT modality. Despite early discontinuation of the offending drugs that were suspected to be the cause of AKI, together with the use of PD, both patients showed rather slow recovery of renal function and remained dialysis-dependent after being discharged from the hospital for a few months. Since there were no repeated hemodynamic collapse, infective complications, or other episodes of AKI, the delayed renal recovery in these patients was likely contributed by severity of the AKI itself. In this scenario of AKI with late renal recovery requiring extended RRT, there is no data whether HD or PD will have superior benefit. Technically, PD put patients at a lower risk of hemodynamic instability as the fluid and metabolites removal occurs slowly, and with no need for using hemodialyser membrane as in HD, performing PD has less inflammation due to bioincompatibility, both of which may promote recovery of renal function. Both of our cases finally attained partial recovery of renal function and became dialysis independent. However, some kidney damage remained, putting them in CKD status. Finally, choosing PD for acute RRT may help decrease financial burden of healthcare systems especially in cases of prolonged AKI as in our cases.

4. Conclusion

AKI is common in HIV-infected patients and associated with poor outcomes. Performing PD in HIV-infected patients with AKI provides not only similar efficacy in fluid and metabolic control as other extracorporeal treatments, but also potentially superior ability to increase the likelihood of renal recovery, particularly in those with prolonged course requiring extended RRT. Moreover, PD in HIV-infected patients lowers exposure of healthcare worker to contaminated blood and decreases financial burden of healthcare systems especially in cases of delayed recovery. In summary, PD possesses several advantages and is a suitable RRT option for HIV-infected patients presenting with AKI.

Acknowledgments

The authors thank all PD nurses, technicians, and staff in the Department of Medicine, Faculty of Medicine, Chulalongkorn University and King Chulalongkorn Memorial Hospital, for their contributions. This report was supported by (1) Rachadaphiseksompot Endorcement Fund (GCURS_59_12_30_03), Chulalongkorn University, Thailand, (2) the National Research Council of Thailand (2558-113), and (3) the Thailand Research Foundation (IRG5780017).

References

[1] A. I. Choi, Y. Li, C. Parikh, P. A. Volberding, and M. G. Shlipak, "Long-term clinical consequences of acute kidney injury in the HIV-infected," *Kidney International*, vol. 78, no. 5, pp. 478–485, 2010.

[2] B. Cullis, M. Abdelraheem, and G. Abrahams, "Peritoneal dialysis for acute kidney injury," *Peritoneal Dialysis International*, vol. 34, no. 5, pp. 494–517, 2014.

[3] D. Ponce, M. Gobo-Oliveira, and A. L. Balbi, "Peritoneal dialysis treatment modality option in acute kidney injury," *Blood Purification*, vol. 43, no. 1-3, pp. 173–178, 2017.

[4] P. Tam, "Peritoneal dialysis and preservation of residual renal function," *Peritoneal Dialysis International*, vol. 29, supplement 2, pp. S108–S1010, 2009.

[5] D. P. Gabriel, J. T. Caramori, L. C. Martim, P. Barretti, and A. L. Balbi, "High volume peritoneal dialysis vs daily hemodialysis: a randomized, controlled trial in patients with acute kidney injury.," *Kidney international. Supplement*, no. 108, pp. S87–93, 2008.

[6] S. Kalim, L. A. Szczech, and C. M. Wyatt, "Acute kidney injury in HIV-infected patients," *Seminars in Nephrology*, vol. 28, no. 6, pp. 556–562, 2008.

[7] J. A. Lopes, M. J. Melo, A. Viegas, M. Raimundo, I. Câmara, F. Antunes et al., "Acute kidney injury in hospitalized HIV-infected patients: a cohort analysis," *Nephrology Dialysis Transplantation*, vol. 26, no. 12, pp. 3888–3894, 2011.

[8] S. Huraib, W. Al Khudair, G. Al Ghamdi, and A. Iqbal, "Post transplant acute tubular necrosis - how long you can wait?: a case report," *Saudi Journal of Kidney Diseases and Transplantation*, vol. 13, no. 1, pp. 50–54, 2002.

[9] D. Ponce, M. N. Berbel, J. M. G. Abrão, C. R. Goes, and A. L. Balbi, "A randomized clinical trial of high volume peritoneal dialysis versus extended daily hemodialysis for acute kidney injury patients," *International Urology and Nephrology*, vol. 45, no. 3, pp. 869–878, 2013.

[10] S. M. Lang, A. Bergner, M. Topfer, and H. Schiffl, "Preservation of residual renal function in dialysis patients: effects of dialysis-technique-related factors," *Peritoneal Dialysis International*, vol. 21, no. 1, pp. 52–57, 2002.

Discontinuation of Hemodialysis in a Patient with Anti-GBM Disease by the Treatment with Corticosteroids and Plasmapheresis despite Several Predictors for Dialysis-Dependence

Yoshihide Fujigaki,[1,2] Chikayuki Morimoto,[1] Risa Iino,[1] Kei Taniguchi,[1] Yosuke Kawamorita,[1] Shinichiro Asakawa,[1] Daigo Toyoki,[1] Shinako Miyano,[1] Wataru Fujii,[1] Tatsuru Ota,[1] Shigeru Shibata,[1] and Shunya Uchida[1]

[1]Department of Internal Medicine, Teikyo University School of Medicine, Itabashi-ku, Tokyo, Japan
[2]Central Laboratory, Teikyo University School of Medicine, Itabashi-ku, Tokyo, Japan

Correspondence should be addressed to Yoshihide Fujigaki; fujigakiyoshihide@gmail.com

Academic Editor: Kouichi Hirayama

A 26-year-old man highly suspected of having antiglomerular basement membrane (GBM) disease was treated with corticosteroid pulse therapy 9 days after initial infection-like symptoms with high procalcitonin value. The patient required hemodialysis the next day of the treatment due to oliguria. In addition to corticosteroid therapy, plasmapheresis was introduced and the patient could discontinue hemodialysis 43 days after the treatment. Kidney biopsy after initiation of hemodialysis confirmed anti-GBM disease with 86.3% crescent formation. Physician should keep in mind that active anti-GBM disease shows even high procalcitonin value in the absence of infection. To pursue recovery of renal function, the challenge of the immediate and persistent treatment with high-dose corticosteroids plus plasmapheresis for highly suspected anti-GBM disease is vitally important despite the presence of reported predictors for dialysis-dependence including oliguria and requiring hemodialysis at presentation.

1. Introduction

Antiglomerular basement membrane (GBM) disease is rare condition usually with rapidly progressive glomerulonephritis (RPGN) and is known as Goodpasture's syndrome when it combines with pulmonary hemorrhage [1]. All patients with anti-GBM disease have circulating and deposited anti-GBM antibody. An early aggressive immunosuppressive treatment to inhibit production of anti-GBM antibody and/or attenuating the antibody-mediated glomerular inflammation and plasmapheresis to reduce or remove anti-GBM antibody are necessary [2, 3], as a recovery of renal function rarely occurs in patients with advanced stage where predictors of dialysis-dependence such as oliguria, requiring hemodialysis and high percentage of crescent formation, were seen [4–6]. However, the patients with anti-GBM disease with severe renal dysfunction are immunocompromised and often show fever, positive C-reactive protein (CRP), and positive procalcitonin (PCT) [7, 8] as an indicator of infection. These factors usually become an obstacle in an early aggressive immunosuppressive therapy.

We present a patient with anti-GBM disease who showed high PCT value and all reported predictors for dialysis-dependence but could discontinue hemodialysis by introducing immunosuppressive therapy plus plasmapheresis. In this case, we add some personal opinions to the recommendation for anti-GBM disease in Kidney Disease Improving Global Outcomes (KDIGO) clinical practice guideline for glomerulonephritis [9].

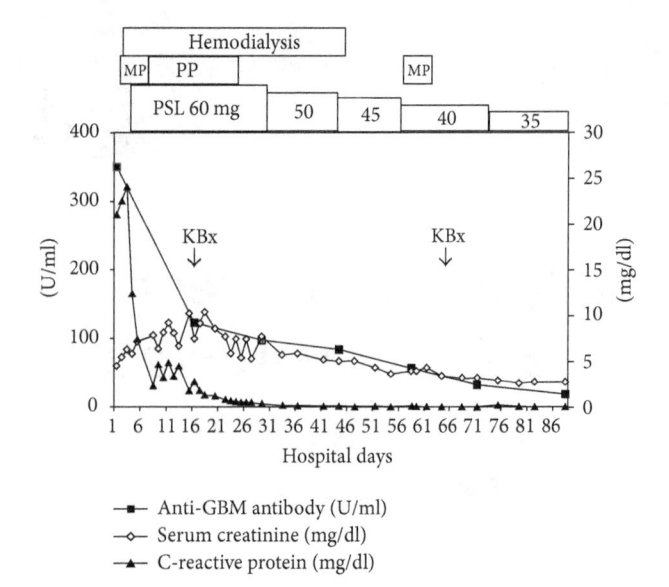

FIGURE 1: Clinical course. MP, methylprednisolone pulse therapy (1 g per day for 3 successive days); PP, plasmapheresis 7 times; PSL, prednisolone; KBx, kidney biopsy.

2. Clinical Presentation

A 26-year-old Japanese man visited a clinic complaining about fever and coral-colored urine 7 days previously. Antihypertensive drug and antibiotics were prescribed for high blood pressure and suspected urinary tract infection, respectively. He was admitted to local hospital 4 days previously because of high fever, general fatigue, nausea, abnormal urinalysis (2+ protein and 3+ occult blood), renal dysfunction (serum creatinine (SCr) of 1.66 mg/dl), and C-reactive protein (CRP) of 15 mg/dl. Since SCr was further increased to 3.39 mg/dl, he was transferred to our hospital.

On admission, he showed body temperature of 37.9°C, blood pressure of 142/84 mmHg, pulse rate of 101/minute, and SpO_2 of 98% and no other abnormal physical examination. He had no smoking and past medical history. Anti-GBM antibody examined in the previous hospital was reported to be positive. Laboratory examination showed proteinuria, hematuria, SCr of 4.49 mg/dl, CRP of 21.04 mg/dl, PCT of 0.62 ng/dl (normal range < 0.05), normocomplementemia, and anti-GBM antibody of 350.0 U/ml (normal range < 3). Myeloperoxidase- and proteinase 3-antineutrophil cytoplasmic antibodies, other autoantibodies, and cryoglobulin were negative. Chest X-ray did not show pulmonary hemorrhage. He was diagnosed as RPGN most likely due to anti-GBM disease. He was given antibiotics after hospitalization for 1 week because both CRP and PCT were high with fever, but he had no apparent focus of infection.

Clinical course after admission was shown in Figure 1. The patient was treated with methylprednisolone pulse therapy (1 g per day for 3 successive days) from 2nd day after admission and then with oral prednisolone 60 mg/day. Coral-color urine and high-grade fever disappeared at 3rd day. However, he was introduced to hemodialysis at 3rd day because of oliguria, further increased SCr of 6.3 mg/dl, severe metabolic acidosis, and hyperkalemia. Plasmapheresis (3,840 ml of plasma with fresh frozen plasma of 32 units as the substitution) through the polyethylene plasma separator OP-05W (Asahi Kasei Medical, Co., Ltd., Tokyo, Japan) began from 5th day seven times.

Kidney biopsy at 16th day showed cellular or fibrocellular crescents with or without necrotic glomerular capillary walls in 19 of 22 glomeruli (86.3%) (Figure 2(a)). There were diffuse inflammatory cell infiltration, patchy tubular injury, and mild fibrosis in the tubulointerstitial areas (Figure 2(a)). Immunofluorescence for IgG showed 2+ linear staining along the glomerular capillary walls (Figure 2(b)). The findings confirmed anti-GBM disease.

Blood pressure during the hemodialysis period was around 150/80 mmHg using doxazosin mesilate. Under high-dose prednisolone urine volume began to increase at 30th day and he could discontinue hemodialysis at 44th day. Methylprednisolone pulse therapy was added (1 g per day for 3 successive days) from 57th day because of the presence of active urinalysis and anti-GBM antibody of 56.6 U/ml. The second kidney biopsy at 65th day revealed 16 glomeruli with global sclerosis and 7 glomeruli with fibrous crescents out of 24 glomeruli and diffuse tubulointerstitial fibrosis with mononuclear cell infiltration and tubular atrophy (Figure 2(c)), indicating no active glomerular lesions. Prednisolone was tapered to 35 mg/day and he was discharged with SCr of 2.74 mg/dl and anti-GBM antibody of 18.2 U/ml at 88th day.

After the discharge, blood pressure had been controlled at around 140/80 mmHg with doxazosin mesilate and nifedipine. 1.0 to 1.5 g/gCr of proteinuria and mild degree of hematuria persisted. Estimated glomerular filtration rate (eGFR) was stable at about 25 ml/min/1.73 m^2 for 4 months after the discharge. However, eGFR began to decrease after that and anti-GBM antibody titer slightly rose; thus methylprednisolone pulse therapy was performed again. Anti-GBM antibody became negative at the dose of 30 mg/day of prednisolone, which was further tapered. The patient did not have any side effects during the immunosuppressive therapy. However, eGFR decline slope was almost constant without additional factors triggering GFR decline and hemodialysis was introduced again 15 months after his discharge.

3. Discussion

In anti-GBM disease, the early, aggressive immunosuppressive therapy and plasmapheresis before progression of severe glomerular damage are essential for recovery of renal function [1]. However, there are some factors that cause delaying the treatment. One is the differentiation of infection from active anti-GBM disease and another is a presence of predictors for dialysis-dependence. As for the former factor, it is reported that the majority of patients at presentation had fever with respiratory tract infections, which needs further investigation to reveal their pathophysiological role in anti-GBM disease [10]. However, it is noteworthy that elevation of PCT, which is thought to be indicator for infection, together with elevation of CRP is often seen in patients with anti-GBM disease in the absence of infection [8] like in patients with

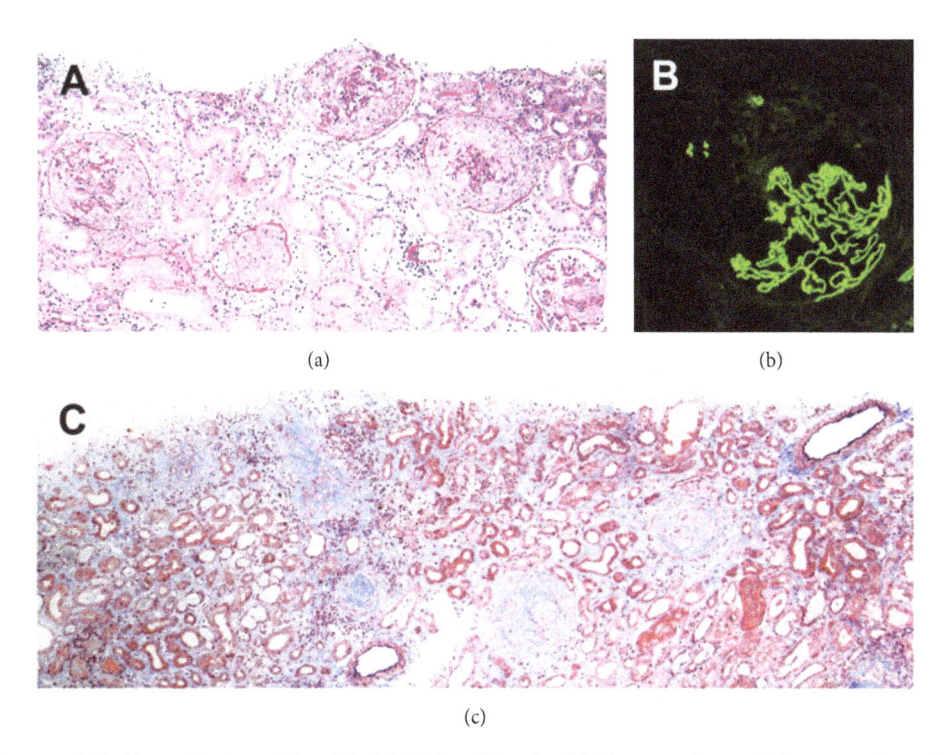

FIGURE 2: Light microscopic findings of 1st (a and b) and 2nd (c) kidney biopsies. (a) There are glomeruli demonstrating cellular or fibrocellular crescents with or without focal segmental necrosis and diffuse inflammatory cell infiltration, patchy tubular injury, and mild fibrosis in the tubulointerstitial areas (PAS staining, ×200). (b) Immunofluorescent staining for IgG shows linear staining along with glomerular capillary walls, ×400. (c) There are globally sclerotic glomeruli and diffuse tubulointerstitial fibrosis with mononuclear cell infiltration and tubular atrophy (Elastica-Masson staining, ×200).

other autoimmune diseases [7]. The mechanisms of elevation of PCT are not well known, but it is suggested that high PCT values in Goodpasture's syndrome might rather reflect severe organ damage of lungs and/or kidneys compared to infection [8]. Thus, physicians can start immunosuppressive therapy immediately after screening of the infection. On the other hand, it is reported that predictors for dialysis-dependence in anti-GBM disease include level of SCr ≥ 600 μmol/L, oliguria, requiring dialysis at presentation, and more than 80–100% of crescent formation [5, 6, 11–13]. Levy et al. [5] reported that, among anti-GBM disease patients treated with immunosuppressants and plasma exchange, patients presenting dialysis-dependence showed only 8% renal survival at 1 year. The aggressive therapy might bring just the increased risk of immunosuppression compared to the likelihood of benefit to the patients with these predictors but without pulmonary hemorrhage. It is also reported that anti-GBM antibody titer could decrease spontaneously with time after introducing dialysis [13] and relapse of anti-GBM disease is rare [1]. KDIGO clinical practice guideline for glomerulonephritis [9] stated that "we recommend initiating immunosuppression with cyclophosphamide and corticosteroids plus plasmapheresis in all patients with anti-GBM glomerulonephritis except those who are dialysis-dependent at presentation and have 100% crescents in an adequate biopsy sample, and do not have pulmonary hemorrhage" and that "start treatment for anti-GBM glomerulonephritis without delay once the diagnosis is confirmed. If the diagnosis is highly suspected, it would be appropriate to begin high-dose corticosteroids and plasmapheresis while waiting for confirmation."

KDIGO guideline does not recommend aggressive therapy to the patients who are dialysis-dependent at presentation. However, in accordance with this guideline half of the patients will not receive immunosuppressive therapy plus plasmapheresis because approximately half of the patients require hemodialysis at the point of initial presentation in large series [5]. Our patient could discontinue hemodialysis despite having all the reported predictors for dialysis-dependence in anti-GBM disease. Kidney biopsy for definitive diagnosis of anti-GBM disease has a potential risk for hemorrhage, which causes difficulty and delay to initiate hemodialysis when necessary. Therefore, to not miss the therapeutic windows, it is worth challenging the treatment with high-dose corticosteroids plus plasmapheresis immediately after screening of the infection before kidney biopsy irrespective of any predictors for dialysis-dependence if the diagnosis of anti-GBM disease is highly suspected.

The effectiveness of plasmapheresis for improving renal function in anti-GBM disease has been reported [14, 15]. Johnson et al. demonstrated a much more rapid fall in circulating anti-GBM antibodies and improved kidney function in patients receiving plasmapheresis when compared with immunosuppressant alone [14]. Plasma exchange of 4 L of plasma for 5% albumin was commonly performed daily for 14 days or until the circulating anti-GBM antibodies were

TABLE 1: The immunofluorescent findings of 1st and 2nd kidney biopsies.

	IgA	IgG	IgM	C1q	C3	κ	λ	IgG1	IgG2	IgG3	IgG4
1st	−	++	−	−	±	+	++	++	−	−	−
2nd	−	++	−	−	±	++	−	++	−	−	−

κ: light chain κ; λ: light chain λ; −: negative; ±: faint staining; +: weak staining in a linear pattern; ++: strong staining in a linear pattern. The tubular basement membrane was negative for all immunoreactants examined.

no longer detected [16]. We used fresh frozen plasma as the substitution for plasma for fear of pulmonary hemorrhage. Due to the limitation of medical insurance in Japan, plasmapheresis could not be performed in our patient until anti-GBM antibody disappeared. Double-filtration plasmapheresis for selectively removing the immunoglobulin fraction from serum [17] combined with immunosuppressive therapy was reported to be effective and a good removal efficacy of anti-GBM antibody in one case with Goodpasture's syndrome [18]. Small series using immunoadsorption for the removal of pathogenic autoantibody in anti-GBM disease [19] documented comparable outcomes when compared with plasma exchange therapy [20, 21].

The 2nd kidney biopsy showed the progression of irreversible glomerular damage 7 weeks after the therapy. The difference of immunofluorescence microscopy result between two kidney biopsies was shown in Table 1. Unfortunately, renal specimen for electron microscopy included only sclerotic glomerulus in the second biopsy. The deposited immunoglobulin in our case was of IgG1 subclass, though the predominant IgG subclass was reported to be IgG3 [22]. Linear deposition of κ and λ light chains, with λ staining being more intense than κ, was found in the first biopsy, but linear deposition of only κ light chain was found in the second biopsy. The mechanism of this difference is not known, but the modification of the antigenicity of the deposited antibodies by either natural course or the treatment might have contributed to the result. Although our patient started the therapy only 9 days after initial symptoms, he had to undergo permanent hemodialysis 15 months after the discontinuation of dialysis. Since a regimen of combination therapy using corticosteroid, cyclophosphamide, and plasmapheresis is used as standard treatment in patients with anti-GBM disease [9], additional treatment with cyclophosphamide with modification of dosage and timing of hemodialysis [23] might have been more effective in preventing progression of glomerular damage in our patient.

In summary, physicians should keep in mind that active anti-GBM disease can show high PCT value in the absence of infection. To pursue recovery of renal function, it is practically important to immediately challenge starting and continuing high-dose corticosteroid therapy plus plasmapheresis in the patients with highly suspected anti-GBM disease despite having predictors for dialysis-dependence. In addition to introduction of every possible early treatment, the treatment to inhibit glomerular damage should be established especially in patients undergoing dialysis therapy.

Acknowledgments

The authors would like to thank Ms. Hiromi Yamaguchi for her technical assistance.

References

[1] S. P. McAdoo and C. D. Pusey, "Anti-Glomerular Basement Membrane Disease," *Clinical Journal of the American Society of Nephrology*, vol. 12, no. 7, pp. 1162–1172, 2017.

[2] J. P. Johnson, W. Whitman, W. A. Briggs, and C. B. Wilson, "Plasmapheresis and immunosuppressive agents in antibasement membrane antibody-induced Goodpasture's syndrome," *The American Journal of Medicine*, vol. 64, no. 2, pp. 354–359, 1978.

[3] C. Savage, C. D. Pusey, C. Bowman, A. J. Rees, and C. M. Lockwood, "Antiglomerular basement membrane antibody mediated disease in the British Isles 1980-4," *British Medical Journal (Clinical research ed.)*, vol. 292, no. 6516, pp. 301–304, 1986.

[4] C. R. K. Hind, C. M. Lockwood, D. K. Peters, H. Paraskevakou, D. J. Evans, and A. J. Rees, "Prognosis after immunosuppression of patients with crescentic nephritis requiring dialysis," *The Lancet*, vol. 321, no. 8319, pp. 263–265, 1983.

[5] J. B. Levy, A. N. Turner, A. J. Rees, and C. D. Pusey, "Long-term outcome of anti-glomerular basement membrane antibody disease treated with plasma exchange and immunosuppression," *Annals of Internal Medicine*, vol. 134, no. 11, pp. 1033–1042, 2001.

[6] B. Alchi, M. Griffiths, M. Sivalingam, D. Jayne, and K. Farrington, "Predictors of renal and patient outcomes in anti-GBM disease: clinicopathologic analysis of a two-centre cohort," *Nephrology Dialysis Transplantation*, vol. 30, no. 5, pp. 814–821, 2015.

[7] I. Buhaescu, R. A. Yood, and H. Izzedine, "Serum procalcitonin in systemic autoimmune diseases—where are we now?" *Seminars in Arthritis and Rheumatism*, vol. 40, no. 2, pp. 176–183, 2010.

[8] C. Morath, J. Sis, G. M. Haensch, M. Zeier, K. Andrassy, and V. Schwenger, "Procalcitonin as marker of infection in patients with Goodpasture's syndrome is misleading," *Nephrology Dialysis Transplantation*, vol. 22, no. 9, pp. 2701–2704, 2007.

[9] Kidney Disease Improving Global Outcomes (KDIGO), "clinical practice guideline for glomerulonephritis," *Kidney International*, Suppl 2, pp. 139–274, 2012.

[10] Q. Gu, L. Xie, X. Jia et al., "Fever and prodromal infections in anti-glomerular basement membrane disease," *Nephrology*, 2017.

[11] F. Merkel, O. Pullig, M. Marx, K. O. Netzer, and M. Weber, "Course and prognosis of anti-basement membrane antibody (anti-BM-Ab)-mediated disease: report of 35 cases," *Nephrology Dialysis Transplantation*, vol. 9, no. 4, pp. 372–376, 1994.

[12] M. Herody, G. Bobrie, C. Gouarin, J. P. Grunfeld, and L. H. Noel, "Anti-GBM disease: Predictive value of clinical, histological and serological data," *Clinical Nephrology*, vol. 40, no. 5, pp. 249–255, 1993.

[13] J. C. Flores, C. O. S. Savage, C. M. Lockwood et al., "Clinical and immunological evolution of oligoanuric anti-gbm nephritis treated by haemodialysis," *The Lancet*, vol. 327, no. 8471, pp. 5–8, 1986.

[14] J. P. Johnson, J. Moore, H. A. Austin, J. E. Balow, T. T. Antonovych, and C. B. Wilson, "Therapy of anti-glomerular basement membrane antibody disease: Analysis of prognostic significance of clinical, pathologic and treatment factors," *Medicine*, vol. 64, no. 4, pp. 219–227, 1985.

[15] Z. Cui, J. Zhao, X.-Y. Jia et al., "Anti-glomerular basement membrane disease: Outcomes of different therapeutic regimens in a large single-center chinese cohort study," *Medicine*, vol. 90, no. 5, pp. 303–311, 2011.

[16] C. M. Lockwood, A. J. Rees, T. A. Pearson, D. J. Evans, D. K. Peters, and C. B. Wilson, "Immunosuppression and plasma exchange in the treatment of Goodpasture's syndrome," *Lancet*, vol. 1, no. 7962, pp. 711–715, 1976.

[17] K. Tanabe, "Double-filtration plasmapheresis," *Transplantation*, vol. 84, supp 12, no. 12, pp. S30–S32, 2007.

[18] N. Hajime, A. Michiko, K. Atsunori et al., "A case report of efficiency of double filtration plasmapheresis in treatment of goodpasture's syndrome," *Therapeutic Apheresis and Dialysis*, vol. 13, no. 4, pp. 373–377, 2009.

[19] K. Laczika, S. Knapp, K. Derfler, A. Soleiman, W. H. Hörl, and W. Druml, "Immunoadsorption in Goodpasture's syndrome," *American Journal of Kidney Diseases*, vol. 36, no. 2, pp. 392–395, 2000.

[20] P. Biesenbach, R. Kain, K. Derfler et al., "Long-term outcome of anti-glomerular basement membrane antibody disease treated with immunoadsorption," *PLoS ONE*, vol. 9, no. 7, article e103568, 2014.

[21] Y.-Y. Zhang, Z. Tang, D.-M. Chen, D.-H. Gong, D.-X. Ji, and Z.-H. Liu, "Comparison of double filtration plasmapheresis with immunoadsorption therapy in patients with anti-glomerular basement membrane nephritis," *BMC Nephrology*, vol. 15, no. 1, article no. 128, 2014.

[22] Z. Qu, Z. Cui, G. Liu, and M.-H. Zhao, "The distribution of IgG subclass deposition on renal tissues from patients with anti-glomerular basement membrane disease," *BMC Immunology*, vol. 14, no. 1, article no. 19, 2013.

[23] M. Haubitz, F. Bohnenstengel, R. Brunkhorst, M. Schwab, U. Hofmann, and D. Busse, "Cyclophosphamide pharmacokinetics and dose requirements in patients with renal insufficiency," *Kidney International*, vol. 61, no. 4, pp. 1495–1501, 2002.

Rifampicin in Nontuberculous Mycobacterial Infections: Acute Kidney Injury with Hemoglobin Casts

Rishi Kora,[1] Sergey V. Brodsky,[2] Tibor Nadasdy,[2] Dean Agra,[3] and Anjali A. Satoskar[2]

[1]*Mount Carmel West Hospital, Columbus, OH, USA*
[2]*Ohio State University Wexner Medical Center, Columbus, OH, USA*
[3]*Columbus Nephrology, Columbus, OH, USA*

Correspondence should be addressed to Anjali A. Satoskar; anjali.satoskar@osumc.edu

Academic Editor: Rumeyza Kazancioglu

Rifampicin is a key component of multidrug regimens not only for tuberculosis, but also nontuberculous mycobacterial infections (NTM) which are on the rise worldwide. Knowledge of the toxicity profile is important. Hepatotoxicity is a well-known side effect of Rifampicin necessitating regular liver function monitoring during therapy. Acute kidney injury (AKI) is a relatively rare complication, usually resulting from allergic interstitial nephritis (AIN). Rifampicin-induced intravascular hemolysis resulting in hemoglobinuria and AKI is even more uncommon, especially in Western countries with low prevalence of mycobacterial infections. Rifampicin-induced antibodies are implicated and this complication preferentially occurs during intermittent drug treatment protocols or when Rifampicin is restarted after a long drug-free interval. Awareness of this drug complication and its unique timing is important especially among emergency room physicians where patients with AKI may first present. It is equally important for nephrologists and pathologists. We describe one such case with detailed clinical course of the patient and interesting biopsy findings of ATN with intratubular hemoglobin casts.

1. Introduction

This is a case of an elderly female with recurrent Mycobacterium avium-intracellulare (MAI) pneumonia, who was restarted on Rifampicin-containing triple drug regimen (after a 16-month drug-free interval) and presented with acute kidney injury (AKI) and blood in the urine ten days after starting treatment with Rifampicin. Serum creatinine was normal before presentation and there was no history of other nephrotoxic insults. A kidney biopsy was performed to identify the etiology of AKI and to look for potentially treatable causes.

2. Case

2.1. Clinical History. Patient is a 65-year-old Caucasian female with past medical history of hypothyroidism and gastroesophageal reflux disease. MAI pneumonia was diagnosed two years ago based on symptoms of shortness of breath, wheezing, and mild hemoptysis; chest CT findings of diffuse bilateral centrilobular nodular ground glass opacities; and bronchoalveolar lavage (BAL) fluid cultures revealing MAI complex. Lung biopsy showed chronic bronchiolitis and rare nonnecrotizing granulomas. She was started on a three-drug regimen with Azithromycin (600 mg), Ethambutol (1800 mg), and Rifampicin (600 mg) three times per week [1]. Patient reported adherence and tolerance to her therapeutic regimen for 8 months. After that, she stopped treatment because of insurance issues.

Sixteen months later, she was found to have recurrent MAI pneumonia, confirmed on bronchoscopy and BAL fluid culture. She was resumed on the same regimen of Azithromycin, Ethambutol, and Rifampicin. Ten days later, she developed nausea, vomiting, weakness, fever, diarrhea, and decreasing urine output.

On admission, she had AKI with serum creatinine of 6.6 mg/dl and blood urea nitrogen of 68 mg/dl. Baseline

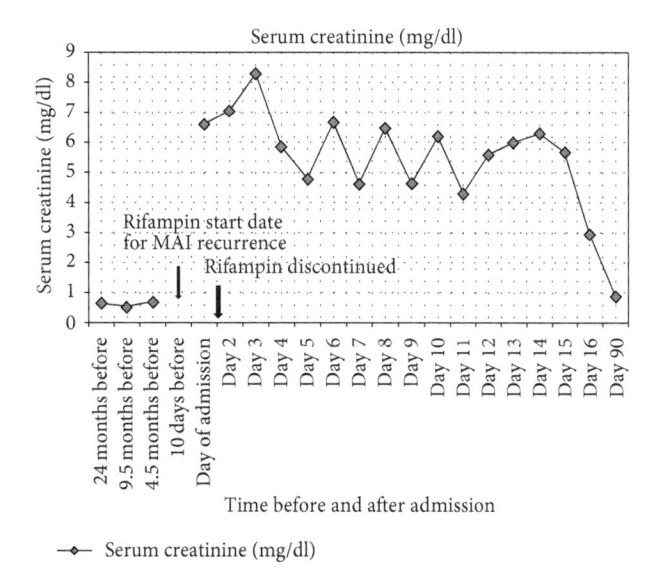

FIGURE 1: Graph with patient's serum creatinine over time, before and after admission for AKI.

TABLE 1: Laboratory testing for serum metabolites at admission.

Comprehensive metabolic profile	Measured value	Reference value
Sodium	131 mMol/L	136–145 mMol/L
Potassium	4.4 mMol/L	3.6–5.1 mMol/L
Chloride	98 mMol/L	98–107 mMol/L
Bicarbonate	17 mMol/L	22–32 mMol/L
Anion gap	16 mMol/L	6–18 mMol/L
Glucose	84 mg/dl	70–110 mg/dl
BUN	68 mg/dl	8–20 mg/dl
Creatinine	6.61 mg/dl	0.6–1.30 mg/dl
Alkaline phosphatase	160 units/L	32–91 units/L
ALT/SGPT	19 units/L	14–63 units/L
AST/SGOT	80 units/L	15–41 units/L
Bilirubin total	2.1 mg/dl	0.3–1.2 mg/dl
Bilirubin direct	1.0 mg/dl	0.1–0.5 mg/dl
Bilirubin indirect	1.1 mg/dl	0.0–1.0 mg/dl
C3	122 mg/dl	79–152 mg/dl
C4	25 mg/dl	16–38 mg/dl
Haptoglobin	225 mg/dl	36–195 mg/dl
Lactate dehydrogenase	232 units/L	98–192 units/L
Hemoglobin	11.4 gm/dl	12–16 gm/dl

TABLE 2: Urinalysis results at admission.

Urinalysis	Measured value	Reference value
Urine color	Yellow	Yellow
Urine appearance	Turbid	Clear
Urine specific gravity	1.012	1.002–1.030
Urine pH	6	4.5–8.0
Urine glucose	Normal	Normal
Urine ketones	Negative	Negative
Urine bilirubin	Negative	Negative
Urine blood	300/UL	Negative
Urine urobilinogen	Normal	Normal
Urine leukocyte esterase	500/UL	Negative
Urine nitrite	Negative	Negative
Urine protein	200 mg/dl	Negative
WBC urine	183/hpf	0–5/hpf
RBC urine	10/hpf	0–5/hpf
Squamous epithelial cells urine	Moderate	Few/hpf
Transitional epithelial cells urine	Few	None/hpf
Urine bacteria	Moderate	None/hpf
Urine mucous	Rare	None/lpf
Microalbumin creatinine ratio	1300 mg/gram	<30 mg/gram
Protein/creatinine ratio	2400 mg/gram	<150 mg/gram

serum creatinine was 0.7 mg/dl three months prior to this presentation (Figure 1) and eGFR was 91 ml/min by CKD-EPI creatinine equation [2]. Laboratory results are shown in Table 1. Patient was anemic with anion gap metabolic acidosis. Urinalysis showed blood, subnephrotic proteinuria (Table 2). Renal ultrasound displayed normal size kidneys measuring 12.9 cm and 12.1 cm, without increased echogenicity, hydronephrosis, masses, or calculus. Patient denied recent use of nonsteroidal anti-inflammatory medications or recent exposure to radiographic contrast.

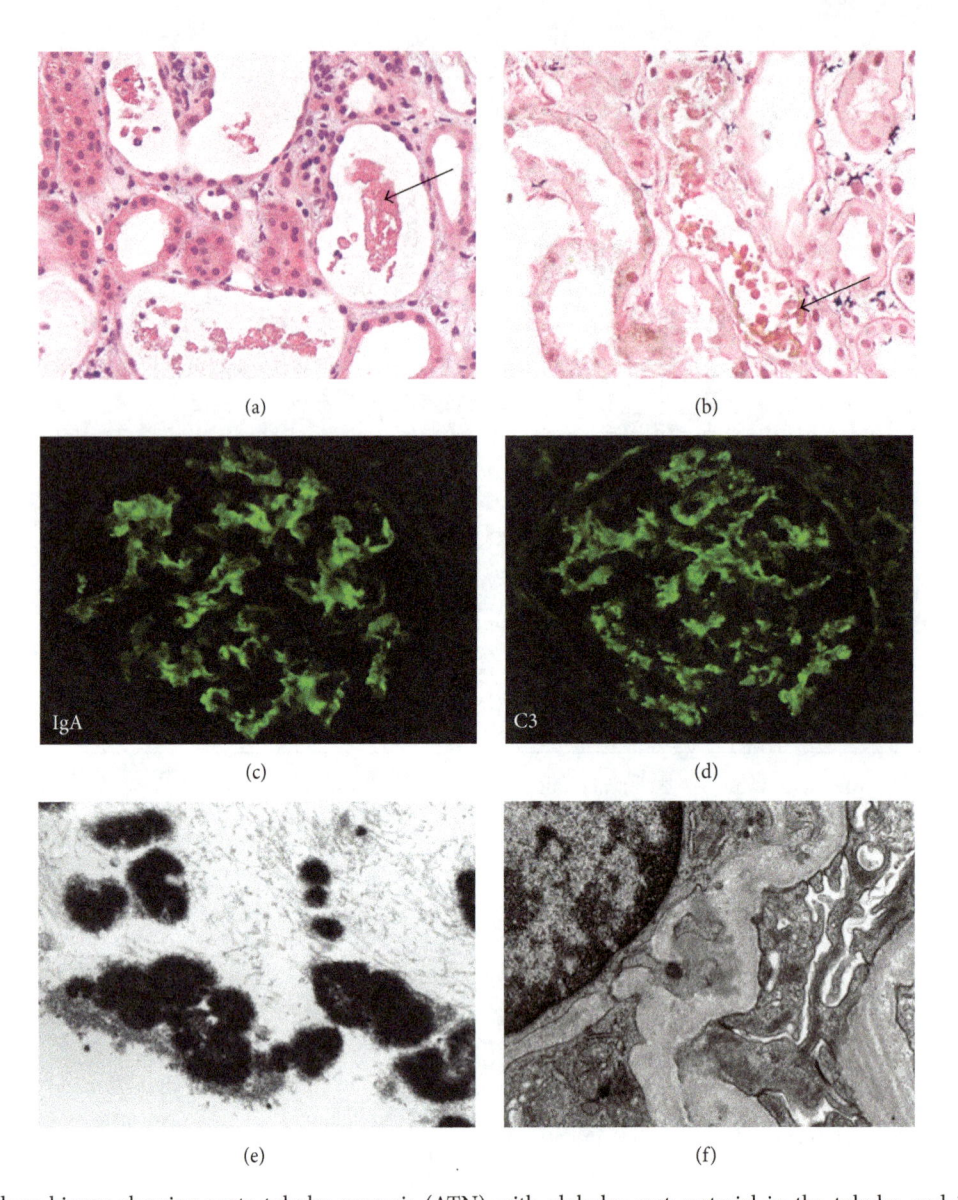

FIGURE 2: (a) Kidney biopsy showing acute tubular necrosis (ATN) with globular cast material in the tubules and interstitial edema (hematoxylin and eosin stained 200x). (b) Special stain for hemoglobin highlights yellow staining in the globular cast material (200x). ((c) and (d)) Direct immunofluorescence staining for IgA and C3 shows granular mesangial staining, respectively (400x). (e) Ultrastructural examination shows osmophilic globular hemoglobin casts in tubular lumen (uranyl acetate and lead citrate fixation, 10,000x). (f) Ultrastructural examination shows small scattered paramesangial electron dense immune-type deposits (uranyl acetate and lead citrate fixation, 12,000x).

2.2. Kidney Biopsy. The biopsy processed per routine protocol (light microscopy, direct immunofluorescence, and electron microscopy) had 23 glomeruli with mild focal mesangial hypercellularity, diffuse acute tubular necrosis (ATN), interstitial edema, and granular/globular casts in scattered tubules (Figure 2(a)). Immunoperoxidase stain for myoglobin was negative, but hemoglobin stain showed yellow-green staining in the globular tubular casts (Figure 2(b)). Interstitial inflammation was mild and patchy. Interstitial fibrosis and tubular atrophy were mild, involving less than 20% of the renal cortex. Direct immunofluorescence study showed mild (1+) mesangial IgA and complement C3 (Figures 2(c) and 2(d)). Electron microscopic examination showed tubules with globular casts and few scattered mesangial electron dense immune-type deposits (Figures 2(e) and 2(f)). In the absence of recent/resolving bacterial infection, the mesangial IgA immune complex deposits suggested mild underlying chronic IgA nephropathy. But there were no active proliferative glomerular lesions and the patient had normal renal function prior to this episode of AKI. Also, this may represent coincidental IgA deposits which can be seen in 3% of the population in the Western countries [3]. IgA nephropathy causes hematuria, but usually not hemoglobinuria (which this patient had). The AKI was attributed primarily to the ATN, which can be multifactorial. The presence of hemoglobin-containing tubular casts however suggested the possibility of ongoing intravascular hemolysis and hemoglobinuria as the plausible cause of the ATN. Since the patient was not receiving any other medications implicated in hemolysis, Rifampicin was considered the likely culprit [4].

2.3. Clinical Management and Followup. Rifampicin and the other antimycobacterial drugs were discontinued. Patient remained anuric for 3 days despite intravenous hydration followed by Lasix challenge. She was initiated on hemodialysis and underwent seven sessions during her 14-day hospital stay and five subsequent sessions as an outpatient. Antimycobacterial treatment was held for 6 weeks after discharge and subsequently resumed on Ethambutol and Azithromycin. Renal function slowly recovered to 1.94 mg/dl at one month and 0.7 mg/dl at three months (eGFR > 60 ml/minute).

3. Discussion

Rifampicin is used in multidrug treatment regimens not only for tuberculosis, but also for NTM infections, leprosy, and Staphylococcal infections [1, 5, 6]. Rifampicin is designated as an essential drug by the WHO [7]. Hepatotoxicity is well-known side effect and liver function monitoring during treatment is routinely performed with the use of this drug [8]. However, AKI is a less common complication of Rifampicin. Despite published reports [9–13], regular renal function monitoring is not routine practice. So patients may present unexpectedly to urgent care facilities with AKI. In this setting, it may not be so intuitive to identify Rifampicin as the trigger for the AKI. Additionally, the patient may be on several other commonly prescribed medications such as antibiotics, proton-pump inhibitors and herbal supplements that are also implicated in the causation of ATN and interstitial nephritis. All these confounding factors may preclude the correct diagnosis. Another important confounding factor is the unique temporal relation between start of Rifampicin-based therapy and the development of AKI. It usually occurs in the setting of reintroduction of therapy after a long drug-free interval and typically few weeks after the start of the day (in contrast to 24 to 48 hours in a typical allergic reaction), [5, 9–13]. Clinical symptoms frequently reported include nausea and vomiting (72%), fever (45%), chills (43%), abdominal pain (40%), diarrhea (26%), jaundice (19%), lumbar pain (17%), and anemia (96%) [12]. Duration of anuric phase is on average 11.4 days +/− 7 days. An average of 4.8 +/− 4.6 hemodialysis sessions is required [12]. Our patient displayed nearly all of the aforementioned features except jaundice.

The mechanisms of rifampicin-induced AKI may be multiple and attributed to type II or III hypersensitivity reactions. Development of anti-Rifampicin antibodies has been described [5, 12]. These antibodies however bind to Rifampicin and these immune complexes are cleared from the circulation. On daily regimens, continuous formation of antigen-antibody complexes prevents rise in free antibody titer to dangerous levels. Rise in titers however does occur with intermittent drug regimen or after prolonged discontinuation and reinstitution of treatment. Unfortunately however, testing for Rifampicin antibodies was not performed in our patient since this is not a routine laboratory test and was unlikely to alter management significantly.

Rifampicin is one of the few drugs known to cause hemolysis [4]. One way is through cross-reaction of Rifampicin antibodies with the blood group I antigen on red blood cells leading to complement-mediated hemolysis. Hemolytic anemia and positive antiglobulin test has been described during Rifampicin treatment [5]. Although antiglobin testing was not performed in our patient, the kidney biopsy did demonstrate hemoglobin-containing tubular casts. Hemoglobin casts are usually small in size, containing globular fragments, more coarse than the usual granular ATN casts, and with targetoid morphology on electron microscopy (Figure 2). They may sometimes be confused with red blood cells (RBCs); in contrast, the hemoglobin globules are uneven in size unlike RBCs. Urinalysis revealed blood on dipstick examination but not RBCs, supportive of hemoglobinuria. Additionally, the patient had low serum hemoglobin level with mildly elevated serum LDH (lactate dehydrogenase) (Table 1), supportive of intravascular hemolysis. But it was not massive hemolysis, since haptoglobin was not low. The most common histologic findings in Rifampicin-associated AKI are interstitial nephritis and associated ATN [13]. Minimal change disease has also been reported [14]. However, our case is unique in that it showed predominantly ATN with hemoglobin-containing tubular casts due to Rifampicin-induced hemolysis (not interstitial nephritis). Although hemoglobin is a normal body pigment, its presence in the tubules is toxic to the tubular epithelial cells [15].

Although Ethambutol also has been reported to cause AKI [16], it is more commonly known to cause ocular optic neuropathy [17]. Most of the published reports suggest Rifampicin as the major culprit for AKI [9–13]. Covic et al. [10] reported AKI in 60 out of 120,132 patients (0.05%) receiving Rifampicin. A much higher prevalence has been reported by Chang et al. [9] in Taiwan (7.1%) probably because of a large population of elderly patients afflicted by tuberculosis in that region. In this large case series by Chang et al., out of 1,394 patients treated with Rifampicin, 99 patients developed AKI. Rifampicin was discontinued in 34 patients. Among them, a rechallenge was performed in 21 patients, with six developing a second episode of AKI. Recovery rate following AKI was reported to be 73%.

In conclusion, our patient developed AKI following reintroduction of Rifampicin-based therapy for recurrent MAI after a prolonged drug-free period. It was followed by slow but complete renal recovery after dialysis and cessation of the drug. Rifampicin is used not only for treatment of mycobacterium tuberculosis infection, but also in nontuberculous mycobacterial infections (NTM) which are prevalent worldwide. Since there is no official recommendation to regularly monitor patient's renal function during Rifampicin therapy, patients may present unexpectedly with AKI. So awareness of renal toxicity of Rifampicin and the unique timing of occurrence is important not only among infectious disease physicians but also among emergency room physicians and nephrologists who are often consulted. It is also important to understand the different mechanisms of rifampicin-induced AKI. In AKI due to ATN alone (without interstitial nephritis), steroid therapy is not warranted in this patient. For the pathologists who evaluate the kidney biopsy, procuring detailed clinical history from the physician and attention to morphologic details in the biopsy are crucial. One should be particularly aware of this subtle histologic finding of small intratubular hemoglobin casts and understand the utility of the hemoglobin stain. This provides an important clue to identify the cause of ATN, which otherwise can be difficult, especially in the presence of several other confounding factors such as recent bacterial infections and concomitant use of other potentially nephrotoxic drugs.

References

[1] D. E. Griffith, T. Aksamit, B. A. Brown-Elliott et al., "An official ATS/IDSA statement: diagnosis, treatment, and prevention of nontuberculous mycobacterial diseases," *American Journal of Respiratory and Critical Care Medicine*, vol. 175, no. 4, pp. 367–416, 2007.

[2] L. A. Stevens, S. Padala, and A. S. Levey, "Advances in glomerular filtration rate-estimating equations," *Current Opinion in Nephrology and Hypertension*, vol. 19, no. 3, pp. 298–307, 2010.

[3] R. Sinniah, "Occurrence of mesangial IgA and IgM deposits in a control necropsy population," *Journal of Clinical Pathology*, vol. 36, no. 3, pp. 276–279, 1983.

[4] K. Manika, K. Tasiopoulou, L. Vlogiaris et al., "Rifampicin-associated acute renal failure and hemolysis: A rather uncommon but severe complication," *Renal Failure*, vol. 35, no. 8, pp. 1179–1181, 2013.

[5] A. S. De Vriese, D. L. Robbrecht, R. C. Vanholder, D. P. Vogelaers, and N. H. Lameire, "Rifampicin-associated acute renal failure: Pathophysiologic, immunologic, and clinical features," *American Journal of Kidney Diseases*, vol. 31, no. 1, pp. 108–115, 1998.

[6] C.-Y. Chen, H.-Y. Chen, C.-H. Chou, C.-T. Huang, C.-C. Lai, and P.-R. Hsueh, "Pulmonary infection caused by nontuberculous mycobacteria in a medical center in Taiwan, 2005–2008," *Diagnostic Microbiology And Infectious Disease*, vol. 72, no. 1, pp. 47–51, 2012.

[7] E. F. T Hoen, H. V. Hogerzeil, J. D. Quick, and H. B. Sillo, "A quiet revolution in global public health: The world health organization's prequalification of medicines programme," *Journal of Public Health Policy*, vol. 35, no. 2, pp. 137–161, 2014.

[8] P. Berthelot, "Isoniazid-rifampicin: an exemplary hepatotoxicity," *Gastroentérologie Clinique et Biologique*, vol. 2, no. 2, pp. 129–132, 1978.

[9] C.-H. Chang, Y.-F. Chen, V.-C. Wu et al., "Acute kidney injury due to anti-tuberculosis drugs: A five-year experience in an aging population," *BMC Infectious Diseases*, vol. 14, no. 1, article no. 23, 2014.

[10] A. Covic, D. J. A. Goldsmith, L. Segall et al., "Rifampicin-induced acute renal failure: A series of 60 patients," *Nephrology Dialysis Transplantation*, vol. 13, no. 4, pp. 924–929, 1998.

[11] T. Muthukumar, M. Jayakumar, E. M. Fernando, and M. A. Muthusethupathi, "Acute renal failure due to rifampicin: A study of 25 patients," *American Journal of Kidney Diseases*, vol. 40, no. 4, pp. 690–696, 2002.

[12] G. Poole, P. Stradling, and S. Worlledge, "Potentially Serious Side Effects of High-Dose Twice-Weekly Rifampicin," *British Medical Journal*, vol. 3, no. 5770, pp. 343–347, 1971.

[13] J. T. Park, S. Lee, W. Kim, S. K. Park, and K. P. Kang, "A Case of Acute Tubulointerstitial Nephritis Associated with Rifampin Therapy Presenting as Fanconi-like Syndrome," *Chonnam Medical Journal*, vol. 53, no. 1, p. 81, 2017.

[14] D. H. Park, S. A. Lee, H. J. Jeong, T.-H. Yoo, S.-W. Kang, and H. J. Oh, "Rifampicin-induced minimal change disease is improved after cessation of rifampicin without steroid therapy," *Yonsei Medical Journal*, vol. 56, no. 2, pp. 582–585, 2015.

[15] M. A. Khalighi, K. J. Henriksen, A. Chang, and S. M. Meehan, "Intratubular hemoglobin casts in hemolysis-associated acute kidney injury," *American Journal of Kidney Diseases*, vol. 65, no. 2, pp. 337–341, 2015.

[16] S. H. Kwon, J. H. Kim, J. O. Yang, E. Lee, and S. Y. Hong, "Ethambutol-induced acute renal failure," *Nephrology Dialysis Transplantation*, vol. 19, no. 5, pp. 1335-1336, 2004.

[17] K. Aouam, A. Chaabane, C. Loussaïef, F. Ben Romdhane, N.-A. Boughattas, and M. Chakroun, "Adverse effects of antitubercular drugs: epidemiology, mechanisms, and patient management," *Médecine et Maladies Infectieuses*, vol. 37, no. 5, pp. 253–261, 2007.

Cisplatin-Induced Nephrotoxicity and HIV Associated Nephropathy: Mimickers of Myeloma-Like Cast Nephropathy

Muhammad Siddique Khurram, Ahmed Alrajjal, Warda Ibrar, Jacob Edens, Umer Sheikh, Ameer Hamza, and Hong Qu

St. John Hospital and Medical Center, Detroit, MI, USA

Correspondence should be addressed to Muhammad Siddique Khurram; siddiqueshaikh80@hotmail.com

Academic Editor: Yoshihide Fujigaki

Myeloma cast nephropathy is an obstructing disorder of renal tubules, caused by precipitation of Bence Jones proteins. Myeloma-like cast nephropathy (MLCN) has been reported in the literature to occur in various primary renal and nonrenal diseases. We present a series of three rare cases of cast nephropathy, two of which are HIV patients, and the third patient is receiving cisplatin-based chemotherapy. However, in all three patients plasma cell dyscrasia has been ruled out. A 30-year-old male was admitted to the hospital with facial cellulitis. The second patient is a 31-year-old male who presented with *Pneumocystis jiroveci* pneumonia. The third patient was treated with cisplatin-based chemotherapy for carcinoma. First two cases revealed foci of diffuse tubular dilatation containing hyaline casts and interstitial inflammatory infiltrate, in addition to globally sclerotic glomeruli with ultrastructural foot process fusion and mesangium expansion. The third case showed acute tubular injury and cast formation of irregular casts composed of amorphous or granular material of low density admixed with scattered high electron-dense globules. Myeloma-like cast nephropathy and true myeloma cast nephropathy pose similar destructive effects on renal parenchyma. This new pattern of HIV-related nephropathy should be considered in HIV patients with MLCN, once monoclonal gammopathy is ruled out.

1. Introduction

Myeloma cast nephropathy (MCN) is the most common pattern of renal injury found in plasma cell dyscrasia and more specifically multiple myeloma (MM). It commonly presents as acute renal injury, which prompts the physician to perform renal biopsy. The pathophysiology of MCN is precipitation of monoclonal immunoglobulins and Tamm-Horsfall glycoproteins in distal tubules and collecting ducts. The histologic hallmark of MCN is the presence of tubular casts, which appear eosinophilic and brittle and usually instigate an intense inflammatory response (cellular reaction) in kidney leading to acute renal failure (ARF); if untreated it can lead to irreversible damage [1, 2].

Myeloma-like cast nephropathy (MLCN) has been reported in the literature to occur in various primary renal and nonrenal diseases including some neoplastic processes, such as pancreatic carcinoma [3]. Some reports also suggested an association of MLCN with antimicrobial therapy [4].

Human immunodeficiency virus associated nephropathy (HIVAN) is the most common disease delineated in biopsy series of patients with HIV infection and renal disease [5, 6]. Two patterns of HIV kidney disease have emerged: HIV associated nephropathy (HIVAN) and HIV immune complex kidney disease (HIVCKD). HIVAN is suggested to be caused directly by HIV-1 infection, possibly via disruption of the normal homeostatic function of mature podocytes caused by HIV proteins Nef, Vpr, and Tat [7]. HIVAN itself is a collapsing glomerulopathy and the most common renal complication amongst patients with HIV-1 infection. HIVCKD is an immunoglobulin related glomerulonephritis. HIVCKD is characterized by immune complex deposition that includes complement, HIV-1 antigens, and reactive antibodies. Typically it is also associated with concurrent infections such as hepatitis C [8]. Immune responses are central to the development of HIVCKD, being associated with the concurrent infections and the deposition of HIV antigen antibody complexes within the glomerulus. For both HIVAN and HIVCKD, hyperplasia within the glomerulus and podocyte injury is central to pathogenesis [9].

We present three patients with MLCN. Two of them were associated with HIV infection while the third patient was treated with cisplatin-based chemotherapy.

2. Methods and Materials

2.1. Case Number 1. A 30-year-old African American male was admitted to the hospital who sustained a laceration a year ago for which he required stitches, and at that time he had some facial swelling. Physician suspected the fungus and antifungal was prescribed at that time. He was doing fine when he presented to our hospital with recurrent painful swelling and yellowish discharge. Comprehensive blood profile along with renal functions tests, CT orbits, and HIV testing were performed. He had an elevated BP and creatinine. HIV was positive and CT showed preseptal swelling. Skin biopsy came positive for coccidiosis. Nephrology consultation for suspected acute renal failure, with mild proteinuria (2.2 g/24 h), was done and a left renal needle biopsy was performed.

2.2. Case Number 2. A 31-year-old African American male came to ER with complaints of progressive difficulty breathing for 4 months and unintentional weight loss of about 50 lbs. Chest X-ray was done which showed reticular nodular pattern. Infectious disease consultation was sought. Comprehensive blood profile along with renal functions tests and HIV testing were performed. He had an elevated BP and creatinine. HIV was positive. Nephrology consultation was done for an elevated creatinine (17 mg/dl) and proteinuria (3.7 g/24 h) with microscopic hematuria, and hemodialysis was initiated. CT scan showed bilateral ground-glass opacities. Bronchoalveolar lavage was done which confirmed *Pneumocystis carinii* pneumonia (PCP). A right renal needle biopsy was performed.

2.3. Case Number 3. A 65-year-old male with history of squamous cell carcinoma of tongue was being treated with cisplatin and radiation therapy. During the second round of chemotherapy he developed acute renal failure with oliguria and markedly elevated serum creatinine levels. The drug history was negative for nonsteroidal anti-inflammatory drugs (NSAIDs). Emergent renal biopsy was performed and appropriately triaged.

3. Results

HIV status for cases I and II was confirmed by ELISA and Western Blot tests.

Myeloma work-up included serum protein electrophoresis and immune-fixation confirmed absence of monoclonal gammopathy.

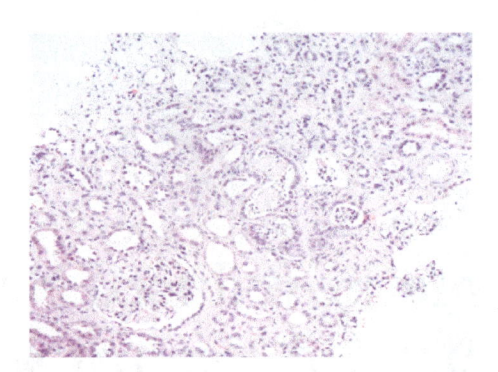

FIGURE 1: H&E section demonstrates fragments of fractured casts with neutrophilic reaction in a tubule. The glomeruli are unremarkable.

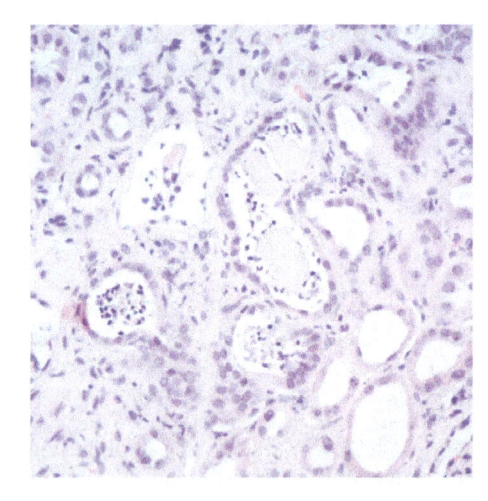

FIGURE 2: Many tubules are dilated with flattening of epithelium. In the adjacent tubules, multiple neutrophilic casts are seen.

3.1. Renal Biopsy Interpretation. All two cases were diagnosed as myeloma-like cast nephropathy. In HIV positive patients biopsy finding confirmed HIV associated changes in addition to myeloma-like cast nephropathy. In all two cases immunofluorescence microscopy failed to demonstrate monoclonal restrictions.

3.2. Light Microscopy. Renal needle biopsy was done showing conventional HIV associated nephropathy with coexisting myeloma-like cast nephropathy. Light microscopy revealed foci of tubular cystic dilatation and diffuse tubular dilatation containing eosinophilic, Periodic Acid–Schiff (PAS) negative casts coupled with segmental collapse of capillary tufts and focal glomerulosclerosis. Multiple casts have intense neutrophilic reaction (Figures 1 and 2). First case has a diffuse focally dense interstitial inflammatory infiltrate including lymphocytes, plasma cells, neutrophils, and rare eosinophils, while second case has focal interstitial infiltrate including lymphocytes and rare neutrophils.

3.3. Electron Microscopy. The ultrastructural findings include podocytes with extensive foot process effacement (Figure 3). The mesangial areas were slightly expended by increased

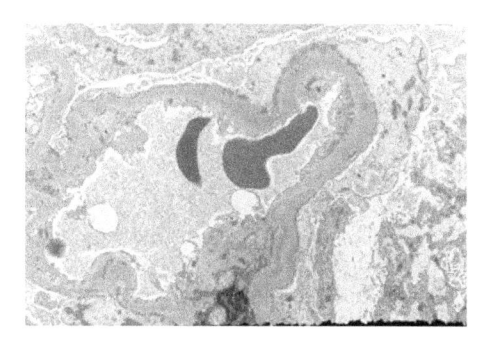

FIGURE 3: Electron micrograph of a glomerular capillary shows thickened glomerular basement membrane and diffuse foot process effacement.

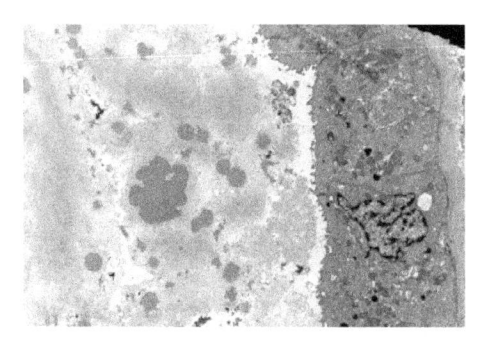

FIGURE 4: Electron micrograph of portion of cast shows light and dark areas with fine granular appearance. The tubular basement membrane seems laminated.

matrix and mesangial cell processes. The glomerular basement membrane was slightly thickened. No well-defined immune complex type or organized protein deposits are identified. Endothelial cells were unremarkable and no tubule-reticular inclusions were identified in cytoplasm of glomerular endothelial cells. The tubular epithelial cells are low cuboidal with luminal cast of variable density. Tubular basement membrane exhibits vague lamination (Figure 4).

3.4. Immunofluorescence Microscopy. Direct immunofluorescence stains were performed using a panel of ten antisera. It failed to demonstrate monoclonal restriction. All glomeruli were negative for albumin, fibrinogen, C1q, C3, C4. IgA, IgM, kappa, and lambda light chain stains.

4. Discussion

Renal disease is one of the major causes of morbidity and mortality in HIV infected patients receiving effective antiretroviral treatment. HIVAN, the classic kidney disease of HIV infection and the most common cause of CKD in HIV infected individuals, is mostly seen in African American descent and is consistent with a strong genetic predisposition. HIV mediates dysregulation of glomerular podocytes, the epithelial cells that maintain the glomerular basement membrane, and apoptosis of renal tubular cells. The resulting lesion of HIVAN is a focal glomerulosclerosis (FGS) and microcytic dilation of the tubules filled with PAS positive casts [10, 11]. HIVAN usually presents as nephritic range proteinuria with a progressive loss of renal function and an interval of <10 months from the time of diagnosis to progression to ESRD [12–16]. Many reports suggest that black race [12–20], Haitian background [21], male gender, injection drug use [12–18, 21], and decreased CD4 cell count [21] are risk factors for the development of HIVAN. Interpretation of these reports is limited by the unknown effects of selection bias introduced through the methods by which patients were identified for inclusion. Several studies have included only those patients who were seen by nephrologists during admissions to the hospital for other diagnoses [17, 20, 22].

It appears that HIVAN occurs in the setting of specific host genes and it has been widely accepted that the gene encoding a non-myosin A heavy chain (MYH9) is associated with FGS, HIVAN, and end-stage kidney disease (ESKD) due to hypertension in individuals of African descent [23, 24]. The interaction of HIV with renal cells has not been clarified. Renal cells lack the classic receptors for HIV, CD4, and the chemokine receptors CCR5 and CXCR4. However, HIV-mRNA has been detected in renal epithelial cells, and HAART slows progression of HIVAN to renal failure [25]. Nonconventional receptors on renal cells such as C-type lectins including DC-Sign and lipid rafts have been suggested as portals of entry of HIV into renal cells [26]. Renal cell infection by HIV, however, is nonproductive [27].

The MLCN, as described earlier, has similar histomorphological features to MCN and both can lead to renal damage. CD4, a receptor for HIV-1 on lymphocyte and macrophages, is the main culprit involved in the pathogenesis of renal cast formation. The renal lesion, MLCN, caused by HIV-1 bears a similarity to the nephropathy seen in cases of myeloma kidney, and it is also quite similar to the lesions seen in experimental Bence Jones protein nephropathy [28]. The lesions are characterized intratubular protein cast formation that are weakly positive for PAS, associated with multinucleated giant cells and neutrophils mostly affecting the cortical collecting ducts, though the distal convoluted tubules are also seen to be affected. It has also been suggested in some experimental models that the targeted expression of viral genes in lymphocytes and lymphoid tissue recapitulates some of the pathologic findings that are observed in the Tg26 mouse model and in human HIVAN, suggesting that HIV-1 gene expression may play a role in the development of HIVAN in both renal and nonrenal tissues [29].

Cisplatin, a chemotherapeutic agent that has been well recognized as a nephrotoxic agent, primarily causes tubulointerstitial lesions and in spite of extreme efforts of finding less toxic alternatives, cisplatin yet is prescribed widely. The nephrotoxicity related to cisplatin involves multiple pathways including apoptotic cascades activation, endonucleases, and oxidant stress. Most of these pathways share the same mechanisms for the cytotoxic effects of cisplatin on neoplastic cells; hence the strategies to reduce the nephrotoxic effects of cisplatin may reduce the antineoplastic effects of cisplatin [30]. Despite all side effects and development of new drugs, its efficacy against neoplastic cells is vital and is still part of many chemotherapeutic regimens because its benefits outweigh the side effects.

Cisplatin is cleared by the kidney by both glomerular filtration and tubular secretion and its concentrations within the kidney exceed those in blood suggesting an active accumulation of drug by renal parenchymal cells. It damages the proximal tubules, specifically the S3 segment of the outer medullary stripe, while the mitochondrial swelling and nuclear pallor occur in the distal nephron. The glomerulus has no obvious morphologic changes. The site of injury involves both the distal tubule and collecting ducts or the proximal and distal tubules. The predominant lesion in patients with acute renal failure is acute necrosis and is located mostly in the proximal convoluted tubules. The severity of necrosis is dependent on dose, concentration, and duration. Patients with chronic nephrotoxicity have focal acute tubular necrosis characterized by cystic dilated tubules lined by a flattened epithelium showing atypical nuclei and atypical mitotic figures with hyaline casts. Long-term cisplatin treatment and injury may cause cyst formation and interstitial fibrosis. Two different membrane transporters capable of transporting cisplatin are Ctr1, a copper transporter, and OCT2, an organic cation transporter. Downregulation of Ctr1 expression in kidney decreases both cisplatin uptake and cytotoxicity [31], while loss of the OCT2 gene reduces urinary cisplatin excretion leading to nephrotoxicity [6].

5. Conclusion

The hallmark of MLCN histologically is the presence of tubular cast associated with intense inflammatory response. Although this is not a typical presentation of an acute renal failure caused by HIV infection, MLCN could be a form of renal injury seen on HIV patients. Based on the histologic evaluation of the two cases we presented, we noticed remarkable similarities in the histologic features of typical myeloma cast nephropathy and myeloma-like cast nephropathy, despite using the standard diagnostic tools to rule out the presence of monoclonal gammopathy or any other condition that could cause MLCN. The cause of the underlying pathology that is causing kidney damage could be obscured, and an incorrect diagnosis of MLCN can set the treating physician on the wrong path seeking diagnosis. Accordingly, having MLCN on the differential diagnosis list of typical myeloma cast nephropathy is advisable.

Authors' Contributions

All authors have contributed significantly, and all authors are in agreement with the content of the manuscript.

References

[1] N. Leung, "Treating myeloma cast nephropathy without treating myeloma," *Journal of Clinical Investigation*, vol. 122, no. 5, pp. 1605–1608, 2012.

[2] S. Stringer, K. Basnayake, C. Hutchison, and P. Cockwell, "Recent Advances in the Pathogenesis and Management of Cast Nephropathy (Myeloma Kidney)," *Bone Marrow Research*, vol. 2011, pp. 1–9, 2011.

[3] K. Reducka, G. W. Gardiner, J. Sweet, A. Vandenbroucke, and R. Bear, "Myeloma-like cast nephropathy associated with acinar cell carcinoma of the pancreas," *American Journal of Nephrology*, vol. 8, no. 5, pp. 421–424, 1988.

[4] J. B. Kopp, M. W. Smith, and G. W. Nelson, "MYII9 is a major risk gene for focal segmentalglomerulosclerosis," *Nature Genetics*, vol. 40, no. 10, Article ID 117584, 2008.

[5] V. DAgati and G. B. Appel, "HIV infection and the kidney," *Journal of the American Society of Nephrology*, vol. 8, pp. 138–152, 1997.

[6] P. E. Klotman, "HIV-associated nephropathy," *Kidney International*, vol. 56, no. 3, pp. 1161–1176, 1999.

[7] L. A. Bruggeman and P. J. Nelson, "Controversies in the pathogenesis of HIV-associated renal diseases," *Nature Reviews Nephrology*, vol. 5, no. 10, pp. 574–581, 2009.

[8] C. M. Wyatt, P. E. Klotman, and V. D. D'Agati, "HIV-associated nephropathy: clinical presentation, pathology, and epidemiology in the era of antiretroviral therapy," *Seminars in Nephrology*, vol. 28, no. 6, pp. 513–522, 2008.

[9] V. DAgati and G. B. Appel, "HIV infection and the kidney," *Journal of the American Society of Nephrology*, pp. 138–152, 1997.

[10] I. Gopalakrishnan, S. S. Iskandar, P. Daeihagh et al., "Coincident idiopathic focal segmental glomerulosclerosis collapsing variant and diabetic nephropathy in an african american homozygous for MYH9 risk variants," *Human Pathology*, vol. 42, no. 2, pp. 291–294, 2011.

[11] J. Mikulak and P. C. Singhals, "HIV-1 and kidney cells: better understanding of viral interaction," *Nephron—Experimental Nephrology*, vol. 115, no. 2, pp. e15–e21, 2010.

[12] A. Valeri and A. J. Neusy, "Acute and chronic renal disease in hospitalized patients," *Clinical Nephrology*, vol. 35, pp. 110–118, 1991.

[13] C. Langs, G. R. Gallo, R. G. Schacht, G. Sidhu, and D. S. Baldwin, "Rapid renal failure in AIDS-associated focal glomerulosclerosis," *Archives of Internal Medicine*, vol. 150, no. 2, pp. 287–292, 1990.

[14] T. K. Rao, E. J. Filippone, A. D. Nicastri et al., "Associated focal and segmental glomerulosclerosis in the acquired immunodeficiency syndrome," *New England Journal of Medicine*, vol. 310, no. 11, pp. 669–673, 1984.

[15] T. K. Sreepada Rao, E. A. Friedman, and A. D. Nicastri, "The types of renal disease in the acquired immunodeficiency syndrome," *New England Journal of Medicine*, vol. 316, no. 17, pp. 1062–1068, 1987.

[16] L. Carbone, V. D'Agati, J. Cheng, and G. B. Appel, "Course and prognosis of human immunodeficiency virus-associated nephropathy," *The American Journal of Medicine*, vol. 87, pp. 389–395, 1989.

[17] J. J. Bourgoignie, R. Meneses, C. Ortiz, D. Jaffe, and V. Pardo, "The clinical spectrum of renal disease associated with human immunodeficiency virus," *American Journal of Kidney Diseases*, vol. 12, no. 2, pp. 131–137, 1988.

[18] E. S. Cantor, P. L. Kimmel, and J. P. Bosch, "Effect of race on expression of acquired immunodeficiency syndrome-associated nephropathy," *Archives of Internal Medicine*, vol. 151, no. 1, pp. 125–128, 1991.

[19] L. Frassetto, P. Y. Schoenfeld, and M. H. Humphreys, "Increasing incidence of human immunodeficiency virus-associated nephropathy at San Francisco General Hospital," *American Journal of Kidney Diseases*, vol. 18, no. 6, pp. 655–659, 1991.

[20] V. Pardo, R. Meneses, L. Ossa et al., "AIDS-related glomerulopathy: occurrence in specific risk groups," *Kidney International*, vol. 31, no. 5, pp. 1167–1173, 1987.

[21] G. W. Nelson, B. I. Freedman, D. W. Bowden et al., "Dense mapping of MYH9 localizes the strongest kidney disease associations to the region of introns 13 to 15," *Human Molecular Genetics*, vol. 19, no. 9, Article ID ddq039, pp. 1805–1815, 2010.

[22] S. A. Mazbar, P. Y. Schoenfeld, and M. H. Humphreys, "Renal involvement in patients infected with HIV: experience at San Francisco general hospital," *Kidney International*, vol. 37, no. 5, pp. 1325–1332, 1990.

[23] M. Murea and B. I. Freedman, "Essential hypertension and risk of nephropathy: a reappraisal," *Current Opinion in Nephrology and Hypertension*, vol. 19, no. 3, pp. 235–241, 2010.

[24] L. A. Szczech, "Tackling the unknowns in HIV-related kidney diseases," *New England Journal of Medicine*, vol. 363, no. 21, pp. 2058-2059, 2010.

[25] J. Mikulak, S. Teichberg, S. Arora et al., "DC-specific ICAM-3-grabbing nonintegrin mediates internalization of HIV-1 into human podocytes," *American Journal of Physiology—Renal Physiology*, vol. 299, no. 3, pp. F664–F673, 2010.

[26] A. K. Khatua, H. E. Taylor, J. E. K. Hildreth, and W. Popik, "Nonproductive HIV-1 infection of human glomerular and urinary podocytes," *Virology*, vol. 408, no. 1, pp. 119–127, 2010.

[27] P. J. Bugelski, H. A. Solleveld, K.-L. L. Fong, A. M. Klinkner, T. K. Hart, and D. G. Morgan, "Myeloma-like cast nephropathy caused by human recombinant soluble CD4 (sCD4) in monkeys," *American Journal of Pathology*, vol. 140, no. 3, pp. 531–537, 1992.

[28] P. Dickie, A. Roberts, R. Uwiera, J. Witmer, K. Sharma, and J. B. Kopp, "Focal glomerulosclerosis in proviral and c-fms transgenic mice links Vpr expression to HIV-associated nephropathy," *Virology*, vol. 322, no. 1, pp. 69–81, 2004.

[29] R. P. Miller, R. K. Tadagavadi, G. Ramesh, and W. B. Reeves, "Mechanisms of cisplatin nephrotoxicity," *Toxins*, vol. 2, no. 11, pp. 2490–2518, 2010.

[30] N. Pabla, R. F. Murphy, K. Liu, and Z. Dong, "The copper transporter Ctr1 contributes to cisplatin uptake by renal tubular cells during cisplatin nephrotoxicity," *American Journal of Physiology: Renal Physiology*, vol. 296, no. 3, pp. F505–F511, 2009.

[31] K. K. Filipski, R. H. Mathijssen, T. S. Mikkelsen, A. H. Schinkel, and A. Sparreboom, "Contribution of organic cation transporter 2 (OCT2) to cisplatin-induced nephrotoxicity," *Clinical Pharmacology and Therapeutics*, vol. 86, no. 4, pp. 396–402, 2009.

Multiple Electrolyte and Metabolic Emergencies in a Single Patient

Caprice Cadacio,[1] Phuong-Thu Pham,[2] Ruchika Bhasin,[1] Anita Kamarzarian,[1] and Phuong-Chi Pham[1]

[1]Olive View-UCLA Medical Center, 14445 Olive View Drive, 2B-182, Sylmar, CA 91342, USA
[2]Ronald Reagan UCLA Medical Center, 200 Medical Plaza, Los Angeles, CA 90095, USA

Correspondence should be addressed to Phuong-Chi Pham; pctp@ucla.edu

Academic Editor: Yoshihide Fujigaki

While some electrolyte disturbances are immediately life-threatening and must be emergently treated, others may be delayed without immediate adverse consequences. We discuss a patient with alcoholism and diabetes mellitus type 2 who presented with volume depletion and multiple life-threatening electrolyte and metabolic derangements including severe hyponatremia (serum sodium concentration [S_{Na}] 107 mEq/L), hypophosphatemia ("undetectable," <1.0 mg/dL), and hypokalemia (2.2 mEq/L), moderate diabetic ketoacidosis ([DKA], pH 7.21, serum anion gap [S_{AG}] 37) and hypocalcemia (ionized calcium 4.0 mg/dL), mild hypomagnesemia (1.6 mg/dL), and electrocardiogram with prolonged QTc. Following two liters of normal saline and associated increase in S_{Na} by 4 mEq/L and serum osmolality by 2.4 mosm/Kg, renal service was consulted. We were challenged with minimizing the correction of S_{Na} (or effective serum osmolality) to avoid the osmotic demyelinating syndrome while replacing volume, potassium, phosphorus, calcium, and magnesium and concurrently treating DKA. Our management plan was further complicated by an episode of significant aquaresis. A stepwise approach was strategized to prioritize and correct all disturbances with considerations that the treatment of one condition could affect or directly worsen another. The current case demonstrates that a thorough understanding of electrolyte physiology is required in managing complex electrolyte disturbances to avoid disastrous outcomes.

1. Introduction

Managing various electrolyte and metabolic disturbances is generally a simple task for nephrologist. However, in complex cases, one must be vigilant of potentially life-threatening interactions among multiple simultaneous treatment plans and cautiously formulate a comprehensive treatment algorithm to prevent disastrous outcomes.

2. Case Report

Clinical History. A 33-year old male with known alcohol abuse and diabetes mellitus type 2 presented with a two-day history of nausea, vomiting, watery diarrhea, and light headedness. Patient denied fevers and chills but endorsed mild midepigastric dull pain and poor oral intake.

Physical Exam. Temperature was 37.2°C, blood pressure 114/85 mmHg, heart rate 109 beats per minute, respiratory rate 22 per minute, and oxygen saturation 98%. Patient was acutely ill-appearing, slow in verbal responses, alert and oriented, and free of stigmata of advanced liver disease. Oral mucosa was dry. Heart exam was notable for tachycardia. Lungs were clear bilaterally. Abdomen had hypoactive bowel sounds and mild midepigastric tenderness without guarding or rebound. Extremities were significant for a few ecchymoses. Neurological exam was nonfocal.

Initial Laboratory Data. Serum chemistries at presentation and hospital course are presented in Table 1. Most notable abnormalities included serum sodium (S_{Na}) 107 mEq/L, potassium (S_K) 2.8 mEq/L, total CO_2 12 mEq/L, glucose 331 mg/dL, and anion gap (S_{AG}) 37 mEq/L. Others were

TABLE 1: Clinical data.

Serum chemistry	Admission	After 2 L normal saline (renal service was consulted)	12 to 14 hours after admission	8 hours after insulin administration (30 to 32 hours after admission)	Discharge (12 days after admission)	Total amount replaced during hospitalization	Electrolyte concentrations of fluids administered
Sodium (mEq/L)	107	111	113	117	132	2 liters of normal saline at presentation	154 mEq/L
Potassium (mEq/L)	2.8	2.2	2.9 to 3.2	2.7	4.5	480 mEq KCl	100 mEq/L
Total CO_2 (mEq/L)	12	11	6	14	25	Corrected with insulin	—
Serum anion gap (mEq/L)	37	31	30	19	10	Corrected with insulin	—
Glucose (mg/dL)	331	248	250	108	217	Corrected with insulin	
Phosphorus (mg/dL)	Not done	<1.0	<1.0	<1.0	5.5	240 mmol KPO_4	15 mmol mixed in 200 mL normal saline or free water as needed to achieve sodium correction goal
Total calcium (mg/dL)	7.2	6.9	6.8	6.8	8.4	4 g calcium gluconate (9.3 mmol)	10% solution
Ionized calcium (mg/dL) [normal 4.6–5.4]	4.1	Not done	4.0	Not done	Not done		
Magnesium (mg/dL)	1.6	Not done	3.1	Not done	1.7	8 g	4 g mixed in 250 mL normal saline

mild transaminitis, mildly elevated lipase, and hemoglobin 12 g/dL.

Renal service was consulted following the increase in S_{Na} from 107 to 111 mEq/L over one hour (effective serum osmolality [S_{osm}] increase of 2.4 mosm/Kg) with the administration of two liters of normal saline.

Additional Investigations. Renal service requested STAT serum phosphorus and magnesium which resulted as <1 mg/dL and 1.6 mg/dL, respectively. *Other findings* were moderate serum ketones, lactic acid 1 mmol/L, and S_{osm} 255 mosm/Kg (serum osmolality gap 6 mosm/Kg).

Venous Blood Gas at Six Hours following Presentation to Emergency Department (ED). pH was 7.40, pCO$_2$ 17 mmHg, and HCO$_3$ 10 mEq/L (S_{AG} 31 mEq/L), and *at thirteen hours*, pH was 7.21, pCO$_2$ 14 mmHg, and HCO$_3$ 6 mEq/L (S_{AG} 30 mEq/L). *Urine studies* show osmolality 450 mosm/Kg, sodium 25 mEq/L, and potassium 25 mEq/L.

Diagnoses. Diagnoses included volume depletion, diabetic ketoacidosis (DKA) (with initial concurrent metabolic and respiratory alkaloses), severe hyponatremia, hypokalemia, hypophosphatemia, mild to moderate hypocalcemia, and mild hypomagnesemia.

Clinical Follow-Up. Patient received emergent potassium chloride (KCl) infusion via a central line (200 mL/hr of 100 mEq/L KCl solution [total 480 mEq KCl]) and potassium phosphate (KPO$_4$) (total 240 mmol), magnesium sulfate (total 8 g), and calcium gluconate (total 4 g) via peripheral lines. Oral thiamine and folate were given daily. All net fluid and effective solutes (sodium and potassium) were closely monitored. Calculations were performed (based on CurbsideConsultant.com) every six hours to readjust all fluid rates as needed to ensure a goal sodium correction rate of 4–6 mEq/L/24 hours. Treatment of DKA was intentionally delayed until S_K reached 2.9 mEq/L to avoid insulin-driven intracellular potassium uptake, exacerbation of hypokalemia, and precipitation of life-threatening arrhythmias. On hospital day 3, patient developed significant aquaresis with approximated free water clearance of 230 to 300 mL/hr (urine output of 3140 mL over 8 hour; urine studies: osmolality 186 mosm/Kg, sodium 13 mEq/L and potassium 16 mEq/L; S_{Na} 122 mEq/L). Two micrograms of desmopressin (DDAVP) and two liters of electrolyte-free water were given intravenously to slow urine output and prevent rapid overcorrection of S_{Na}, respectively. Over the first four hospital days, S_{Na} corrected at an average of 5 mEq/L/day. Additionally, patient also underwent upper gastroendoscopy for gastrointestinal bleed and nausea which revealed diffuse gastritis, presumed to be induced by his chronic alcohol consumption. His nausea resolved with proton pump inhibitor and supportive care.

3. Discussion

The current case was challenged by multiple concurrent problems including the need for continuing volume support and substantial administration of both KCl and KPO$_4$ without rapidly correcting hyponatremia, optimization of all treatable osmotic demyelinating syndrome (ODS) risks, correction of DKA to prevent respiratory decompensation without worsening the life-threatening hypokalemia, and intermittent infusions of magnesium sulfate and calcium gluconate while anticipating and managing any significant aquaresis without derailing the planned S_{Na} correction rate. The algorithm for the comprehensive management of current patient is summarized in Figure 1.

Hypokalemia was the most life-threatening and one of first abnormalities to be treated emergently. Etiologies likely included poor dietary intake, renal wasting given recent vomiting and poorly controlled diabetes, and diarrhea. Immediate life-saving interventions included KCl infusion via a central line along with instructions to avoid alkalinization or administration of insulin or glucose-containing fluids, the latter because of endogenous insulin secretion, and to prevent intracellular K$^+$-shift and worsening hypokalemia.

While aggressive potassium administration was critical, S_{Na} level had to be closely monitored because potassium effectively increases S_{Na}. Serum sodium concentration has been shown to be directly proportional to the sum of total exchangeable Na$^+$ and K$^+$ content [1]. Mechanisms whereby K$^+$ administration can raise S_{Na} include the following [2]:

(1) intracellular K$^+$-uptake induces an equivalent extracellular Na$^+$-movement and hence increased S_{Na},

(2) parallel K$^+$-Cl- intracellular uptake leads to increased intracellular osmolality which leads to intracellular free water shift and lower extracellular free water volume and hence increased S_{Na}, or

(3) intracellular K$^+$-uptake induces an equivalent extracellular H$^+$-movement to maintain electrical neutrality. While H$^+$ can bind to the extracellular buffer system and not perturb extracellular osmolality, the intracellular K$^+$-gained increases intracellular osmolality and hence intracellular free water shift. The lower extracellular free water volume increases extracellular S_{Na}.

Given the direct effect of K$^+$ on S_{Na}, both sources of potassium, KCl and KPO$_4$, were accounted for in all calculations for expected changes in S_{Na}. Further sodium administration was withheld because potassium supplement alone was determined to be sufficient to correct hyponatremia. Failure to recognize this fact and unwarranted infusion of sodium-containing solutions could have easily led to rapid hyponatremia overcorrection.

Hypophosphatemia may be a risk factor for ODS [3]. Our routine hyponatremia treatment protocol requested a STAT level, which was likely life-saving. Patient's severe hypophosphatemia could arise from poor oral intake, renal wasting, hypomagnesemia-induced skeletal resistance to parathyroid hormone (PTH 161 pg/mL, 1,25 (OH)$_2$ vitamin D 146 pg/mL), and possibly some degree of intracellular uptake associated with primary respiratory alkalosis at presentation [4]. The latter could induce intracellular alkalemia and associated increased glycolysis and intracellular uptake of phosphorus for ATP production [5]. Phosphorus replacement was given

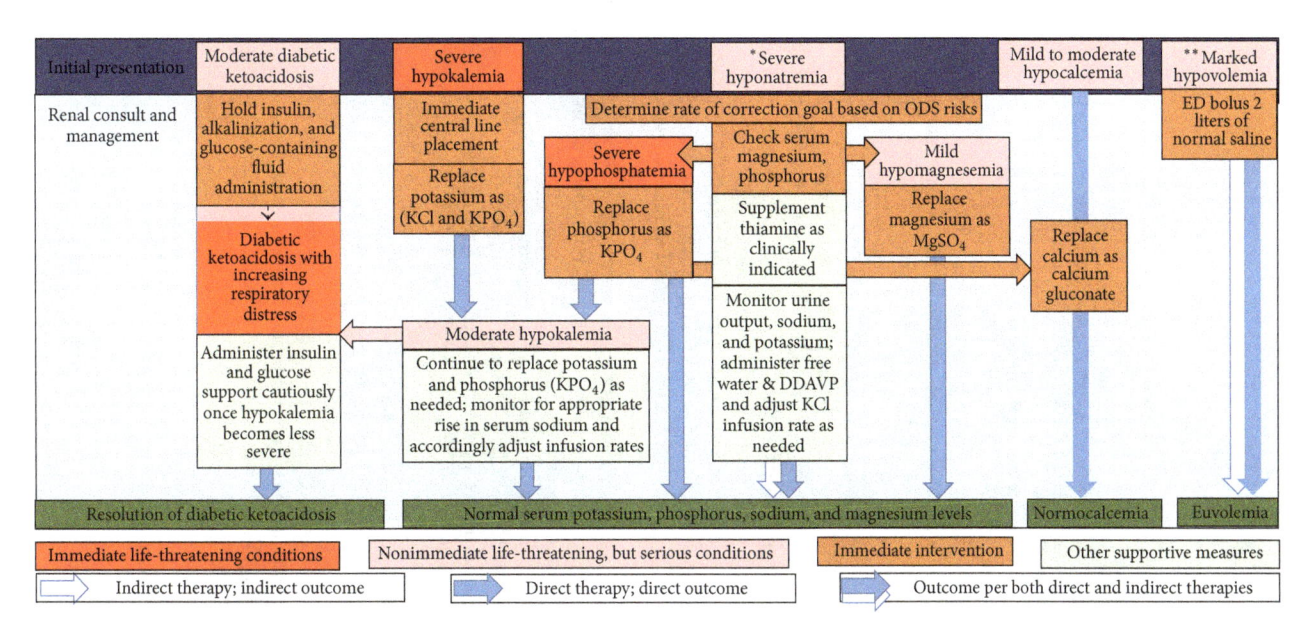

FIGURE 1: Algorithm for the treatment of multiple concurrent life-threatening disturbances. *For hyponatremia, correction resulted from both potassium infusion (indirect therapy) and fine adjustment with intermittent free water infusion and single administration of desmopressin (direct therapy) to achieve rate of correction goal during an episode of aquaresis. **For volume depletion, patient received two liters of normal saline on presentation to the emergency department (direct therapy) and continuous KCl infusion at 200 mL/hour (indirect therapy, i.e., the main purpose for KCl infusion, was potassium replacement, but patient benefited from the infusion as maintenance intravenous fluid) over the following 2 to 3 days while his oral intake was poor. ODS: osmotic demyelination syndrome; ED: emergency department; DDAVP: desmopressin.

emergently to avoid respiratory and cardiac arrest among other potential serious complications.

Volume depletion is typically managed with normal saline (NS), but not in current case. Patient received predominantly K^+-containing fluids (200 mL/hour of 100 mEq/L KCl solution and 25 to 50 mL/hour of KPO_4 solution [15 mmol KPO_4 mixed in 200 mL of either normal saline or sterile water as indicated by S_{Na}]). Since K^+ is an effective solute, either K^+ or Na^+-containing solutions that are relatively isotonic to patient's effective osmolality will effectively expand intravascular volume. With the exception of two liters of NS given in the ED, patient's total body volume was repleted and maintained with the infusion of K^+-containing fluids intended for potassium and phosphorus repletion. Failure to recognize the volume expansion capacity of relatively isotonic KCl-containing fluid and unwarranted infusion of NS for the sole purpose of volume support would have complicated the treatment of hyponatremia. Additionally, high volume infusions of multiple fluids would have led to excess urinary loss of ketone bodies necessary for bicarbonate production with insulin administration [6].

Hypocalcemia was likely due to poor nutrition, malabsorption, and hypomagnesemia-induced hypoparathyroidism [7, 8]. Given prolonged QTc, patient received low dose calcium gluconate intravenously following the initiation of KPO_4 administration to avoid any potential calcium-induced worsening of severe hypophosphatemia via calcium phosphate precipitation.

Diabetic ketoacidosis was potentially life-threatening, but not the most serious derangement. Insulin administration was intentionally delayed to avoid worsening of hypokalemia.

Patient's respiratory status, however, was closely monitored. Once S_K reached 2.9 mEq/L, insulin was cautiously given to avoid respiratory failure as patient exerted high work of breathing to compensate for the metabolic acidosis. Within 12 hours of insulin administration, S_{AG}, likely all reflecting ketone bodies, decreased from 30 mEq/L to 19 mEq/L with a parallel increase in total CO_2 from 6 to 14 mEq/L. The rapid inverse change in S_{AG} and total CO_2 demonstrates perfectly how *sufficient* fluid resuscitation, *not excessive* fluid administration with resultant urinary loss of serum ketone bodies, can allow for preservation of serum ketone bodies, where rapid hepatic conversion to bicarbonate occurs with insulin administration [6]. Patient's respiratory status also improved significantly with correction of metabolic acidosis.

Hyponatremia was likely multifactorial and includes continuing free water intake in the presence of enhanced secretion of antidiuretic hormone (ADH) with volume depletion and/or inappropriate ADH secretion in the setting of nausea, "beer potomania," and small degree of hyperglycemia-induced extracellular free water shift. The major goal in hyponatremia correction is ODS prevention. This requires both setting an appropriate correction goal and recognizing and optimizing any concurrent factors that could potentiate the risk of developing ODS [3, 9]. The correction goal was determined to be 4 to a maximum of 6 mEq/L/day because of patient's ODS risks including severe hyponatremia, hypokalemia, alcoholism, hypophosphatemia, hypomagnesemia, glucose intolerance, and presumed thiamine deficiency [3, 9]. Routine assessment of reversible ODS risk factors is warranted because electrolytes such as phosphorus and magnesium are not routinely measured at many institutions, including our own (Table 2).

TABLE 2: Teaching points box.

General teaching points	Comments pertinent to current case
Treatment of one electrolyte or metabolic abnormality can critically worsen another. In a patient with multiple disturbances, a comprehensive management plan must *prioritize* the most to least life-threatening disturbance and treat accordingly. Additionally, consideration must be made for all possible *treatment interactions*, particularly when the treatment of a less critical problem can exacerbate a life-threatening condition	(i) Hypokalemia and hypophosphatemia were the two most life-threatening conditions in current patient. Since the treatment of diabetic ketoacidosis (DKA) with insulin with or without glucose support could have exacerbated the severe hypokalemia and precipitate cardiac arrest, such treatment was intentionally delayed. Aggressive potassium replacement with both KCl and KPO_4 to achieve a safer serum potassium level was done PRIOR to the treatment of DKA
Comprehensive protocol for the management of hyponatremia: (i) Determine osmotic demyelination risks (ODS) and appropriate rate of correction (ii) Assess and treat all correctable ODS risks (hypokalemia, hypomagnesemia, hypophosphatemia, altered glucose metabolism, and clinical need for thiamine) (iii) Understand that potassium can increase serum sodium exactly as if the same amount of sodium is being administered (iv) Monitor urine output and its content of sodium and potassium for any possible aquaretic phase	(i) While hyponatremia was being corrected with KCl and KPO_4 infusions, the immediate plan to monitor and correct factors [hypophosphatemia and hypomagnesemia] associated with high ODS risks led to the prompt recognition of severe and life-threatening hypophosphatemia (ii) In addition to the correction of concurrent electrolyte disturbances, thiamine supplementation should be considered in patients with malnutrition or alcoholism as thiamine deficiency has been implicated in increasing the risk for ODS (iii) Current patient's serum sodium concentration improved as planned with only potassium-containing fluids (iv) Aggressive monitoring of both urine output and content of effective electrolytes (sodium and potassium) allows for prompt intervention and thus prevention of rapid over correction of hyponatremia
KCl is as effective as NaCl solution as a volume expander and may be preferred or even required when potassium is critically deficient	(i) The substitution of KCl for NaCl solution for volume expansion can only be given in cases of severe hypokalemia. The rate and concentration of the KCl solution MUST be adjusted to assure a safe rate of increase in serum sodium (ii) Note that a maximum of 20 mEq of KCl may be continuously infused per hour through a central venous catheter
Respiratory hyperventilation and metabolic acidosis associated with diabetic ketoacidosis alone may be easily and promptly reversed with the administration of insulin. Persistent abnormalities should thus prompt an evaluation for other underlying etiologies	(i) Following the administration of insulin, our patient's respiratory status improved from a respiratory rate up to mid-30's breaths per minute down to mid-20's within 24 hours (ii) Similarly, patient's serum total CO_2 improved from 6 to 14 mEq/L within 8 hours (iii) Note, however, close monitoring of potassium must be done following insulin and glucose support therapy. With the initiation of insulin therapy, patient's serum potassium decreased from a high of 3.2 mEq/L to 2.7 mEq/L within 7 hours

In terms of actual hyponatremia correction, the infusion of potassium-containing solutions alone was sufficient. Patient's S_{Na} improved daily at expected rates from the predominant infusions of KCl and KPO_4 solutions (Table 1). Additionally, as per our routine hyponatremia management protocol, monitoring of urine output, sodium, and potassium was done at regular intervals. Patient indeed developed a significant aquaretic phase when electrolyte-free water and DDAVP were promptly given to divert hyponatremia overcorrection. Significant aquaresis during the treatment of hyponatremia may occur in multiple clinical settings and generally stems from the rapid cessation of ADH secretion following the correction of underlying stimuli that induced ADH secretion like correction of volume depletion, nausea, pain, among others [10]. In current case, the aquaretic phase was likely due to the correction of volume depletion and nausea.

Hypomagnesemia was likely due to poor oral intake, gastrointestinal malabsorption, and possibly urinary loss associated with diabetes mellitus [11]. Patient was monitored closely for hypomagnesemia and treated as needed.

Thiamine was also supplemented given history of alcoholism to minimize ODS risk [4].

Respiratory and metabolic alkalosis on presentation were likely due to pain/anxiety and volume depletion, respectively. Both conditions resolved with comprehensive supportive care.

4. Conclusions

We present a complex case involving multiple life-threatening electrolyte and metabolic disturbances which demonstrates the critical need for prioritization for the treatment of each abnormality and considerations for all interactions among multiple concurrent treatment plans.

Aggressive potassium replacement prior to the administration of insulin for the DKA is vital to prevent worsening of life-threatening hypokalemia.

Both sodium and potassium are equivalent effective solutes. Hyponatremia can be corrected with the predominant infusion of potassium. Similarly, volume expansion with relatively isotonic KCl solution is as effective as NaCl in current case of severe hypokalemia.

The treatment of hyponatremia must incorporate correction rate, monitoring, and treatment of all factors (potassium, phosphorus, magnesium, glucose, and thiamine) associated with increased ODS risks. Additionally, during the treatment of hyponatremia, transient aquaresis may arise for various reasons and must be anticipated and immediately treated to avoid rapid overcorrection [11].

Insulin effectively converts ketone bodies to bicarbonate if the former have not been lost in the urine with excessive fluid administration.

Despite multiple life-threatening electrolyte and metabolic disturbances, patient was discharged within twelve days in good condition and continued to do well at one month follow-up.

Teaching points are summarized in Table 2.

References

[1] I. S. Edelman, J. Leibman, M. P. O'Meara, and L. W. Birkenfeld, "Interrelations between serum sodium concentration, serum osmolarity and total exchangeable sodium, total exchangeable potassium and total body water," *The Journal of Clinical Investigation*, vol. 37, no. 9, pp. 1236–1256, 1958.

[2] B. D. Rose, Ed., *Clinical Physiology of Acid-Base and Electrolyte Disorders*, McGraw-Hill, New York, NY, USA, 4th edition, 1994.

[3] P.-M. T. Pham, P.-A. T. Pham, S. V. Pham, P.-T. T. Pham, P.-T. T. Pham, and P.-C. T. Pham, "Correction of hyponatremia and osmotic demyelinating syndrome: have we neglected to think intracellularly?" *Clinical and Experimental Nephrology*, vol. 19, no. 3, pp. 489–495, 2015.

[4] J. J. Freitag, K. J. Martin, M. B. Conrades et al., "Evidence for skeletal resistance to parathyroid hormone in magnesium deficiency. Studies in isolated perfused bone," *Journal of Clinical Investigation*, vol. 64, no. 5, pp. 1238–1244, 1979.

[5] N. Brautbar, H. Leibovici, and S. G. Massry, "On the mechanism of hypophosphatemia during acute hyperventilation: evidence for increased muscle glycolysis," *Mineral and Electrolyte Metabolism*, vol. 9, no. 1, pp. 45–50, 1983.

[6] P. Felig, "Diabetic ketoacidosis," *New England Journal of Medicine*, vol. 290, no. 24, pp. 1360–1363, 1974.

[7] L. R. Chase and E. Slatopolsky, "Secretion and metabolic efficacy of parathyroid hormone in patients with severe hypomagnesemia," *Journal of Clinical Endocrinology and Metabolism*, vol. 38, no. 3, pp. 363–371, 1974.

[8] R. K. Rude, S. B. Oldham, and F. R. Singer, "Functional hypoparathyroidism and parathyroid hormone end–organ resistance in human magnesium deficiency," *Clinical Endocrinology*, vol. 5, no. 3, pp. 209–224, 1976.

[9] J. G. Verbalis, S. R. Goldsmith, A. Greenberg et al., "Diagnosis, evaluation, and treatment of hyponatremia: expert panel recommendations," *The American Journal of Medicine*, vol. 126, no. 10, supplement 1, pp. S1–S42, 2013.

[10] P. C. Pham, P. V. Chen, and P. T. Pham, "Overcorrection of hyponatremia: where do we go wrong?" *American Journal of Kidney Diseases*, vol. 36, no. 2, article no. E12, 2000.

[11] P.-C. T. Pham, P.-M. T. Pham, S. V. Pham, J. M. Miller, and P.-T. T. Pham, "Hypomagnesemia in patients with type 2 diabetes," *Clinical Journal of the American Society of Nephrology*, vol. 2, no. 2, pp. 366–373, 2007.

Bilateral Testicular Infarction from IgA Vasculitis of the Spermatic Cords

Mazen Toushan,[1] Ashka Atodaria,[2] Stephen D. Lynch,[2] Hassan D. Kanaan,[1] Limin Yu,[1] Mitual B. Amin,[1] Mamon Tahhan,[2] Ping L. Zhang,[1] Paul S. Kellerman,[3] and Abhishek Swami[3]

[1]Division of Anatomic Pathology, Department of Pathology, Beaumont Health, Royal Oak, MI, USA
[2]Department of Internal Medicine, Beaumont Health, Royal Oak, MI, USA
[3]Division of Nephrology, Department of Internal Medicine, Beaumont Health, Royal Oak, MI, USA

Correspondence should be addressed to Abhishek Swami; abhishek.swami@beaumont.edu

Academic Editor: Ze'ev Korzets

A 51-year-old man with type 2 diabetes mellitus and chronic obstructive pulmonary disease presented to the emergency room with increasing bilateral leg pain, rash, and scrotal swelling with pain. Skin biopsy from his thigh revealed IgA-associated vasculitis. Due to hematuria, a renal biopsy was performed and showed an IgA glomerulonephritis with focal fibrinoid necrosis and neutrophil accumulation. Bilateral orchiectomies were performed in two separate procedures ten and thirteen days after the renal biopsy, as a result of uncontrolled abscess formation in testicles. Microscopically, both testicles revealed large abscess formation destroying almost the entire testicular parenchyma without tumor cells. Spermatic cord margins were further scrutinized microscopically to show bilateral vasculitis in many small size vessels, confirmed by positive endothelial staining for IgA. Some of the affected arteries revealed central organizing thrombi with recanalization features, highly suggestive of vasculitis-associated thrombi formation, resulting in testicular ischemic infarction and abscess formation. We conclude that this adult patient developed a severe form of Henoch-Schönlein purpura, with vasculitis affecting multiple organs, including the most serious and unusual complication of bilateral testicular infarction.

1. Introduction

Henoch-Schönlein purpura (HSP) is a systematic vasculitis presenting primarily in children, but less so in adults, often resulting in IgA-associated vasculitis in skin and IgA nephritis [1, 2]. HSP can also present with arthritis, gastrointestinal bleeding, and orchitis with symptoms of testicular pain and swelling in up to 20% of affected boys clinically [3–9], but there has been no pathologically proven IgA-associated vasculitis of the testicles documented even in patients with testicular pain. In addition, IgA-associated orchitis has not been previously described in adults. We report an unusual case in a 51-year-old man who developed IgA-associated vasculitis involving the skin, kidneys, and bilateral spermatic cords resulting in bilateral testicular infarction. This is the first report of histologically proven IgA-associated orchitis in the literature.

2. Case Presentation

A 51-year-old male with uncontrolled diabetes (type II) presented to the hospital with severe lower extremity and scrotal edema, associated with pain, and extremity rash. The rash began 3 weeks prior to presentation and involved his lower abdomen, bilateral lower extremities, and scrotum. He reported intermittent painful edema of his legs and scrotum for the past year which had been attributed to neuropathic pain related to uncontrolled diabetes and chronic venous stasis. Patient also reported fatigue, malaise, 50-pound weight loss over the past one year, intermittent bloody bowel movements, and dysuria but denied any fevers, chills, hematuria, history of sexually transmitted infections, HIV, or malignancy.

Two weeks prior to presentation at our hospital, the patient had presented to an outside hospital with syncope and was found to be hypoglycemic. Biopsy of the rash from his calf was positive for leukocytoclastic vasculitis. Autoimmune workup was negative except for elevated C-reactive protein (CRP). Bilateral lower extremity Doppler study was negative for thromboembolism. Patient was treated with Vancomycin followed by clindamycin for cellulitis. He left against medical advice before presenting to our hospital.

The patient's past medical history was positive for uncontrolled diabetes type II with peripheral neuropathy, peripheral vascular disease with chronic lower extremity ulcers, chronic obstructive pulmonary disease, and opioid dependence. His past surgeries included amputation of a digit on his right hand due to osteomyelitis with gangrene and lumbar spinal fusion. Family history was positive for breast cancer in his sister. There was no family history of autoimmune disease. He is a current smoker with a 40-pack-year history and denied any current alcohol or drug use. His medications included basal-bolus insulin, glipizide 10 mg twice daily, furosemide 40 mg twice daily, pregabalin, and methadone maintenance.

At presentation, the patient was found to be afebrile with blood pressure of 151/105 mmHg, heart rate of 88/per minute, respiratory rate of 20/per minute, SpO2 of 94%, and BMI of 22.8. His laboratory indices are presented in Table 1. The patient appeared to be cachectic with peripheral wasting. Exam revealed tachycardia with regular rhythm and no murmurs. Lung exam revealed wheezes bilaterally. His abdomen was distended and tender to palpation. There was tender scrotal edema as well as severe pitting edema of his lower extremities. He had a diffuse purpuric rash over his lower extremities, genitalia, and abdomen. Smaller petechiae were found on his hands and arms. He also had multiple healing lesions on his legs, a chronic healing ulcer under the left heel, and a large ulcer with eschar without drainage or odor on the right lower leg.

Records from his previous admission showed elevated CRP serology, and autoimmune work was negative. A skin biopsy of the lower extremity rash done at an outside hospital was positive for leukocytoclastic vasculitis.

His chest X-ray was negative and ECG was unremarkable. Scrotal ultrasound showed bilateral wall edema with inguinal lymphadenopathy. CT of the abdomen and pelvis also showed anasarca with bilateral inguinal and para-aortic and external iliac lymphadenopathy. CT and ultrasound of the kidneys were unremarkable. Lower extremity Doppler was negative for deep vein thrombosis.

Repeat rheumatological workup revealed positive ANA with a titer of 1:320 and negative anti-dsDNA, Smith, RNP, Sjogren SSA, and SSB. C3 and C4 levels were normal. Serum immunoglobulins revealed elevated IgA level at 431 mg/dL with normal IgG and IgM. Serum protein electrophoresis showed elevated kappa and lambda light chains and low albumin with elevated alpha 1 and beta globulins, suggestive of active inflammation. Blood, urine, and stool cultures were negative. The patient tested positive for *C. difficile* stool antigen. EGD and colonoscopy were performed which were negative for malignancy and hemolytic workup was negative.

Patient was initially started on IV Vancomycin for sepsis, scrotal elevation, glucose control with basal-bolus insulin, and local wound management. Vancomycin was held upon negative cultures. Patient was started on intravenous solumedrol 30 mg every 8 hours for vasculitis. Pain control with pregabalin, patient controlled analgesia (PCA) pump, and total parenteral nutrition (TPN) were initiated.

The patient's purpuric rash improved significantly and rapidly with intravenous solumedrol, but his scrotal pain and edema persisted and patient developed painful penile ulcer. A repeat skin biopsy was performed from his left thigh which showed leukocytoclastic vasculitis. Immunofluorescence was positive for IgA, IgM, and C3 in the vessel wall of the superficial dermis, consistent with IgA-associated leukocytoclastic vasculitis (Figures 1(a) and 1(b)).

His serum creatinine levels were at 0.83 to 1.1 mg/dL, but his urine analysis revealed 3+ blood and 2-3+ protein, and the protein/creatinine ratio was 1.6. A subsequent 24-hour urine protein was 2338 mg/24 hours. He was evaluated by nephrologist and a renal biopsy was performed. Light microscopy revealed two cores of renal tissue. Eleven glomeruli were identified without evidence of diffuse proliferation, crescents, and global or segmental sclerosis. Many of the glomeruli showed an increase in mesangial cellularity with focal neutrophilic infiltration as well as fibrinoid necrosis. The glomerular basement membrane showed no significant microscopic abnormality (Figure 1(c)). Masson trichrome stain revealed minimal to mild interstitial fibrosis. The blood vessels were mildly thickened without vasculitis or thrombi. Immunofluorescence study showed 3+ positive granular IgA staining in the mesangial and peripheral loop of the glomeruli (Figure 1(d)). There was mesangial and peripheral granular staining for IgM at 1+, C3 at 1+, kappa at 1+, and lambda at 2+, while IgG and C1q stained negatively in the glomeruli. Ultrastructurally, there was focal effacement of foot processes. The basement membranes were slightly thickened. Scattered immune complex deposits were identified in the mesangial areas but not in subendothelial spaces or subepithelial areas. The overall findings supported a diagnosis of IgA glomerulonephritis. Because there were no history of staphylococcal infection and no diffuse proliferative pattern in the glomeruli, with no "humps" identified at subepithelial spaces, a potential differential diagnosis of IgA dominant postinfectious glomerulonephritis was excluded [10, 11].

Repeat ultrasound of the scrotum with Doppler was done due to persistent scrotal pain, which revealed hypoperfusion of the left testicle without evidence of torsion. Left orchiectomy was performed 3 weeks after admission. Grossly the cut surface of the testicle revealed the entire testicular parenchyma to be brown-red, partially liquefied, and necrotic. In the area of the epididymis and rete testes there was yellow-green soft discoloration. The microscopy sections revealed testicular infarction with testicular/paratesticular abscess that involved the epididymis and spermatic cord.

Pain in his right testicle persisted, and, four days later, orchiectomy of the right testicle was also performed. Both gross and microscopic findings in the right testicle were similar to those in the left orchiectomy specimen. Testicular abscess was identified (Figure 1(e)). Spermatic cord margins from bilateral orchiectomy specimens were further analyzed to show diffuse vasculitis in small arteries with scattered

Table 1: Patient's laboratory values upon admission.

Component	Value	Ref range & units
Complete blood count with differential		
WBC	5.7	3.5–10.1 bil/L
RBC	3.56 (L)	4.31–5.48 tril/L
Hemoglobin	9.5 (L)	13.5–17.0 g/dL
Hematocrit	32.0 (L)	40.1–50.1%
MCV	90	80–100 fL
MCH	27 (L)	28–33 pg
RDW CV	17 (H)	12–15%
Platelets	395	150–400 bil/L
Neutrophils	4.4	1.6–7.2 bil/L
Lymphocytes	0.7 (L)	1.1–4.0 bil/L
Monocytes	0.4	0.0–0.9 bil/L
Immature granulocytes	0.07 (H)	0.00–0.04 bil/L
Urine analysis		
Color	Yellow	
Clarity	Clear	
Glucose	+3	Negative
Protein	+2	Negative
Blood	trace	Negative
Ketones	negative	Negative
RBCs	4–10/hpf	0–3/hpf
WBCs	5–10/hpf	0–5/hpf
Casts, hyaline	0–2/lpf	0–2/lpf
Urine protein to creatinine ratio	1.6	0–0.2
Blood chemistries		
Sodium	127 (L)	135–145 mmol/L
Potassium	6.0 (H)	3.5–5.2 mmol/L
Chloride	96 (L)	98–110 mmol/L
Carbon dioxide (CO2)	22	22–32 mmol/L
Anion gap	9	5–17
Glucose	700 (HH)	60–99 mg/dL
Blood urea nitrogen (BUN)	33 (H)	8–22 mg/dL
Creatinine	1.18	0.60–1.40 mg/dL
Calcium	7.0 (L)	8.4–10.4 mg/dL
Protein total	5.2 (L)	6.4–8.6 g/dL
Albumin	1.7 (L)	3.5–5.1 g/dL
Globulin	3.5	2.2–4.0 g/dL
Albumin/globulin ratio	0.5	
Alkaline phosphatase (ALP)	71	30–110 U/L
Aspartate aminotransferase (AST)	38 (H)	10–37 U/L
Alanine aminotransferase (ALT)	23	9–47 U/L
Bilirubin total	0.9	0.3–1.2 mg/dL
Bilirubin direct	0.3	0–0.3 mg/dL
GFR non-African American	71	>59 mL/min/1.73 m2
GFR African American	82	>59 mL/min/1.73 m2
ESR	46 (H)	0–15 mm/hr
Lactic acid	3.1	0.5–2.2 mmol/L
Lipase	10	7–60 U/L
Beta hydroxybutyrate	0.10	0.02–0.27 mmol/L
BNP	51	0–100 pg/mL

(a) Skin biopsy

(b) IgA positive in vessels and epithelium

(c) Renal biopsy

(d) IgA positive in glomerulus

(e) Spermatic cord margin

(f) Vasculitis in spermatic cord

(g) Organizing thrombosis

(h) Positive IgA staining in small arteries

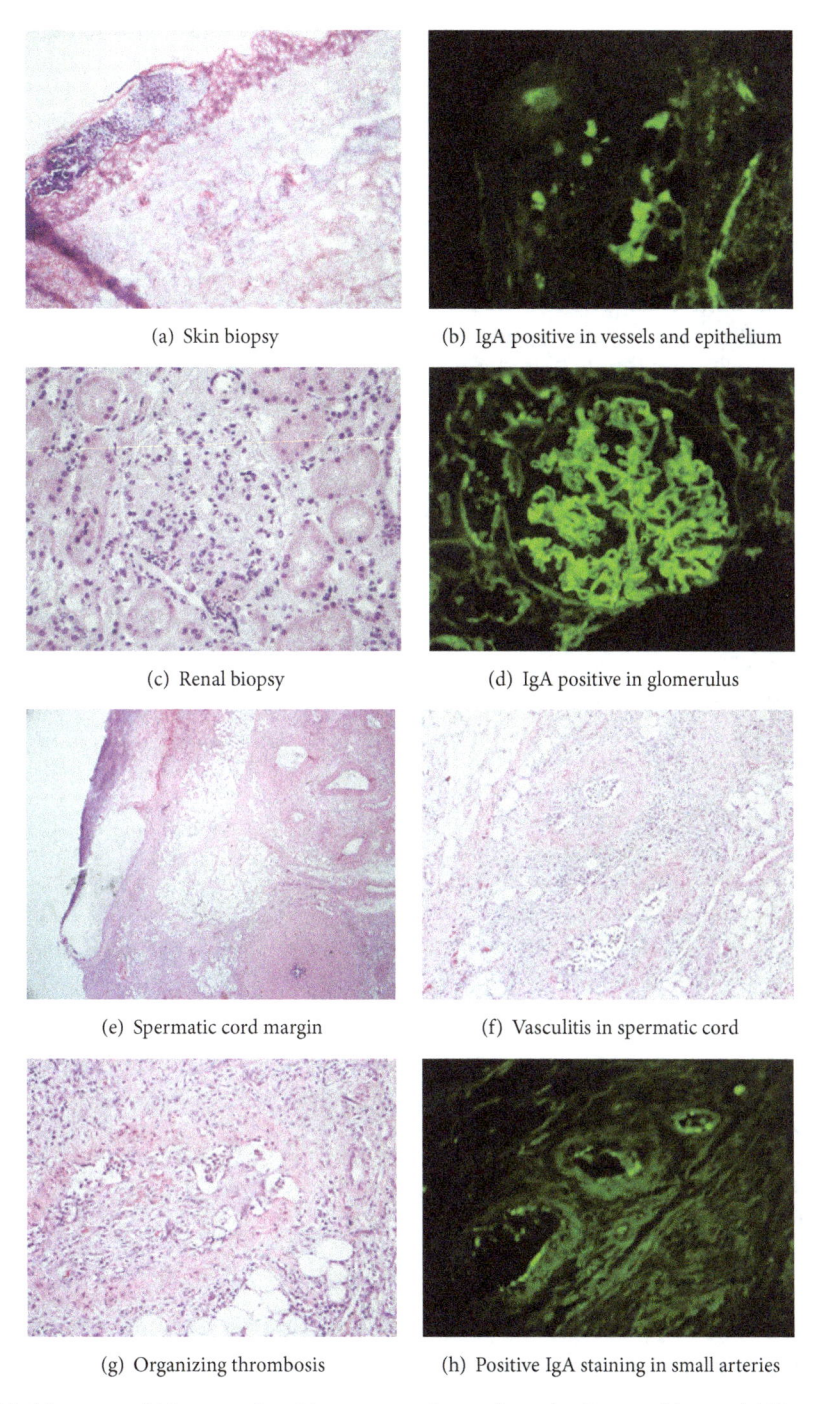

FIGURE 1: Evaluation of skin biopsy, renal biopsy, and orchiectomy specimens from the 51-year-old man. (a) Hematoxylin and eosin stained section revealed surface ulceration in the skin. (b) IgA immunofluorescence was positive in epidermis and vessels of dermis. (c) Hematoxylin and eosin stained section revealed mesangial expansion with focal neutrophil aggregation in the glomerulus. (d) IgA immunofluorescence was positive mainly in the mesangium and some along the glomerular capillary loops. (magnifications ×400 in (a)–(d)). (e) A low power view (×40) revealed the unremarkable vas deferens at the right lower corner and necrosis and abscess in the testicular parenchyma at the left upper corner. (f) Vasculitis was seen in multiple small arteries of spermatic cord at medium power view (×200). (g) High power view (×400) revealed organizing thrombus in a small artery causing nearly total occlusion of the vessel in the spermatic cord. (h) IgA immunofluorescence (×200) was positive (green granular staining) at the endothelium of multiple inflamed small arteries. Hematoxylin and eosin stains were performed in (e)–(g).

organizing thrombi in some (Figures 1(f) and 1(g)). Paraffin embedded sections of bilateral spermatic cords were digested and stained for IgA by direct immunofluorescent method (as previously reported) [12]. The immunofluorescent section revealed strongly positive IgA staining along the endothelium of inflamed small arteries (Figure 1(h)), confirming the IgA vasculitis of the spermatic cords as the cause of the testicular ischemic infarction. His scrotal edema gradually improved with wound care and nutritional support. In addition to steroids, dapsone was started per Rheumatology.

His hospital course was complicated by persistent diarrhea, drug-seeking behavior, bacteremia, persistent hyperglycemia, and ischemia of multiple digits requiring amputations. His rash did not recur while on the steroids, and he was discharged to a long-term acute care facility with close follow-up.

3. Discussion

Scrotal manifestations of HSP are overwhelmingly described in pediatric populations, based solely on clinical evaluations [3–9]. No histologically proven cases of IgA-associated orchitis have been reported in any pediatric study. Furthermore scrotal disease due to IgA vasculitis is easily missed or misdiagnosed due to low level of suspicion and its propensity to manifest later in the course of disease, sometimes after initial signs and symptoms of HSP have resolved. HSP in adults is usually associated with worse outcomes compared to children [1, 2]. It is unclear whether IgA-associated orchitis in adults would have worse outcomes compared to children. In this patient the involvement was severe leading to tissue necrosis and required bilateral orchiectomies despite high dose steroid therapy. Due to initial lack of awareness the etiology for the patient's scrotum swelling had remained uncertain and was felt to be part of generalized edema and nephrotic syndrome. Patient developed *Klebsiella* bacteremia and the source of this bacteremia was felt to be from extremity ulcers and soft tissue infections. Later it was realized only after orchiectomy that the source of bacteremia was most likely from testicular infarction.

During the examination of the spermatic cords, vasculitis, characterized by edematous changes in vessel walls and infiltration of inflammatory cells, was seen in small arteries with occasional organizing thrombi. In addition, we reprocessed the paraffin embedded tissue for immunofluorescent staining of IgA, and IgA positivity was only present along endothelium of inflamed vessels, confirming that the IgA-associated vasculitis was the etiology causing thrombotic obstruction in the vessels with subsequent ischemic pain in the scrotum, testicular infarction, abscess formation, and possible overgrowth of bacteria.

In summary, this 51-year-old male patient developed a systemic IgA vasculitis involving the skin of the extremities, kidneys, and bilateral testicles with the most serious complication of testicular infarctions and subsequent abscess formation. This is the first report of histologically proven IgA-associated orchitis in the literature. This case illustrates the need for low threshold of suspicion for vasculitic scrotal involvement when caring for adult patients with HSP who develop scrotal pain and swelling. Scrotal involvement may be more prevalent than reported. Genital examination is often not performed; also scrotal pain may be mislabeled, which may lead to diagnosis being missed. Genital examination should be routinely carried out in these patients for early detection of scrotal involvement. Scrotal swelling, pain, and tenderness should prompt immediate diagnostic evaluation and urology consultation where needed.

References

[1] R. Blanco, V. M. Martinez-Taboada, V. Rodriguez-Valverde et al., "Henoch-Schonlein purpura in adulthood and childhood: two different expressions of the same syndrome," *Arthritis Rheum*, vol. 40, no. 5, pp. 859–864, 1997.

[2] P. S. Kellerman, "Henoch-Schönlein Purpura in Adults," *American Journal of Kidney Diseases*, vol. 48, no. 6, pp. 1009–1016, 2006.

[3] F. T. Saulsbury, "Henoch-Schönlein purpura in children. Report of 100 patients and review of the literature," *Medicine*, vol. 78, no. 6, pp. 395–409, 1999.

[4] A. A. Lardhi, "Henoch-Schonlein purpura in children from the eastern province of Saudi Arabia," *Saudi Med*, vol. 33, no. 9, pp. 973–978, 2012.

[5] K. Masarweh, Y. Horovitz, A. Avital, and R. Spiegel, "Establishing hospital admission criteria of pediatric Henoch-Schonlein purpura," *Rheumatology International*, vol. 34, no. 11, pp. 1497–1503, 2014.

[6] P. Davol, J. Mowad, and C. M. Mowad, "Henoch-Schonlein purpura presenting with orchitis: a case report and review of the literature," *Cutis*, vol. 77, pp. 89–92, 2006.

[7] T.-S. Ha and J.-S. Lee, "Scrotal involvement in childhood Henoch-Schönlein purpura," *Acta Paediatrica*, vol. 96, no. 4, pp. 552–555, 2007.

[8] LH. Huang, CY. Yeung, SD. Shyur, HC. Lee, FY. Huang, and NL. Wang, "Diagnosis of Henoch-Schonlein purpura by sonography and radionuclear scanning in a child presenting with bilateral acute scrotum," *J Microbiol Immunol Infect*, vol. 37, no. 3, 2004.

[9] O. Jauhola, J. Ronkainen, O. Koskimies et al., "Clinical course of extrarenal symptoms in Henoch-Schönlein purpura: A 6-month prospective study," *Archives of Disease in Childhood*, vol. 95, no. 11, pp. 871–876, 2010.

[10] S. H. Nasr, G. S. Markowitz, M. B. Stokes, S. M. Said, A. M. Valeri, and V. D. D'Agati, "Acute postinfectious glomerulonephritis in the modern era: experience with 86 adults and review of the literature," *Medicine*, vol. 87, no. 1, pp. 21–32, 2008.

[11] S. H. Nasr and V. D. D'Agati, "IgA-dominant postinfectious glomerulonephritis: A New twist on an old disease," *Nephron Clinical Practice*, vol. 119, no. 1, pp. c18–c25, 2011.

[12] N. C. Messias, P. D. Walker, and C. P. Larsen, "Paraffin immunofluorescence in the renal pathology laboratory: More than a salvage technique," *Modern Pathology*, vol. 28, no. 6, pp. 854–860, 2015.

Acute Renal Failure due to a Tobramycin and Vancomycin Spacer in Revision Two-Staged Knee Arthroplasty

Ronak A. Patel, Hayden P. Baker, and Sara B. Smith

College of Medicine, University of Illinois at Chicago, Chicago, IL, USA

Correspondence should be addressed to Hayden P. Baker; baker66@uic.edu

Academic Editor: Anja Haase-Fielitz

Two-stage revision total knee arthroplasty (TKA) is the standard of care for prosthetic joint infections. The first stage involves removal of the infected prosthesis and placement of an antibiotic impregnated cement spacer; following a period ranging from 4 weeks to 6 months, the spacer is then removed and replaced with a permanent prosthesis. The advantage to this approach is that antibiotic impregnated spacers provide supratherapeutic levels in the joint without toxic accumulation in serum. However, it remains important for physicians and pharmacists to be aware of antibiotic associated complications in knee revisions. We present a case of a two-stage revision total knee arthroplasty in which a cement antibiotic spacer caused acute renal failure and ultimately resulted in persistent chronic kidney disease without hemodialysis at 2 months' follow-up. Our case reports the third highest serum tobramycin (13.7 mcg/ml) and second highest serum creatinine (8.62 mg/dl) for patients experiencing ARF due to an antibiotic spacer in two-stage revision TKA.

1. Introduction

Periprosthetic joint infections (PJI) are a common complication of arthroplasty, with an incidence of 1-3% [1, 2]. Typical treatment involves a two-staged revision total knee arthroplasty, whereby the infected prosthesis is removed and replaced with a temporary antibiotic impregnated spacer. Parenteral antibiotics are also administered in order to create supratherapeutic levels [3]. Following a period ranging from 4 weeks to 6 months, the spacer is removed and replaced with a permanent prosthesis [4–7]. Using this method, literature describes success in approximately 90% of patients, demonstrating the efficacy of the procedure [1, 5, 8]. However, complications may include acute kidney injury (AKI) and reinfection [1, 4–6].

Nephrotoxic antibiotics are mixed with bone cement in the creation of temporary spacers to treat PJI [5, 6]. As a result, multiple studies show that AKI during two-stage revision TKA is both a common and underreported complication, with an incidence of 4.8-26% [5, 6, 9]. The AKI is often mild and transient [5, 6]. However, there have been case reports and case series detailing progression of AKI to acute renal failure (ARF) requiring hemodialysis in the setting of a two-stage revision TKA [5]. Most cases resolve with kidney function returning to baseline [5]. We present a case of a tobramycin and vancomycin spacer causing ARF requiring hemodialysis with resultant Stage IV CKD at 2 months' follow-up. Our case reports the third highest serum tobramycin and second highest serum creatinine for patients experiencing ARF due to an antibiotic spacer in two-stage revision TKA.

2. Case Description

A 65-year-old male with a history of multiple periprosthetic infections of the left knee presented for the first stage of his revision TKA. His past medical history included diabetes, obstructive sleep apnea, congestive heart failure, and gastroesophageal reflux disease. Previous surgeries included a lumbar spinal fusion and multiple failed revision two-stage TKAs to treat his periprosthetic infection. Medications at the time included furosemide, gabapentin, carvedilol, lansoprazole, docusate, and enalapril. There was no documented history of allergies or complications with anesthesia.

On the operative day, the patient was brought to the operating room and cephalexin 2 mg was administered. Upon

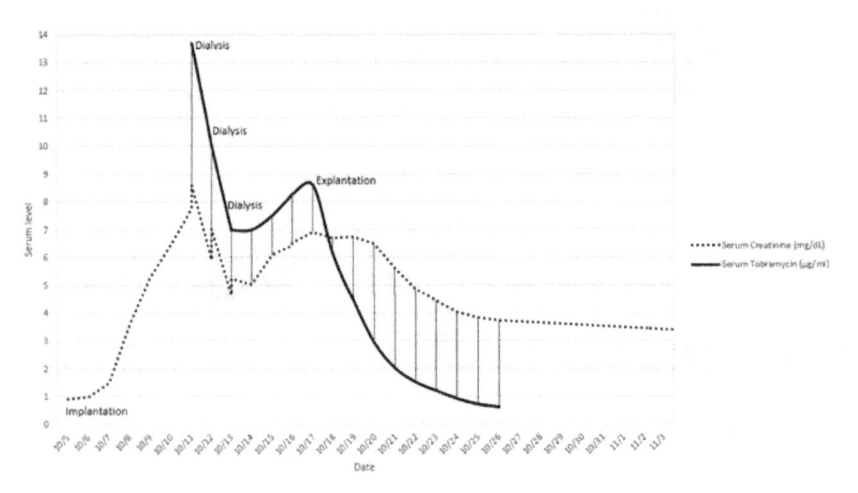

FIGURE 1: *Serum Tobramycin and Creatinine Levels.* Serum tobramycin and creatinine levels trended from surgical implantation of the antibiotic spacer on 10/5, to 3 sessions of dialysis on 10/11, 10/12, and 10/13, to explanation and replacement with a 4 g cephazolin spacer on 10/17.

opening the left knee, cloudy fluid was appreciated and sent for culture and sensitivities. Both the infected cement spacers on the femur and tibia were debrided and irrigated. Tobramycin and vancomycin cement mixture formed the new spacer. A total of 5 bags of Simplex P (Stryker, Mahwah, NJ) cement were mixed with 26.4 g of tobramycin and 9 g of vancomycin. Intraoperatively, records showed brief episodes of hypotension on induction requiring 3 pressors. For the duration of the case, he required intermittent pressure support with a total of phenylephrine 360 mcg, epinephrine 30 mcg, and norepinephrine 36 mcg. He was extubated and transferred to the recovery room in stable condition. His medications postoperatively included celecoxib 200 mg BID and aspirin 325 mg BID, and he was continued on lansoprazole.

Vancomycin 2 g IV every 12 hours and piperacillin-tazobactam 3.375 g IV every 6 hours were started. Cultures revealed the joint to be infected with *Corynebacterium striatum*, and as a result IV piperacillin-tazobactam was discontinued.

On postoperative day (POD) 2, he developed a nonoliguric AKI from a baseline creatinine of 0.9 mg/dl to 1.5 mg/dl. As the AKI progressed, on subsequent days, the consulting nephrology team speculated that the etiology was multifactorial, likely secondary to ATN from intraoperative hypotension and nephrotoxic medication side effects from his celecoxib, lansoprazole, or IV vancomycin. On POD 3, a random vancomycin level was drawn at 53.8 mcg/ml with subsequent discontinuation of IV vancomycin and celecoxib. He was then started on doxycycline 100 mg BID. On POD 6, his AKI progressed to a peak creatinine of 8.62 mg/dl and hyperkalemia at 6.3 mmol/L with marked ECG changes prompting administration of calcium gluconate and kayexalate with emergent hemodialysis and ICU transfer. Tobramycin levels were drawn, and results showed 13.7 mcg/ml. Hemodialysis was repeated on POD 7 and 8 and tobramycin levels downtrended as seen in Figure 1. Following the 3 total sessions of hemodialysis, the patient was able to produce adequate volumes of urine, and hemodialysis was discontinued. Following the cessation of hemodialysis, tobramycin levels began to uptrend. At that time, the decision was made to explant the antibiotic impregnated spacer containing vancomycin and tobramycin.

The antibiotic spacer was subsequently explanted on POD 13 with a reimplantation of a spacer containing 4 g cefazolin. In the following days, he experienced a marked reduction in creatinine to 3.72 mg/dl and tobramycin level to 0.6 mcg/ml upon discharge. At two months' follow-up, his serum creatinine downtrended and stabilized to 2.28 mg/dl without evidence of hyperkalemia or oliguria.

3. Discussion

PJI is a common complication among patients undergoing TKA [5, 6]. Treatment includes two-stage TKA with an antibiotic spacer followed by replacement with a permanent prosthesis and is successful in approximately 90% of patients [1]. However, a two-stage revision TKA bears a significant risk of AKI with potential for progression to ARF [10, 11].

Antibiotic spacers used to treat PJI have their own host of side effects. In our case, both vancomycin and tobramycin have known nephrotoxicity, which most likely contributed to our patient's ARF (Naranjo Score=6) [12–14]. Antibiotic choice within the spacer is a crucial step to successful treatment of PJI. Aminoglycosides alone or in combination with vancomycin are the most frequently used [4, 5, 13]. Although there is little data comparing different mixtures of antibiotics, this combination provides both Gram-negative and Gram-positive coverage to treat PJI [1].

The incidence of AKI in two-stage revision TKA varies from 4.8 to 26% [5, 6, 8, 9]. Data surrounding potential risks are limited but may include increased dosage of tobramycin and vancomycin in the spacer, administration of nephrotoxic IV antibiotics, low hemoglobin, high patient BMI, nonsteroidal use, intraoperative hypotension, and concomitant CKD among other factors [5, 6, 8, 15, 16]. Multiple studies suggest that IV antibiotics and intraoperative hypotension requiring vasopressors are not significant risk factors for the development of AKI in this setting [6, 8, 15]. However, our patient experienced several of the theoretical risk factors including intraoperative hypotension requiring vasopressors, NSAID use, low hemoglobin, high patient BMI, and a high dose antibiotic spacer that may have contributed to his ARF.

The elution characteristics from the spacers depend on a variety of factors including the cement type as well as amounts and types of antibiotics [17, 18]. For there to be clinically relevant elution, greater than 3.6 g of antibiotic per 40 g of cement needs to be present [19]. Various elution curves have been theorized, with a majority suggesting peak values during POD 1-2, followed by a gradual decline to steady state [17]. Increased antibiotic content within spacers may contribute to duration of elution, but other factors are not well studied [18]. Elution duration can range from weeks to months [19].

There are no current standardized recommendations for the quantity of antibiotic in each spacer. Earlier studies by Springer et al. and Evans et al. indicated high dose antibiotics to be both safe and efficacious [9, 20]. More recent studies question the notion, stating the risk of adverse effects increases with increasing doses of antibiotic [6]. Doses of tobramycin >4.8 g increased odds of AKI in patients by 5.87 (95% CI, 1.43-24.19; P = .01) and may be dosage dependent, with every 1 g increase of antibiotic increasing the odds of AKI by 1.24 (95% CI, 1.00-1.52; P = .049) [6]. General guidelines suggest low dose spacers contain <2.0 g of antibiotic per 40 g of cement, and high dose spacers contain >3.6 g of antibiotic per 40 g of cement [14]. There is data to suggest a lower dose spacer increases the risk of reinfection, with Geller et al. suggesting the odds of failure are higher (OR, 0.82; 95% CI, 0.70- 0.96; P = .01) with low dose antibiotics at 1 year and 2 years (OR, 0.83; 95% CI, 0.71-0.96; P = .01) [8]. The dosage our patient received was within recommendations and constituted high dose antibiotics. Overall, he received 26.4 g tobramycin and 9 g vancomycin total in 5 bags of 40 g cement.

It is also unclear whether antibiotics contribute to changes of elution from cement spacers, with the most studied combination being tobramycin and vancomycin [13, 21]. In an in vitro analysis by Klekamp et al., the elution of vancomycin failed to affect the elution of tobramycin and vice versa [13]. In a similar analysis by Penner et al., the combination antibiotic increased elution of tobramycin by 68% and vancomycin by 103% compared to each antibiotic alone [18]. Penner et al. speculated that increased amounts of antibiotic within the cement created porosity and increased surface area, allowing for higher elution rates [18]. In vivo, Masri et al. suggested increasing tobramycin levels provided increased elution of vancomycin [19]. In the context of various conflicting studies, the impact of combination of tobramycin and vancomycin on each antibiotic's elution characteristics in our patient cannot be reliably determined.

Treatment for AKI remains conservative with the determination of fluid status and supportive care [5, 6]. Most patients experience AKI due to reduction in renal blood flow from hypovolemia as opposed to direct nephrotoxicity, and they are often treated with IV fluids to restore flow [5, 6]. Patients experiencing severe AKI may progress to acute tubular necrosis (ATN) and acute renal failure [5, 6]. Our patient may have experienced ATN and progressed to ARF due to direct nephrotoxicity of tobramycin and vancomycin as they reached nephrotoxic levels within the serum [5, 6, 10, 14, 22]. Treatment for ARF includes determining the etiology and treating or removing inciting factors, optimizing fluids and electrolytes and occasionally hemodialysis [5, 6]. In case reports and small series, patients experiencing ARF due to antibiotics spacer toxicity required multiple sessions of dialysis and eventually antibiotic spacer explantation before kidney function was restored [5]. We dialyzed our patient initially for hyperkalemia with ECG changes but repeated it for elimination of tobramycin and vancomycin. Upon the cessation of hemodialysis, tobramycin and creatinine began to reaccumulate in the serum suggesting conservative management would not be adequate. Subsequently the patient underwent surgical explantation of the spacer.

Overall, our patient experienced significant morbidity secondary to his AKI. Many factors may be implicated in this outcome, but it is unclear which are significant. Based on the Naranjo Score (=6), our patient most likely experienced AKI secondary to the vancomycin and tobramycin antibiotic spacer. More studies are needed to further delineate elution profiles of spacers as well as perioperative and patient risk factors contributing to AKI during revision arthroplasty.

4. Conclusion

Uses of tobramycin and vancomycin antibiotic spacers used in two-stage revision arthroplasty have potentially severe complications of acute renal failure. Physicians and pharmacists should have a high level of suspicion of spacers causing AKI and be aware of the risk of ARF during the postoperative period in patients undergoing revision arthroplasty.

Acknowledgments

The authors of this manuscript would like to acknowledge The Research Open Access Publishing Fund of the University of Illinois at Chicago for financial support towards the open access publishing fee for this article.

References

[1] A. L. Lima, P. R. Oliveira, V. C. Carvalho, E. S. Saconi, H. B. Cabrita, and M. B. Rodrigues, "Periprosthetic joint infections," *Interdisciplinary Perspectives on Infectious Diseases*, vol. 2013, Article ID 542796, 7 pages, 2013.

[2] B. N. Patrick, M. P. Rivey, and D. R. Allington, "Acute renal failure associated with vancomycin- and tobramycin-laden cement in total hip arthroplasty," *Annals of Pharmacotherapy*, vol. 40, no. 11, pp. 2037–2042, 2006.

[3] A. James and T. Larson, "Acute renal failure after high-dose antibiotic bone cement: Case report and review of the literature," *Renal Failure*, vol. 37, no. 6, pp. 1061–1066, 2015.

[4] T. N. Joseph, A. L. Chen, and P. E. Di Cesare, "Use of antibiotic-impregnated cement in total joint arthroplasty.," *Journal of the American Academy of Orthopaedic Surgeons*, vol. 11, no. 1, pp. 38–47, 2003.

[5] A. Luu, F. Syed, G. Raman et al., "Two-stage arthroplasty for prosthetic joint infection: a systematic review of acute kidney injury, systemic toxicity and infection control," *The Journal of Arthroplasty*, vol. 28, no. 9, pp. 1490.e1491–1498.e1491, 2013.

[6] T. J. Menge, J. R. Koethe, C. A. Jenkins et al., "Acute kidney injury after placement of an antibiotic-impregnated cement spacer during revision total knee arthroplasty," *The Journal of Arthroplasty*, vol. 27, no. 6, pp. 1221.e1221-1222–1227.e1221-1222, 2012.

[7] I. Vielgut, P. Sadoghi, M. Wolf et al., "Two-stage revision of prosthetic hip joint infections using antibiotic-loaded cement spacers: when is the best time to perform the second stage?" *International Orthopaedics*, vol. 39, no. 9, pp. 1731–1736, 2015.

[8] J. A. Geller, G. Cunn, T. Herschmiller, T. Murtaugh, and A. Chen, "Acute kidney injury after first-stage joint revision for infection: risk factors and the impact of antibiotic dosing," *The Journal of Arthroplasty*, vol. 32, no. 10, pp. 3120–3125, 2017.

[9] B. D. Springer, G.-C. Lee, D. Osmon, G. J. Haidukewych, A. D. Hanssen, and D. J. Jacofsky, "Systemic safety of high-dose antibiotic-loaded cement spacers after resection of an infected total knee arthroplasty," *Clinical Orthopaedics and Related Research*, no. 427, pp. 47–51, 2004.

[10] A. I. Edelstein, K. T. Okroj, T. Rogers, C. J. Della Valle, and S. M. Sporer, "Systemic absorption of antibiotics from antibiotic-loaded cement spacers for the treatment of periprosthetic joint infection," *The Journal of Arthroplasty*, 2018.

[11] T. M. van Raaij, L. E. Visser, A. G. Vulto, and J. A. N. Verhaar, "Acute renal failure after local gentamicin treatment in an infected total knee arthroplasty," *The Journal of Arthroplasty*, vol. 17, no. 7, pp. 948–950, 2002.

[12] J. M. Curtis, V. Sternhagen, and D. Batts, "Acute renal failure after placement of tobramycin-impregnated bone cement in an infected total knee arthroplasty," *Pharmacotherapy*, vol. 25, no. 6, pp. 876–880, 2005.

[13] J. Klekamp, J. M. Dawson, D. W. Haas, D. DeBoer, and M. Christie, "The use of vancomycin and tobramycin in acrylic bone cement: biomechanical effects and elution kinetics for use in joint arthroplasty," *The Journal of Arthroplasty*, vol. 14, no. 3, pp. 339–346, 1999.

[14] S. A. Salim, J. Everitt, A. Schwartz et al., "Aminoglycoside impregnated cement spacer precipitating acute kidney injury requiring hemodialysis," *Seminars in Dialysis*, vol. 31, no. 1, pp. 88–93, 2018.

[15] E. S. Y. Aeng, K. F. Shalansky, T. T. Y. Lau et al., "Acute kidney injury with tobramycin-impregnated bone cement spacers in prosthetic joint infections," *Annals of Pharmacotherapy*, vol. 49, no. 11, pp. 1207–1213, 2015.

[16] G. Z. Kalil, E. J. Ernst, S. J. Johnson et al., "Systemic exposure to aminoglycosides following knee and hip arthroplasty with aminoglycoside-loaded bone cement implants," *Annals of Pharmacotherapy*, vol. 46, no. 7-8, pp. 929–934, 2012.

[17] K. Anagnostakos, P. Wilmes, E. Schmitt, and J. Kelm, "Elution of gentamicin and vancomycin from polymethylmethacrylate beads and hip spacers in vivo," *Acta Orthopaedica*, vol. 80, no. 2, pp. 193–197, 2009.

[18] M. J. Penner, B. A. Masri, and C. P. Duncan, "Elution characteristics of vancomycin and tobramycin combined in acrylic bone-cement," *The Journal of Arthroplasty*, vol. 11, no. 8, pp. 939–944, 1996.

[19] B. A. Masri, C. P. Duncan, and C. P. Beauchamp, "Long-term elution of antibiotics from bone-cement: an in vivo study using the prosthesis of antibiotic-loaded acrylic cement (PROSTALAC) system," *The Journal of Arthroplasty*, vol. 13, no. 3, pp. 331–338, 1998.

[20] R. P. Evans, "Successful treatment of total hip and knee infection with articulating antibiotic components: a modified treatment method," *Clinical Orthopaedics and Related Research*, no. 427, pp. 37–46, 2004.

[21] V. Mounasamy, P. Fulco, P. Desai, R. Adelaar, and G. Bearman, "The successful use of vancomycin-impregnated cement beads in a patient with vancomycin systemic toxicity: a case report with review of literature," *European Journal of Orthopaedic Surgery and Traumatology*, vol. 23, no. 2, pp. S299–S302, 2013.

[22] S. Dovas, V. Liakopoulos, L. Papatheodorou et al., "Acute renal failure after antibiotic-impregnated bone cement treatment of an infected total knee arthroplasty," *Clinical Nephrology*, vol. 69, no. 3, pp. 207–212, 2008.

A Case of Hepatic Glomerulosclerosis with Monoclonal IgA1-κ Deposits

Yusuke Okabayashi,[1,2] Nobuo Tsuboi,[1] Naoko Nakaosa,[1] Kotaro Haruhara,[1] Go Kanzaki,[1] Kentaro Koike,[1] Akihiro Shimizu,[1] Akira Fukui,[1] Hideo Okonogi,[1] Yoichi Miyazaki,[1] Tetsuya Kawamura,[1] Makoto Ogura,[1] Akira Shimizu,[2] and Takashi Yokoo[1]

[1]*Division of Nephrology and Hypertension, Department of Internal Medicine, The Jikei University School of Medicine, Tokyo, Japan*
[2]*Department of Analytic Human Pathology, Nippon Medical School, Tokyo, Japan*

Correspondence should be addressed to Nobuo Tsuboi; tsuboi-n@jikei.ac.jp

Academic Editor: Kouichi Hirayama

Glomerular immunoglobulin A (IgA) deposition is a common finding in hepatic glomerulosclerosis; thus, this disease is also called hepatic IgA nephropathy. However, only a small number of patients with hepatic IgA nephropathy have active glomerular lesions, so functional decline is slow in most cases. In this report, we describe a 60-year-old man who developed nephrotic syndrome and progressive renal impairment during follow-up for alcoholic liver cirrhosis. A renal biopsy showed a membranoproliferative glomerulonephritis-like pattern; diffuse double-contours of the glomerular basement membrane and focal active glomerular lesions with moderate-to-severe endocapillary proliferation and fibrocellular crescents. Immunofluorescence findings revealed granular staining for monoclonal IgA1-κ and C3 on the peripheral capillary walls. Laboratory examinations did not reveal any definitive evidence of myeloproliferative disorders. Therefore, this case may represent a previously unrecognized etiology of renal injury in relation to liver cirrhosis that is characterized by monoclonal IgA1-κ deposits and proliferative glomerulonephritis.

1. Introduction

Hepatic glomerulosclerosis is a form of glomerulopathy found in patients with liver cirrhosis [1–3]. The histopathological findings of hepatic glomerulosclerosis include increased mesangial matrices, subendothelial and paramesangial deposits, and diffuse double-contours in the glomerular basement membrane. Reflecting the ischemic changes associated with hepatorenal syndrome, hepatic glomerulosclerosis is typically accompanied by relatively advanced chronic lesions such as glomerulosclerosis, interstitial fibrosis, and renal tubular atrophy [1–3]. Because this disease state is often accompanied by immunoglobulin A (IgA) deposits in glomeruli, it is also termed hepatic IgA nephropathy. Although liver injury and/or a portal venous shunt may cause significant loss of IgA clearance from the liver, the pathogenesis of this disease is not well understood [4–6]. Unlike patients with primary IgA nephropathy, hepatic glomerulosclerosis cases with a large amount of proteinuria or active glomerular lesions are rare [1–3].

We report an atypical case of hepatic glomerulosclerosis showing progressive loss of renal function together with nephrotic syndrome and active glomerular lesions. To our knowledge, this is the first case report of hepatic glomerulosclerosis with monoclonal IgA-κ deposits in the glomeruli.

2. Case Report

The patient was a 60-year-old man who was diagnosed with alcoholic liver cirrhosis and type 2 diabetes when he was 50 years old. His drinking history was 540–720 mL Japanese sake per day for 35 years, and his smoking history was 30 cigarettes per day for 30 years. His ascites increased in 2008 when he was 57 years old, and he repeatedly exhibited symptoms of

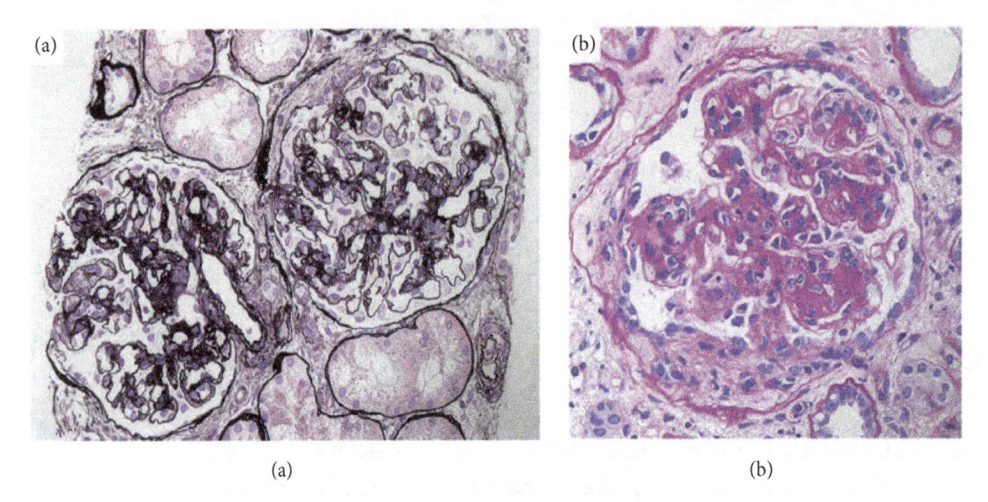

FIGURE 1: Light microscopy findings. In the renal biopsy specimen, glomeruli showed diffuse double-contours in the glomerular basement membrane and moderate to severe focal endocapillary and mesangial hypercellularity (a). Some nonsclerotic glomeruli were accompanied by fibrocellular crescents (b) ((a), periodic acid methenamine silver stain, original magnification 400×; (b), periodic acid-Schiff stain, original magnification 400×).

hepatic encephalopathy. Due to the liver cirrhosis symptoms, the patient was treated with several medications including furosemide, spironolactone, lactulose, and total amino acid preparation. To prevent the complications of liver cirrhosis, coil embolization to a portal venous shunt was performed twice. The patient was admitted to our hospital in June 2012 because of slowly progressive renal impairment and nephrotic syndrome.

Upon admission, the patient's height and weight were 166 cm and 64 kg, respectively. His body temperature was 36.7°C and his blood pressure was 150/60 mmHg. His consciousness was clear. His abdomen was slightly expanded but exhibited no tenderness. The liver and spleen were not palpable. No rash or purpura was noted on the skin. Diabetic and/or hypertensive changes were not observed in the ocular fundus.

The laboratory findings on admission were hemoglobin level of 9.4 g/dL (normal range 13.5–17.6 g/dL), platelet count of $11 \times 10^4/\mu L$ (normal range, $13.1–36.2 \times 10^4/\mu L$), prothrombin time measurement of 68% (normal range, 70–130%), total bilirubin level of 0.9 mg/dL (normal range, 0.3–1.2 mg/dL), NH_3 level of 85 mg/dL (normal range, 30–80 mg/dL), blood urea nitrogen level of 41 mg/dL (normal range, 8–20 mg/dL), serum creatinine concentration of 1.77 mg/dL (normal range, 0.5–1.1 mg/dL), serum total protein level of 5.7 g/dL (normal range, 6.7–8.3 g/dL), serum albumin level of 2.1 g/dL (normal range, 3.5–5.2 g/dL), total cholesterol of 188 mg/dL (normal range, 120–219 mg/dL), and HbA1c of 5.8% (normal range, 4.3–5.8%). The serum levels of IgG were 1558 mg/dL (normal range, 870–1700 mg/dL), of IgA were 481 mg/dL (normal range, 110–410 mg/dL), of IgA1 were 398 mg/dL (normal range, 50–314 mg/dL), of IgA2 were 83 mg/dL (normal range, 10–156 mg/dL), and of IgM were 219 mg/dL (normal range, 35–220 mg/dL). The serum levels of free κ and λ light chains were 149.0 mg/L (normal range, 3.3–19.4 mg/L) and 106.0 mg/L (normal range, 5.7–26.3 mg/L). The serum free light chain ratio was within normal range. The serum level of complement factor C3 was 79 mg/dL (normal range, 65–135 mg/dL), of C4 was 17 mg/dL (normal range, 13–35 mg/dL), and of CH50 was 41.1 U/mL (normal range, 30–50 U/mL). All of the other serology findings including antinuclear antibody, hepatitis B virus surface antigen, hepatitis C virus antibody, anti-neutrophil cytoplasmic antibody, and anti-glomerular basement membrane antibody were negative. There was no M-spike on serum and urine protein electrophoresis. A serum test for a cryoglobulin precipitation was negative.

The urinary sediments showed many red blood cells in high power fields together with granular casts and dysmorphic red blood cells. The urinary protein excretion was 4.7 g/day. The 24-hour creatinine clearance was 45 mL/min. Computed tomography revealed liver deformity with moderate accumulation of ascites. The kidneys were normal in size and there were no signs of urinary tract obstruction.

The renal biopsy specimens contained a total 28 glomeruli, 12 of which were globally sclerotic. The degree of interstitial fibrosis/tubular atrophy was 50–60% of the total biopsy specimen identified. Moderate fibrous intimal hyperplasia was observed in the arcuate artery. Diffuse segmental double-contours of the glomerular basement membrane and mesangial cell hypercellularity were identified in nonsclerotic glomeruli, exhibiting a membranoproliferative glomerulonephritis-like pattern (Figure 1(a)). Some glomeruli showed moderate-to-severe endocapillary hypercellularity, accompanied by fibrocellular crescents (Figure 1(b)). Fluorescent immunostaining showed granular staining of IgA and C3, but not of IgG, IgM, or C1q, on glomerular capillaries and some mesangial areas (Figures 2(a)–2(e)). Among the IgA subtypes, staining of IgA1 (GenWay Biotech, San Diego, CA, USA) was observed, but staining of IgA2 (GenWay Biotech) was not identified (Figures 2(f) and 2(g)). With light chain immunostaining, only κ (SouthernBiotech, Birmingham, AL, USA) was identified and no λ staining (SouthernBiotech) was seen (Figures 2(h) and 2(i)). On electron microscopy, the glomerular capillary

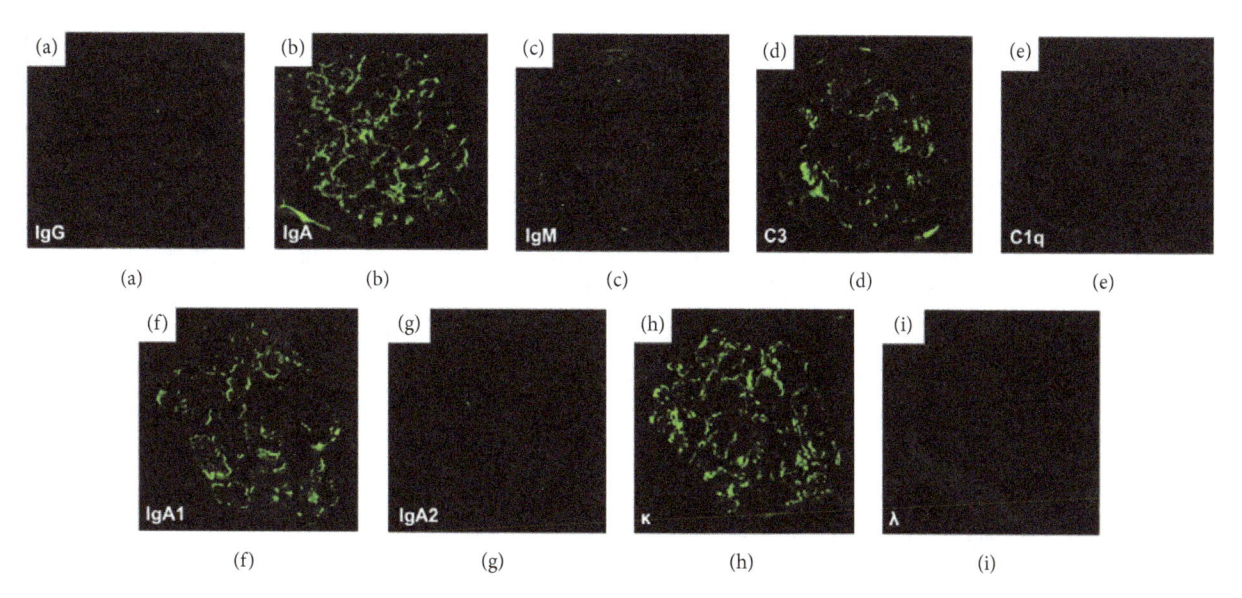

FIGURE 2: Immunofluorescence microscopy findings. Fluorescent immunostaining showed positive staining for IgA and C3, whereas IgG, IgM, and C1q staining were negative. Fluorescent immunostaining of IgA subtypes and light chains showed positive staining for IgA1 and κ light chains, while staining for IgA2 and λ light chains was negative.

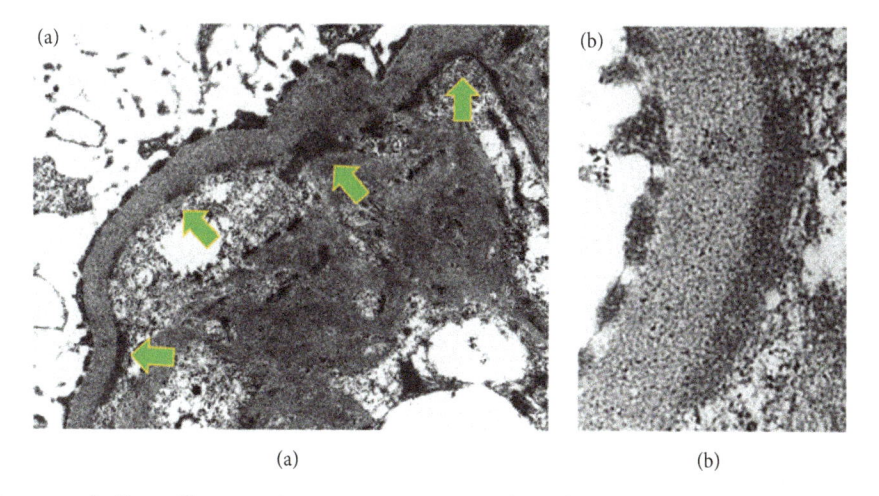

FIGURE 3: Electron microscopy findings. Electron microscopic examination showed nonorganized deposits in the subendothelial area along the glomerular basement membrane and paramesangial area ((a), original magnification 12,000×; (b), original magnification 50,000×). Because no glomeruli were identified in the portion of the biopsy specimen fixed in glutaraldehyde, the formalin-fixed and paraffin-embedded specimen was reprocessed for electron microscopy. Arrows indicate nonorganized deposits.

walls showed double contours. Electron-dense deposits were found in the paramesangium and around the subendothelial space of the glomeruli (Figure 3(a)). No organized structure deposits were identified (Figure 3(b)). Based on these findings, this case was histologically diagnosed as diffuse membranoproliferative glomerulonephritis with monoclonal IgA1-κ deposits.

Because this case was accompanied by moderately advanced decompensated liver cirrhosis, there was a concern that the patient may have serious side effects due to aggressive treatment such as the administration of corticosteroids. Thus, supportive treatment based on medications such as RAS inhibitors/diuretics, in addition to dietary therapy including salt restriction/branched-chain amino acid administration, was selected. Although these treatments led to a modest decrease in the urinary protein excretion, the patient's renal dysfunction slowly progressed and finally resulted in end-stage renal failure and initiation of dialysis therapy.

3. Discussion

Proteinuria and hematuria are found in about 9% of cases of liver cirrhosis, whereas the frequency of nephrotic syndrome is estimated to be about 1.6% [1–3]. An autopsy study has shown that a moderate or high numbers of glomerular lesions are present in about 50% of liver cirrhosis patients [1]. Interestingly, this patient showed typical features of hepatic glomerulosclerosis, including chronic sclerotic and fibrotic changes, upon histological examination. However, this case was also atypical due to the presence of nephrotic syndrome, progressive renal deterioration, and active glomerular lesions along with depositions of monoclonal IgA1-κ in the glomeruli.

The serum increase of IgA1 observed in this case was consistent with what is generally found in hepatic glomerulosclerosis [3]. To our knowledge, however, no previous study has characterized glomerular IgA immunocomplexes in hepatic glomerulosclerosis. Therefore, this case may represent a previously unrecognized etiology of renal injury related to liver cirrhosis that is characterized by monoclonal IgA1-κ deposits and proliferative glomerulonephritis.

There have been some reported cases of glomerulonephritis characterized by monoclonal IgA glomerular deposits [7–12]. The six reported cases and our case occurred with or without clinically apparent myeloproliferative disorders, such as multiple myeloma, monoclonal gammopathy of undetermined significance, or dysproteinemia. Although bone marrow puncture was not performed in our case, no abnormalities in protein electrophoresis of serum and urine or the serum free light chain ratio were observed; therefore, the involvement of myeloproliferative diseases was excluded. In addition, our patient did not have a clinical history or show serological evidence of viral infection or autoimmune disorders. Therefore, these results suggest that factors other than paraprotein diseases, viral infections, or autoimmune diseases are involved in the pathogenesis of glomerulopathy associated with monoclonal IgA1-κ deposits.

Similar to patients with idiopathic IgA nephropathy, recent studies on the glycosylation of serum IgA in patients with hepatic glomerulosclerosis identified abnormalities in the IgA hinge lesion (increase in galactosylation, decrease in sialylation), which indicates that abnormal glycosylation in the IgA hinge lesion may result in glomerular IgA deposition [3]. One study on glomerular light chains in 65 patients with primary IgA nephropathy, but without other potentially contributing diseases, revealed that six cases (9.2%) had monoclonal IgA deposits (5 IgA-λ type cases, 1 IgA-κ case) [13]. However, there was no clear difference in the clinicopathological findings and renal outcomes between the patients with monoclonal IgA deposits and those with polyclonal IgA deposits. Therefore, the pathological significance of monoclonal IgA glomerular deposits is undetermined, even in patients diagnosed with primary IgA nephropathy without background diseases such as liver cirrhosis.

There are no specific treatments for hepatic glomerulosclerosis, and the degree of liver disease is an important predictor of the progression of end-stage renal disease (ESRD). Babbs et al. reported that surgery for portal hypertension resulted in remission of the nephrotic syndrome in a patient with hepatic glomerulosclerosis [14]. In our current case, however, treatment of portal hypertension, such as coil embolization of a portal venous shunt, had no effect on the renal outcome. Considering their adverse events, we did not choose corticosteroid therapy in our case. In comparison, Takeda et al. reported two patients with hepatic glomerulosclerosis who were successfully treated with corticosteroids with no adverse events [15]. Further reports and studies are needed to clarify the clinical utility of corticosteroid therapy for hepatic glomerulosclerosis.

In conclusion, this case suggests that a hepatic glomerulosclerosis subgroup defined by monoclonal deposits of glomerular IgA and active glomerular lesions may exist. The pathogenesis of monoclonal IgA deposits in the glomeruli in this case has yet to be determined. Thus, further studies to evaluate immunoglobulin subclasses and light chain staining in similar cases are needed to elucidate the pathogenesis of this previously unrecognized renal injury etiology in patients with liver cirrhosis.

Disclosure

Parts of this case report were presented at Tokyo Renal Biopsy Conference, July 2014, Tokyo, Japan.

References

[1] Y. Nakamoto, H. Iida, K. Kobayashi et al., "Hepatic glomerulonephritis - Characteristics of hepatic IgA glomerulonephritis as the major part," *Virchows Archiv A: Pathological Anatomy and Histology*, vol. 392, no. 1, pp. 45–54, 1981.

[2] G. C. Newell, "Cirrhotic glomerulonephritis: incidence, morphology, clinical features and pathogenesis," *American Journal of Kidney Diseases*, vol. 9, no. 3, pp. 183–190, 1987.

[3] S. Pouria and J. Barratt, "Secondary IgA Nephropathy," *Seminars in Nephrology*, vol. 28, no. 1, pp. 27–37, 2008.

[4] D. Roccatello, G. Picciotto, M. Torchio et al., "Removal systems of immunoglobulin A and immunoglobulin A containing complexes in IgA nephropathy and cirrhosis patients: The role of asialoglycoprotein receptors," *Laboratory Investigation*, vol. 69, no. 6, pp. 714–723, 1993.

[5] G. Kalambokis, L. Christou, D. Stefanou, E. Arkoumani, and E. V. Tsianos, "Association of liver cirrhosis related IgA nephropathy with portal hypertension," *World Journal of Gastroenterology*, vol. 13, no. 43, pp. 5783–5786, 2007.

[6] R. Coppo, S. Arico, G. Piccoli et al., "Presence and origin of IgA1- and IgA2-containing circulating immune complexes in chronic alcoholic liver diseases with and without glomerulonephritis," *Clinical Immunology and Immunopathology*, vol. 35, no. 1, pp. 1–8, 1985.

[7] T. Naito, H. Yokoyama, Y. Koshino et al., "A Case of Diffuse Panbronchiolitis(DPB) with Benign Monoclonal IgA Gammopathy and IgA Nephropathy with Monoclonal IgA Deposition," *Japanese Journal of Medicine*, vol. 28, no. 4, pp. 503–505, 1989.

[8] D. Birchmore, C. Sweeney, D. Choudhury, M. F. Konwinski, K. Carnevale, and V. D'Agati, "IgA multiple myeloma presenting AS Henoch-Schönlein purpura/polyarteritis nodosa overlap syndrome," *Arthritis & Rheumatology*, vol. 39, no. 4, pp. 698–703, 1996.

[9] S. M. Soares, D. J. Lager, N. Leung, E. N. Haugen, and F. C. Fervenza, "A proliferative glomerulonephritis secondary to a monoclonal IgA," *American Journal of Kidney Diseases*, vol. 47, no. 2, pp. 342–349, 2006.

[10] S. Kaneko, J. Usui, Y. Narimatsu et al., "Renal involvement of monoclonal immunoglobulin deposition disease associated with an unusual monoclonal immunoglobulin A glycan profile," *Clinical and Experimental Nephrology*, vol. 14, no. 4, pp. 389–395, 2010.

[11] K. Setoguchi, Y. Kawashima, T. Tokumoto et al., "Proliferative glomerulonephritis with monoclonal immunoglobulin A light-chain deposits in the renal allograft," *Nephrology (Carlton, Vic.)*, vol. 19, pp. 49–51, 2014.

[12] N. Miura, Y. Uemura, N. Suzuki et al., "An IgA1-lambda-type monoclonal immunoglobulin deposition disease associated with membranous features in a patient with chronic hepatitis C viral infection and rectal cancer," *Clinical and Experimental Nephrology*, vol. 14, no. 1, pp. 90–93, 2010.

[13] H. Nagae, A. Tsuchimoto, K. Tsuruya et al., "Clinicopathological significance of monoclonal IgA deposition in patients with IgA nephropathy," *Clinical and Experimental Nephrology*, vol. 21, no. 2, pp. 266–274, 2017.

[14] C. Babbs, T. W. Warnes, H. B. Torrance, and F. W. Ballardie, "IgA nephropathy in non-cirrhotic portal hypertension," *Gut*, vol. 32, no. 2, pp. 225-226, 1991.

[15] D. Takada, K. Sumida, A. Sekine et al., "IgA nephropathy featuring massive wire loop-like deposits in two patients with alcoholic cirrhosis," *BMC Nephrology*, vol. 18, no. 1, 2017.

Cetuximab-Associated Crescentic Diffuse Proliferative Glomerulonephritis

Sukesh Manthri,[1] Sindhura Bandaru,[1] Anthony Chang,[2] and Tamer Hudali[1]

[1]Southern Illinois University, Springfield, IL, USA
[2]The University of Chicago Medicine, Chicago, IL, USA

Correspondence should be addressed to Tamer Hudali; thudali39@siumed.edu

Academic Editor: Yoshihide Fujigaki

Cetuximab-induced nephrotoxicity is very rare, occurring in less than 1% of colorectal cancer patients and not defined in other populations. We report a rare case of crescentic diffuse proliferative glomerulonephritis (GN) that developed in close temporal association with cetuximab treatment. A 65-year-old female recently completed chemotherapy with cetuximab treatment for moderately differentiated oral squamous cell carcinoma. She was admitted with acute renal failure and nephrotic-range proteinuria. Laboratory data showed serum creatinine of 6.6 mg/dl and urinalysis showed proteinuria, moderate hemoglobinuria, hyaline casts (41/LPF), WBC (28/HPF), and RBC (81/HPF). Serologic studies were negative for ANA, anti-GBM, ANCA, hepatitis B, and hepatitis C. Serum C3 and C4 level were normal. Renal biopsy showed crescentic diffuse proliferative GN with focal features of thrombotic microangiopathy. Patient was started on cyclophosphamide and steroids. Her renal function did not improve on day 8 and she was started on hemodialysis. Previous reports suggest that EGFR-targeting medications can possibly trigger or exacerbate an IgA-mediated glomerular process leading to renal failure. This case suggests that cetuximab therapy may have triggered or exacerbated a severe glomerular injury with an unfavorable outcome. Treating physicians should maintain a high degree of caution and monitor renal function in patients on EGFR inhibitors.

1. Introduction

Cetuximab is a genetically engineered mouse/human chimeric immunoglobulin G1 (IgG1) monoclonal antibody, which specifically binds to epidermal growth factor receptor, and is used for locally advanced, recurrent, and/or metastatic squamous cell carcinoma of the head and neck [1] along with advanced colorectal cancer [2]. Cetuximab-induced nephrotoxicity is rare, occurring in less than 1% in colorectal cancer patients. We report a rare case of crescentic diffuse proliferative glomerulonephritis developed in close temporal association with cetuximab treatment for oral squamous cell cancer.

2. Case Description

A 65-year-old Caucasian female with stage T4aN2b moderately differentiated squamous cell carcinoma of right retromolar trigone was admitted for acute kidney injury. The squamous cell carcinoma was discovered 12 weeks prior to admission and required radical neck dissection and postoperatively she received 7 cycles of cetuximab and 33 sessions of radiation treatment. Her last dose was three weeks prior to kidney injury and nephrotic syndrome (renal function during cetuximab therapy is shown in Table 1). Other pertinent medical history includes asthma and hypertension. Her home medications include Losartan and Ventolin HFA inhaler.

Upon admission, patient complained of nausea and loose stools, at least 4-5 bowel movements per day. She denied any abdominal pain, fever, chills, or vomiting. Due to acute illness, patient was poorly hydrated. She was afebrile and slightly hypertensive (blood pressure, 146/76 mmHg), and physical examination showed 1+ pedal edema but otherwise was unremarkable. Laboratory data on admission showed an increased serum creatinine level at 6.6 mg/dl (estimated GFR, 6 mL/min/1.73 m^2) from baseline of 0.7 mg/dl (estimated GFR, 84 mL/min/1.73 m^2). Complete blood count showed the following values: white blood cells, 11.8×10^3/uL; hemoglobin, 6.0 g/dL (Hgb was around 10.4 g/dL during 7 cycles of

TABLE 1: Patient's sodium (mmol/l), potassium (mmol/l), BUN (mg/dl), creatinine (mg/dl), serum albumin (gm/dl), proteinuria (mg/dl), and hematuria (per hpf) during 7 cycles of cetuximab treatment and 3 weeks later after completing 7th cycle of treatment.

	1st cycle	2nd cycle	3rd cycle	4th cycle	5th cycle	6th cycle	7th cycle	3 weeks later
Sodium	130	133	133	136	133	130	131	134
Potassium	4.5	4.9	4.4	4.6	4.4	4.5	4.3	4.1
BUN	20	24	25	30	19	19	18	*100*
Creatinine	0.8	0.7	0.7	0.7	0.7	0.8	0.8	*6.6*
Serum albumin	3.2	3.7	3.5	3.3	3.0	3.1	2.4	*1.5*
Proteinuria	30	n/a	n/a	n/a	n/a	n/a	n/a	*>500*
Hematuria	1	n/a	n/a	n/a	n/a	n/a	n/a	*81*

chemotherapy); hematocrit, 18%; and platelets, 332×10^3/uL. Serum iron, ferritin, TIBC, and % saturation levels were consistent with anemia of chronic disease. She received 2 units of packed RBC transfusion and later her Hgb was stable at 9 gm/dL. Urinalysis showed proteinuria (>500 mg/dl), moderate hemoglobinuria, hyaline casts (41/LPF), WBC (28/HPF), and RBC (81/HPF). FeNa was 2.6% and urine protein-creatinine ratio was 12.29 g/g (nephrotic-range proteinuria). Serum albumin level was 2.4 g/dL. Serologic studies were negative for antinuclear antibodies, anti-glomerular basement membrane antibodies, anti-neutrophil cytoplasmic antibodies, hepatitis B, and hepatitis C. Serum C3 and C4 levels were normal at 88 mg/dL (reference range, 79–152 mg/dL) and 28 mg/dL (reference range, 13–38 mg/dL), respectively. Serum and urine protein electrophoresis results were negative for monoclonal proteins. Serum-free light chain assay showed elevated free kappa light chains of 477 mg/L (reference range, 3.3–19.4 mg/L) and lambda light chains of 321 mg/L (reference range, 5.7–26.3 mg/L), but ratio was normal. Serum-free light chains can be 20–30-fold above the upper limit of normal in patients with acute kidney injury [3]. Bilateral renal ultrasound showed increased renal parenchymal echogenicity bilaterally, mild bilateral caliectasis, small amount of ascites, and bilateral pleural effusions. She underwent kidney biopsy to determine the cause of acute kidney injury.

Kidney biopsy showed cellular crescents involving up to 63% of the sampled glomeruli (Figure 4), which demonstrated a membranoproliferative pattern of injury with prominent accentuation of the lobular structure and duplication of the glomerular basement membranes (Figure 1). Additional findings of a thrombotic microangiopathic injury were observed in a hilar arteriole with a thrombus (Figure 3). There was also diffuse interstitial edema and inflammation, consisting of lymphocytes, neutrophils, and some eosinophils, which were more prominent in the medulla. The degree of interstitial fibrosis and tubular atrophy was difficult to assess given the degree of tubulointerstitial inflammation. On a 0–4+ scale, immunofluorescence microscopy demonstrated granular capillary wall and mesangial staining for C3 (2+), C4d (1-2+), C1q (1+), and IgG (1+ in a segmental distribution) (Figure 2). A glomerulus with a crescent showed segmental fibrinogen (2-3+) staining. There was no significant glomerular staining for IgA, IgM, or kappa or lambda light chains. Glomeruli were not available in the sample submitted for electron microscopy and an attempt to process the paraffin tissue block for electron microscopy did not yield any additional glomeruli. The final diagnosis was crescentic diffuse proliferative glomerulonephritis with focal features of thrombotic microangiopathy.

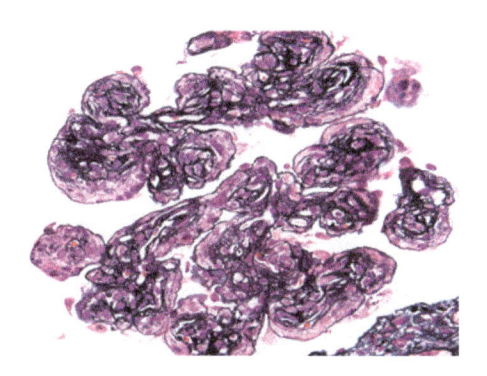

FIGURE 1: This glomerulus demonstrates accentuation of the lobular architecture with associated endocapillary hypercellularity and duplication of the glomerular basement membranes (Jones methenamine silver).

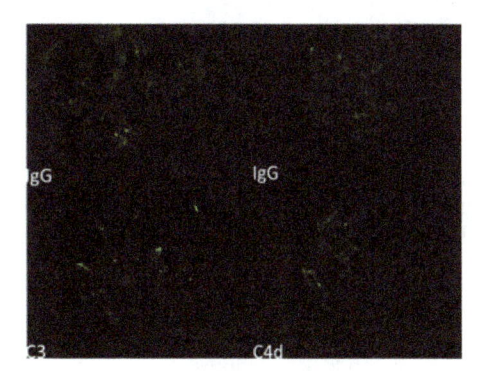

FIGURE 2: There is granular mesangial and capillary wall immunofluorescence staining for the respective immunoglobulins and complement components that range from 1 to 2+ on a scale of 0–4+.

The patient presented with a creatinine of 6.6 mg/dl which did not improve significantly with hydration, resulting in the initiation of hemodialysis after 7 days. Based on the biopsy findings, she was started on cyclophosphamide and pulse methylprednisolone followed by a taper and later discharged home. Unfortunately, she was readmitted to hospital 4 weeks

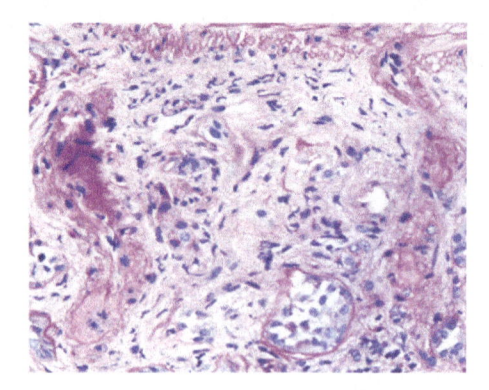

FIGURE 3: Figure demonstrating arteriolar thrombotic microangiopathy.

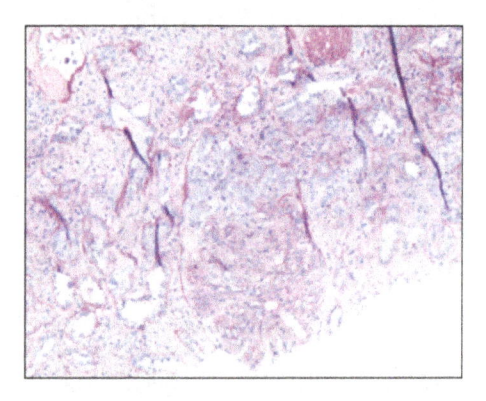

FIGURE 4: A cellular crescent fills Bowman space adjacent to this glomerulus with prominent endocapillary hypercellularity (Periodic acid-Schiff).

later due to acute hypoxic respiratory failure secondary to MRSA pneumonia. She continued to be on scheduled hemodialysis and her immunosuppressive medications were temporarily held due to infection. Given her poor prognosis, the family chose comfort measures and the patient died.

3. Discussion

The number of targeted therapies for advanced cancers is rapidly increasing. While their side effect profiles have been established, the increasing use of these agents will reveal rare complications, such as those in our patient. Checkpoint inhibitors, immunomodulatory antibodies that are group of novel drugs that are used to enhance the immune system, are substantially being used. Cetuximab can frequently cause electrolyte imbalance (hypomagnesemia, hypokalemia, and hypocalcemia) and renal tubular acidosis. Our biopsy represents the third report of glomerular injury associated with cetuximab, given the close temporal association of therapy. The crescentic membranoproliferative pattern of injury with an additional component of a thrombotic microangiopathic injury represents the most severe complication of cetuximab that has been yet reported.

The protein construct for cetuximab consists of Immunoglobulin G1, anti-human epidermal growth factor receptor (human-mouse monoclonal C225 g1-chain), disulfide with human-mouse monoclonal C225 kappa-chain, dimer [4]. The IgG that was detected by immunofluorescence microscopy in the biopsy may represent the recombinant protein itself, even though monoclonal kappa light chain staining was not detected, as the modest degree of IgG staining could be related to the three-week interval since the last administration. This has been demonstrated to occur with eculizumab [5]. Anti-chimeric (or human anti-mouse) antibodies were found in just under 4% of patients being treated with cetuximab in phase 1 trials [6]. It is possible that this patient was one of the rare patients to develop these antibodies and that these were responsible for her renal failure. Unfortunately, we could not test for these antibodies.

Glomerular diseases are associated with many solid and hematologic malignancies. The exact pathogenesis of these glomerular lesions is unclear. Membranous nephropathy and IgA nephropathy are reported glomerular diseases associated with head and neck cancer. Crescentic glomerulonephritis has been associated with renal cell, gastric, and lung cancers [7]. Cancer-associated glomerular diseases have shown that treating the cancer may lead to resolution of the glomerular process. Our patient developed GN after finishing treatment with targeted therapy. She responded very well to cancer treatment and she was in remission. So we suspect her glomerular injury to be in close temporal association with cetuximab treatment.

We are aware of two reports of glomerular injury associated with cetuximab. Sasaki et al. [8] described IgA-dominant proliferative and crescentic glomerulonephritis in a patient treated with cetuximab. In that patient kidney function dramatically improved with cessation of cetuximab and a short course of cyclophosphamide and methylprednisolone. Unlike this case, our patient's renal function did not improve after 4 weeks of immunosuppressive therapy. Koizumi et al. [9] reported a kidney biopsy with glomerular features of TMA due to cetuximab administration. Administration of cetuximab was discontinued and, nine weeks after the discontinuation of cetuximab, the proteinuria decreased.

Our case is unique with both crescentic diffuse proliferative glomerulonephritis associated with focal features of thrombotic microangiopathy (TMA). TMA is usually common to hemolytic uremic syndrome, atypical hemolytic uremic syndrome, and thrombotic thrombocytopenic purpura and can also be induced by various drugs. Radiation treatment could contribute to this injury process, but our patient's radiation was localized to the head and neck region without direct exposure of the kidneys. The possibility of direct endothelial cell toxicity by cetuximab cannot be entirely excluded. Atypical hemolytic uremic syndrome is difficult to exclude, but there was no overt evidence of microangiopathic hemolytic anemia or thrombocytopenia.

Steroids combined with cyclophosphamide is the mainstay of treatment for MPGN reported in case reports. Our patient's renal function did not improve on day 8 of hospitalization and she was started on hemodialysis along with a short course of methylprednisolone and cyclophosphamide.

Although glomerular injury in patients treated with EGFR inhibitors is rare (<0.01%) and no cases were reported in randomized clinical trials using EGFR inhibitors, [10] this may be an underappreciated complication, as kidney biopsies are not often obtained, so increased awareness and close monitoring of kidney function in these patients is warranted.

References

[1] C. G. Azzoli, S. Baker Jr., S. Temin et al., "American society of clinical oncology clinical practice guideline update on chemotherapy for stage IV non-small-cell lung cancer," *Journal of Clinical Oncology*, vol. 27, no. 36, pp. 6251–6266, 2009.

[2] P. F. Engstrom, "Systemic therapy for advanced or metastatic colorectal cancer: National Comprehensive Cancer Network guidelines for combining anti-vascular endothelial growth factor and anti-epidermal growth factor receptor monoclonal antibodies with chemotherapy," *Pharmacotherapy*, vol. 28, no. 11, 2008.

[3] J. M. Abadie, K. H. van Hoeven, and J. M. Wells, "Are renal reference intervals required when screening for plasma cell disorders with serum free light chains and serum protein electrophoresis?" *American Journal of Clinical Pathology*, vol. 131, no. 2, pp. 166–171, 2009.

[4] https://www.fda.gov/drugs/drugsafety/postmarketdrugsafety-informationforpatientsandproviders/ucm113714.htm.

[5] L. C. Herlitz, A. S. Bomback, G. S. Markowitz et al., "Pathology after eculizumab in dense deposit disease and C3 GN," *Journal of the American Society of Nephrology*, vol. 23, no. 7, pp. 1229–1237, 2012.

[6] F. Robert, M. P. Ezekiel, S. A. Spencer et al., "Phase I study of anti-epidermal growth factor receptor antibody cetuximab in combination with radiation therapy in patients with advanced head and neck cancer," *Journal of Clinical Oncology*, vol. 19, no. 13, pp. 3234–3243, 2001.

[7] J. Bacchetta, L. Juillard, P. Cochat, and J.-P. Droz, "Paraneoplastic glomerular diseases and malignancies," *Critical Review in Oncology/Hematology*, vol. 70, no. 1, pp. 39–58, 2009.

[8] K. Sasaki, E. Anderson, S. J. Shankland, and R. F. Nicosia, "Diffuse proliferative glomerulonephritis associated with cetuximab, an epidermal growth factor receptor inhibitor," *American Journal of Kidney Diseases*, vol. 61, no. 6, pp. 988–991, 2013.

[9] M. Koizumi, M. Takahashi, M. Murata, Y. Kikuchi, K. Seta, and K. Yahata, "Thrombotic microangiopathy associated with cetuximab, an epidermal growth factor receptor inhibitor," *Clinical Nephrology*, vol. 87, no. 1, pp. 51–54, 2017.

[10] F. Petrelli, M. Cabiddu, K. Borgonovo, and S. Barni, "Risk of venous and arterial thromboembolic events associated with anti-EGFR agents: A meta-analysis of randomized clinical trials," *Annals of Oncology*, vol. 23, no. 7, Article ID mdr592, pp. 1672–1679, 2012.

Nontraumatic Exertional Rhabdomyolysis Leading to Acute Kidney Injury in a Sickle Trait Positive Individual on Renal Biopsy

Kalyana C. Janga,[1] Sheldon Greenberg,[1] Phone Oo,[1] Kavita Sharma,[2] and Umair Ahmed[1]

[1]Department of Nephrology, Maimonides Medical Center, Brooklyn, NY, USA
[2]Department of Infectious Diseases, Maimonides Medical Center, Brooklyn, NY, USA

Correspondence should be addressed to Kalyana C. Janga; kjanga@maimonidesmed.org

Academic Editor: Yoshihide Fujigaki

A 26-year-old African American male with a history of congenital cerebral palsy, sickle cell trait, and intellectual disability presented with abdominal pain that started four hours prior to the hospital visit. The patient denied fever, chills, diarrhea, or any localized trauma. The patient was at a party at his community center last evening and danced for 2 hours, physically exerting himself more than usual. Labs revealed blood urea nitrogen (BUN) level of 41 mg/dL and creatinine (Cr) of 2.8 mg/dL which later increased to 4.2 mg/dL while still in the emergency room. Urinalysis revealed hematuria with RBC > 50 on high power field. Imaging of the abdomen revealed no acute findings for abdominal pain. With fractional excretion of sodium (FeNa) > 3%, findings suggested nonoliguric acute tubular necrosis. Over the next couple of days, symptoms of dyspepsia resolved; however, BUN/Cr continued to rise to a maximum of 122/14 mg/dL. With these findings, along with stable electrolytes, urine output matching the intake, and prior use of proton pump inhibitors, medical decision was altered for the possibility of acute interstitial nephritis. Steroids were subsequently started and biopsy was taken. Biopsy revealed heavy deposits of myoglobin. Creatinine phosphokinase (CPK) levels drawn ten days later after the admission were found to be elevated at 334 U/dl, presuming the levels would have been much higher during admission. This favored a diagnosis of acute kidney injury (AKI) secondary to exertional rhabdomyolysis. We here describe a case of nontraumatic exertional rhabdomyolysis in a sickle cell trait (SCT) individual that was missed due to findings of microscopic hematuria masking underlying myoglobinuria and fractional excretion of sodium > 3%. As opposed to other causes of ATN, rhabdomyolysis often causes FeNa < 1%. The elevated fractional excretion of sodium in this patient was possibly due to the underlying inability of SCT positive individuals to reabsorb sodium/water and concentrate their urine. Additionally, because of their inability to concentrate urine, SCT positive individuals are prone to intravascular depletion leading to renal failure as seen in this patient. Disease was managed with continuing hydration and tapering steroids. Kidney function improved and the patient was discharged with a creatinine of 3 mg/dL. A month later, renal indices were completely normal with persistence of microscopic hematuria from SCT.

1. Introduction

Rhabdomyolysis is a condition characterized by muscle cell death and the release of muscle cell constituents into the circulation. The causes of rhabdomyolysis include trauma +/− muscle compression; nontraumatic, nonexertional causes (drugs, toxins, or infections); and nontraumatic, exertional rhabdomyolysis [1]. The incidence of exertional rhabdomyolysis is unknown; however, a recent retrospective cohort study revealed that, out of all their rhabdomyolysis cases in a set amount of time, 35% were exertional [2]. Nontraumatic, exertional rhabdomyolysis can occur in extreme exertion or normal physical exertion in addition to risk factors that impair muscle oxygenation, ultimately leading to muscle cell death. One of these risk factors includes individuals with the sickle cell trait (SCT).

Sickle cell trait is the heterozygous state (HBAS) of sickle cell disease [3]. SCT is a benign carrier state; it is by itself

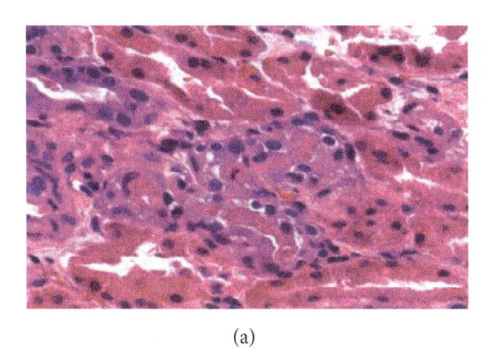

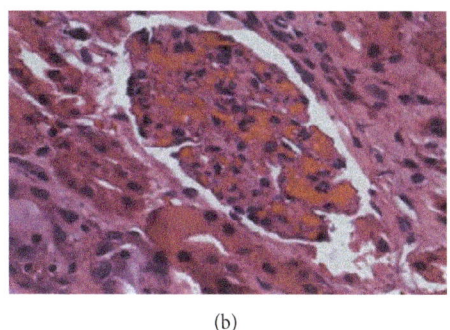

FIGURE 1: H&E stain. (a) Reddish tubular casts. Most tubules are preserved, mild interstitial fibrosis with tubular atrophy. (b) Glomeruli with congestion.

not considered a disease [4]. SCT is present in 7–9% of the African American population. Additionally, a recent cross-sectional study reviewing hemoglobin phenotypes in African Americans with end stage renal disease found that SCT was twice as common among African Americans with end stage renal disease [5]. Although the overall effects of SCT are benign, many studies and case reports have identified that individuals with SCT are at an increased risk for rare conditions including exertional rhabdomyolysis with prolonged physical activity, compartment syndrome, and sudden cardiac death [6]. We report on an SCT patient with symptoms of hematuria and isosthenuria developing stage III nonoliguric AKI from exertional rhabdomyolysis.

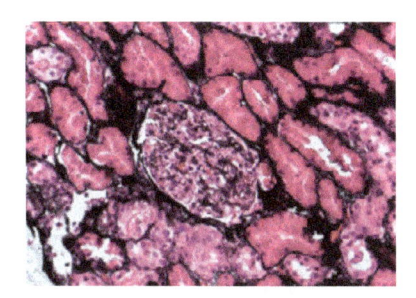

FIGURE 2: PAS stain. PAS stain showing tubular atrophy, glomeruli congestion, and normal capillary loops in the glomerulus.

2. Case Presentation

A 26-year-old African American male with a history of congenital cerebral palsy, sickle cell trait, and intellectual disability presented with abdominal pain that started four hours prior to the hospital visit. His only medication is occasional proton pump inhibitors for indigestion and belching. Abdominal pain was characterized as colicky, constant, and located in the epigastric region and was associated with symptoms including nausea and two episodes of vomiting. The patient denied fever, chills, diarrhea, or any localized trauma. The patient was at a party at his community center last evening and danced for 2 hours, physically exerting himself more than usual. Physical examination revealed mild epigastric tenderness upon palpation; skin was warm and dry with normal turgor. The buccal mucosa was moist. Blood work revealed BUN of 41 mg/dL (reference range: 7–18 mg/dL) and creatinine of 2.8 mg/dL (reference range: 0.6–1.2 mg/dL) which later increased to 4.2 mg/dL while still in the emergency room. Additionally, liver enzymes were minimally elevated. Urinalysis revealed microscopic hematuria with RBC > 50 on high power field. Imaging of the abdomen was benign. Decision was made to admit the patient based on abnormal liver enzymes and worsening kidney injury suggesting signs of nonoliguric acute tubular necrosis.

Over the next couple of days, symptoms of dyspepsia resolved; however, renal indices continued to worsen despite adequate hydration and 1 ml/kg/h bicarbonate infusion,

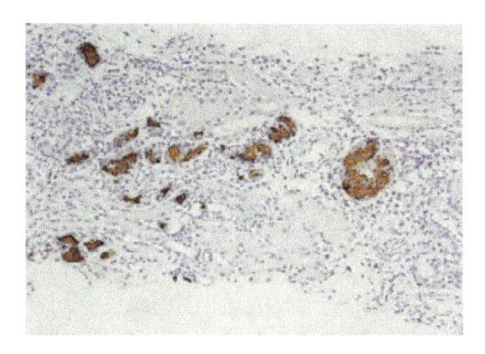

FIGURE 3: Tubular casts are positive for myoglobin immunostain.

reaching a peak of creatinine of 14 mg/dL. Due to these findings, stable electrolytes, urine output matching the intake, and prior use of occasional proton pump inhibitors, medical decision was altered for the possibility of allergic interstitial nephritis. Steroids were subsequently started and biopsy was taken.

Biopsy revealed heavy deposits of myoglobin (Figures 1–3). CPK levels were drawn shortly after the results (day 10) and were found to be elevated at 334 U/L. This favored a diagnosis of AKI secondary to exertional rhabdomyolysis. Decision was made to continue hydration and taper steroids. Kidney function improved and the patient was discharged with a creatinine of 3 mg/dL. A month later, renal indices were completely normal with persistence of microscopic hematuria from SCT.

TABLE 1: Basic investigation for acute renal failure (*tests can be ordered if needed based on history and physical).

Blood tests	Complete blood counts with differentials
	Complete metabolic profile
	Phosphorus
	Uric acid
	Myoglobin
	Creatinine phosphokinase
	Liver function tests
	Brain natriuretic peptide* (BNP)
	Arterial blood gas
Urine tests	Urinalysis with microscopy and culture
	Urine osmolality
	Urine electrolytes
	Urine eosinophils*
	Urine protein/creatinine ratio (PCR)
Radiology tests	Renal and bladder sonogram
	Chest X-ray*

3. Discussion

In this case, the patient initially presented with symptoms of nonoliguric acute tubular necrosis (ATN). The patient had abdominal pain, elevated liver enzymes, elevated BUN/Cr, and FeNa > 3%. Intrarenal AKI is characterized as damage to the major structures of the kidney including the tubules, glomeruli, interstitium, and the intrarenal blood vessels [7]. Damage can be caused by toxins, contrast, drugs, myoglobin, and others (Table 1). Although the patient's symptoms resolved the next day, his BUN/Cr continued to rise with hydration. Medical decision was altered for the possibility of proton pump inhibitor induced acute interstitial nephritis. So, steroids were started and biopsy was taken, which revealed rhabdomyolysis.

Rhabdomyolysis is a condition characterized by muscle cell death and the release of muscle cell constituents into the circulation. Common symptoms of rhabdomyolysis include muscle pain, rashes, weakness, and dark colored urine due to myoglobinuria [8, 9]. Additional symptoms in severe cases include fever, altered mental status, nausea/vomiting, or abdominal pain which our patient had. Physical examination findings may include positive muscle tenderness, muscle swelling, and/or skin discolorations. Laboratory diagnosis is essential based on the measurement of biomarkers of muscle injury, with creatinine phosphokinase being the biochemical "gold standard" for diagnosis and myoglobin the "gold standard" for prognostication, especially in patients with nontraumatic rhabdomyolysis. Serum CPK levels are usually at least 5 times the upper limit of normal at presentation, reaching the peak within 24–72 hours and then declining after 3–5 days with cessation of muscle injury [9]. The CPK levels are more sustained and long-lasting as compared to myoglobin which has a short half-life due to faster elimination kinetics. Most believe that CPK levels correlate with the amount of muscle injury and disease activity. Additional tests such as muscle biopsy, kidney biopsy, MRI, and electromyography are usually not needed [8, 9]. The filtered myoglobin is degraded into a heme pigment which can damage the kidney in three different ways, that is, direct tubular cell injury, vasoconstriction leading to decreased blood flow, and tubular obstruction [10]. However, in contrast to other causes of intrarenal AKI, the fractional excretion of sodium is often <1% and urine sodium is <20. This is possibly due to the vasoconstriction and volume depletion often observed in rhabdomyolysis. Urinalysis may also reveal findings of myoglobinuria, a positive dipstick with the absence of RBCs on urine microscopy.

It may be difficult to differentiate between hematuria and myoglobinuria. Both present with red-brown colored urine and a positive urine reagent strip test. This test is able to detect heme-positive compounds including hemoglobin and myoglobin because heme catalyzes the oxidation of tetramethylbenzidine which produces a color change [11]. The sensitivity of the test decreases with elevated specific gravity or high urinary protein. A microscopic evaluation must be done to detect the presence of RBCs and differentiate between hematuria and myoglobinuria [8, 9]. Other tests to detect myoglobin include qualitative tests such as the precipitation test and capillary electrophoresis [11]. Our patient did have a positive urine dipstick with large amounts of hemoglobin found on microscopic evaluation. This suggested the symptoms of hematuria commonly found in SCT positive patients, rather than myoglobin from rhabdomyolysis.

As discussed above, the causes of rhabdomyolysis include nontraumatic, exertional rhabdomyolysis. Patients may develop exertional rhabdomyolysis with no underlying disease and normal muscle tissue. A recent case report has shown an increasing number of patients diagnosed with exertional rhabdomyolysis after attending a spinning class [12]. None of these patients were on medications, nor did they have any significant past medical history. Although not a prerequisite, most patients that do develop exertional rhabdomyolysis will have some underlying disease or risk factors that impair muscle oxygenation, ultimately leading to muscle cell death. One of these risk factors includes individuals with the sickle cell trait (SCT).

SCT is heterozygous for the sickle hemoglobin (HbS) point mutation and is considered a benign carrier state [4]. Most individuals with SCT are asymptomatic; however, patients may develop symptoms of isosthenuria or episodes of hematuria. Isosthenuria is the inability to concentrate the urine, resulting in symptoms of polyuria, enuresis, and higher incidences of dehydration. Patients may also experience episodes of hematuria spontaneously or with heavy physical exertion. The pathophysiology behind this is due to the microvascular obstruction by rigid erythrocytes, which will lead to tissue necrosis and renal papillary infarcts causing the hematuria [13, 14]. Many studies have identified that patients with SCT are at an increased risk of exertional rhabdomyolysis. It was found that there was a significantly higher risk of exertional rhabdomyolysis in African American US military army soldiers with SCT. Additionally, similar increased risks were observed in obese and tobacco using individuals [15]. In fact, due to the increasing number of published case reports

TABLE 2: Renal biopsy indications.

Isolated glomerular hematuria	Persistent and severe hematuria, hypertension, and elevated creatinine
Isolated nonnephrotic syndrome	Persistent and >1-gram proteinuria
Nephrotic syndrome	Routinely indicated in adults including diabetes, connective tissue disorders, steroid-resistant nephrotic syndrome, and obesity Exception is first attack in children
Nephritic syndrome	Connective tissue disorders, hepatitis, infection-related nephritic syndrome, and rapidly progressive glomerulonephritis
Unexplained acute kidney injury	After clinical diagnosis fails
Unexplained progressive chronic kidney disease	Normal size kidneys and extent of kidney damage
Familial renal diseases	Biopsy of one member can yield the diagnosis of other family members
Renal transplant dysfunction	Acute versus chronic rejection versus drug-induced renal failure
Small localized renal tumors/lesions	Benign renal tumors, metastasis, lymphoma, and focal kidney infection

of sudden death and exertional rhabdomyolysis occurring at a high rate in SCT positive military personnel, the Department of Defense developed screening guidelines in 1972 for the testing of SCT in new recruits [16]. The increased risk of exertional rhabdomyolysis found in SCT individuals may be due to the underlying renovascular changes combined with the inability to concentrate the urine. The pathophysiology behind this is that RBC sickling found in SCT may cause the congestion of the vasa recta. This may lead to ischemia and retention of the medullary interstitium. Since water reabsorption is dependent on interstitial osmolality, there will be a decrease of reabsorption across antidiuretic hormone stimulated collecting ducts [3]. With the inability to concentrate the urine, SCT positive individuals are more inclined to dehydration and are unable flush out renal toxins adequately.

Our patient had nontraumatic exertional rhabdomyolysis due to excessive physical exertion the night before his symptoms began. As discussed above, he was at an increased risk of developing this condition because he had the sickle cell trait. The diagnosis of rhabdomyolysis was missed because of symptoms of hematuria, FeNa > 3%, and failure to order CPK levels initially. Although he received the proper treatment of fluid/electrolyte replacement, his condition took longer to recover because of the underlying renal disease found in SCT patients. Fortunately, this patient was able to recover and his kidney function normalized without the need for hemodialysis. Acute exertional rhabdomyolysis may lead to metabolic acidosis and electrolyte disturbances including hyperkalemia [17]. Severe cases may lead to renal failure and death. Although continued renal replacement therapy and hemodialysis will improve creatinine, BUN, and potassium and reduce the duration of oliguria phase and length of hospital stay, no significant differences were found in mortality rates compared with conventional therapy in rhabdomyolysis. It is important to build awareness and counsel SCT positive patients and families on avoiding excessive physical exertion in order to avoid such complications.

4. Conclusion

This case report describes the occurrence of nontraumatic exertional rhabdomyolysis in individuals that have the sickle cell trait. There is an increased risk of AKI secondary to exertional rhabdomyolysis in these individuals. The rhabdomyolysis was missed here due to no history of trauma, microscopic hematuria, and fractional excretion of sodium > 3%. Classic rhabdomyolysis subjects will have some type of trauma, no microscopic hematuria, and fractional excretion of sodium < 1%. In summary, we recommend checking CPK levels in all unknown causes of acute renal failure and renal biopsy should remain the gold standard in determining the cause of unknown AKI (Table 2). We also recommend screening of African American patients for SCT due to the high prevalence in this population. Early screening as done in military recruits will allow for proper counseling of these individuals in order to prevent complications including exertional rhabdomyolysis, which, through multiple published case reports, have proved to be detrimental in some patients. It is important for physicians to counsel SCT patients on these increased risks of kidney injury and advise them to avoid nephrotoxins, stay hydrated, and avoid excessive physical exertion.

References

[1] M. L. Miller, I. N. Targoff, and M. S. Jeremy, Causes of rhabdomyolysis, in. UpToDate, https://www.uptodate.com/contents/causes-of-rhabdomyolysis.

[2] J. P. Alpers and L. K. Jones, "Natural history of exertional rhabdomyolysis: A population-based analysis," *Muscle & Nerve*, vol. 42, no. 4, pp. 487–491, 2010.

[3] K. A. Nath and R. P. Hebbel, "Sickle Cell Disease: renal manifestations and mechanisms," *Nature Reviews Nephrology*, vol. 11, no. 3, pp. 161–171, 2015, https://www.ncbi.nlm.nih.gov/pubmed/25668001.

[4] R. P. Naik and C. Haywood, "Sickle cell trait diagnosis: clinical and social implications," *International Journal of Hematology*, vol. 2015, no. 1, pp. 160–167, 2015.

[5] V. K. Derebail, P. H. Nachman, N. S. Key, H. Ansede, R. J. Falk, and A. V. Kshirsagar, "High prevalence of sickle cell trait in African Americans with ESRD," *Journal of the American Society of Nephrology*, vol. 21, no. 3, pp. 413–417, 2010.

[6] P. Saxena, C. Chavarna, and J. Thurlow, "Rhabdomyolysis in a Sickle Cell Trait Positive Active Duty Male Soldier," *U.S. Army Medical Department Journal*, vol. 20, no. 3, 2016, https://www.ncbi.nlm.nih.gov/pubmed/26874092.

[7] D. P. Basile, M. D. Anderson, and T. A. Sutton, "Pathophysiology of acute kidney injury," *Comprehensive Physiology*, vol. 2, no. 2, pp. 1303–1353, 2012.

[8] X. Bosch, E. Poch, and J. M. Grau, "Rhabdomyolysis and Acute Kidney Injury," *New England Journal of Medicine*, vol. 361, pp. 61–72, 2009, http://www.nejm.org/doi/full/10.1056/NEJMra0801327.

[9] M. L. Miller, I. N. Targoff, and M. S. Jeremy, Clinical Manifestations and diagnosis of rhabdomyolysis. 2016. In: UpToDate, Post TW, Waltham, MA https://www.uptodate.com/contents/clinical-manifestations-and-diagnosis-of-rhabdomyolysis?source=see_link.

[10] M. A. Perazella, M. Rosner, P. Palevsky, and A. Sheridan, Clinical Features and diagnosis of heme pigment-induced AKI. 2016. In: UpToDate, Post TW, Waltham, MA https://www.uptodate.com/contents/clinical-features-and-diagnosis-of-heme-pigment-induced-acute-kidney-injury?source=see_link.

[11] R. S. Riley and R. McPherson, Basic Examination of Urine. *Henry's Clinical Diagnosis and Management by Laboratory Methods*. Chapter 28, 442-480.e3, https://www.clinicalkey.com/#!/content/book/3-s2.0-B9780323295680000280?scrollTo=%23hl0002163.

[12] D. Kim, E. Ko, H. Cho, P. Hyung, and S. Lee, "Spinning-induced Rhabdomyolysis: Eleven Case Reports and Review of the Literature," *Electrolytes and Blood Pressure*, vol. 13, no. 2, pp. 58–61, 2015, https://www.ncbi.nlm.nih.gov/pmc/articles/PMC4737663/.

[13] E. P. Vichinsky, D. H. Mahoney, and J. Tirnauer, Cell Trait. In: UpToDate, Post TW, Waltham, MA https://www.uptodate.com/contents/sickle-cell-trait?source=search_result&search=sickle%20cell%20trait&selectedTitle=1~108.

[14] U. Khan, L. Kleess, J. Yeh, C. Berko, and S. Kuehl, "Sickle cell trait: not as benign as once thought," *Journal of Community Hospital Internal Medicine Perspectives (JCHIMP)*, vol. 4, no. 5, p. 25418, 2014.

[15] D. A. Nelson, P. Deuster, R. Carter, O. Hill, W. L. Wolcott, and L. Kurina, "Sickle Cell Trait, Rhabdomyolysis, and Mortality among U.S. Army Soldiers," *New England Journal of Medicine*, vol. 375, no. 5, pp. 435–442, 2016, https://www.ncbi.nlm.nih.gov/pmc/articles/PMC5026312/.

[16] N. A. Raju, S. V. Rao, J. Chakravarthy Joel et al., "Predictive value of serum myoglobin and creatine phosphokinase for development of acute kidney injury in traumatic rhabdomyolysis," *Indian Journal of Critical Care Medicine*, vol. 21, no. 12, pp. 852–856, 2017.

[17] J. N. Makaryus, J. N. Catanzaro, and K. C. Katona, "Exertional rhabdomyolysis and renal failure in patients with sickle cell trait: Is it time to change our approach?" *International Journal of Hematology*, vol. 12, no. 4, pp. 349–352, 2007.

Achromobacter xylosoxidans Relapsing Peritonitis and *Streptococcus suis* Peritonitis in Peritoneal Dialysis Patients: A Report of Two Cases

Rafał Donderski,[1] Magdalena Grajewska,[1] Agnieszka Mikucka,[2] Beata Sulikowska,[1] Eugenia Gospodarek-Komkowska,[2] and Jacek Manitius[1]

[1]Department of Nephrology, Hypertension and Internal Medicine, Ludwik Rydygier Collegium Medicum in Bydgoszcz, Nicolaus Copernicus University in Toruń, Poland
[2]Department of Microbiology, Ludwik Rydygier Collegium Medicum in Bydgoszcz, Nicolaus Copernicus University in Toruń, Poland

Correspondence should be addressed to Rafał Donderski; rafdon@o2.pl

Academic Editor: David Mudge

Peritonitis is considered to be the most common complication of peritoneal dialysis (PD). It is usually caused by Gram positive *Staphylococcus epidermidis*. *Achromobacter xylosoxidans* (*A. xylosoxidans*) and *Streptococcus suis* (*S. suis*) are rare pathogens, but there is emerging evidence that they may be also responsible for PD related peritonitis. We described 2 cases of rare peritonitis treated in our center. In our opinion this is the first described case of PD related peritonitis caused by *Streptococcus suis*.

1. Introduction

Peritoneal dialysis (PD) is a worldwide used modality of renal replacement therapy (RRT). Disadvantages of this kind of treatment are infectious complications such as peritonitis, exit site infection (ESI), or tunnel infection. Peritonitis contributes to increased hospitalization rate, technique failure, and increased mortality in PD patients. Nowadays, according to novel connectivity systems and impact on educational training of patients the annual incidence of a new peritonitis episode seems to be decreased [1]. *Achromobacter xylosoxidans* (formerly *Alcaligenes xylosoxidans*) infections are extremely rare in PD patients. This bacterium was first described in 1971 by Yabuuchi and Ohyama in patients with chronic otitis media [2]. It is mostly detected in immunocompromised patients such as diabetic patients, chronic kidney disease (CKD) patients, or individuals undergoing chemotherapy. *S. suis* is a pig pathogen and it is rarely identified in humans. There is emerging evidence of *S. suis* infections such as meningitis, peritonitis, and septic shock in especially immunodeficient patients [3]. In our center we reported a rare case of *A. xylosoxidans* relapsing peritonitis and a case of *S. suis* peritonitis.

2. Patient 1

27-year-old woman who had been on PD because of chronic glomerulonephritis confirmed by renal biopsy (histopathological evaluation revealed focal segmental glomerulosclerosis (FSGS)) and end-stage kidney disease (ESKD) for 2 years was admitted to our center with clinical symptoms of peritonitis. She was complaining of diffuse abdominal pain, fever, and cloudy dialysate. There were no signs of exit site infection (ESI). She was on automated peritoneal dialysis (APD) using Home Choice Pro device delivered by Baxter (USA). Her dialysis regimen was 12.0 liters of 1.36% Dianeal fluid. Her ultrafiltration was approximately 1000ml. Residual diuresis was approximately 1.0 liter daily. She had not had any PD-associated infections in the past. Moreover, she was suffering from chronic hepatitis C, hypertension, reflux esophagitis, and chronic gastritis. She had renal anemia treated with darbepoetin alfa s.c. and chronic kidney disease—mineral

TABLE 1: Laboratory investigation and antibiotics treatment in the first episode of *A. xylosoxidans* peritonitis in patient 1.

Laboratory tests	Antibiotics prescription
WBC – 15.000/mm^3 (N: 4-11x10^3/mm^3)	(1) Ceftazidime 1,0g+cefazoline 1,0 IP∗
CRP -84,5mg/L (N<5,0)	(2) Imipenem 0,5g IV∗
DLC- 7217/mm^3 (N<100)	

N: normal value; WBC: white blood count; CRP: C-reactive protein; DLC: dialysate leukocyte count; IP: intraperitoneally; IV: intravenously. ∗ means once a day.

and bone disorder (CKD-MBD) were treated according to latest updated KDIGO Guidelines 2017 (calcium carbonicum in a dose of 3 x 3,0g daily, cinacalcet in a dose of 30mg daily, paricalcitol 2,0mcg 3 times a week). In 1990 she had episode of hemolytic-uremic syndrome (HUS) and acute kidney injury (AKI stage 3) with need for dialysis (PD was used for a month that time). Her vital signs on admission were as follows: she presented generalized abdominal tenderness, her blood pressure was 130/90mmHg, her temperature was 38°C, heart rate was 100 beats per minute, and respiration rate was 20 per minute. Laboratory test included white blood count (WBC) of 15.000/mm^3, hemoglobin (Hgb) of 12,1g/dl, platelets count of 254.000/mm^3, C-reactive protein (CRP) of 84,5mg/L, blood urea nitrogen (BUN) of 65mg/dl, serum creatinine of 4,15mg/dl, serum albumin of 3,8g/dl, total protein of 6,58g/dl, total cholesterol of 220mg/dl, dialysate leukocyte count (DLC) of 7217/mm^3 (neutrophils/lymphocytes=86% vs 11%), PTH (parathormone) of 984pg/ml, serum calcium of 2,10mmo/l, and phosphorus of 1,86mmo/l. Blood culture and urine culture were both negative. We decided to start initial empiric antibiotics treatment with ceftazidime 1,0g daily and cefazolin 1,0g daily infused intraperitoneally (ip) into Extraneal 2,0-liter bag. Dwell time was 8 hours. Positive culture of *A. xylosoxidans* colonies was isolated from peritoneal fluid (using BD Bactec™ FX Becton Dickinson System, USA). Isolation of bacteria was performed using routine method at the clinical microbiology laboratory. The identification of isolated strain was further confirmed by applying mass spectrometric method (Matrix-Assisted Laser Desorption/Ionization-Time-Of-Flight, MALDI-TOF) using MALDI Biotyper (Bruker, Germany). Antimicrobial susceptibility testing of examined *A. xylosoxidans* strain was performed by the agar dilution method and carried out according to the European Committee on Antimicrobial Susceptibility testing recommendation (version 7.0). According to the antibiogram, the pathogen was sensitive to piperacillin/tazobactam, ceftazidime, and imipenem and was resistant to ciprofloxacin and cefepime. The treatment regimen was changed according to antibiogram results into imipenem+cilastatin intravenously (iv) in a dose of 2 x 0,25g daily. She was given the antibiotic for 2 weeks. Laboratory investigation and antibiotics regimen in the first episode of *A. xylosoxidans* peritonitis are given in Table 1.

We observed improvement in her clinical condition. There was no abdominal pain. Dialysate leukocyte count gradually decreased and control dialysate culture was negative. 3 weeks after the treatment, she was discharged from hospital. 7 days later she was admitted again because of another episode of peritonitis. Dialysate culture was positive and *A. xylosoxidans* colonies were identified again. Pathogen was sensitive to imipenem and ceftazidime and we started these antibiotics in a dose of 2 x 0,25g iv and 1 x 1,0 g intraperitoneally (ip), respectively. This time we decided to perform computed tomography (CT). There were no signs of gut perforation or abdominal abscess. After antibiotics implementation her symptoms disappeared quickly. We continued the treatment in the hospital for another 2 weeks. 2 weeks after being discharged from the hospital, there was another third episode of peritonitis with the same pathogen, *A. xylosoxidans* isolated from peritoneal fluid. In the case of relapsing *A. xylosoxidans* peritonitis, we decided to remove peritoneal catheter and transfer her to hemodialysis. After permanent catheter insertion into right carotid vein and control chest X-ray, she started temporary hemodialysis treatment. She was on 3 hemodialysis sessions per week. The tip of removed peritoneal catheter was sent for microbiological evaluation. Colonization of *A. xylosoxidans* was stated. After 2 months on hemodialysis, we decided to continue PD in her case and she was admitted to Department of Surgery for peritoneal catheter insertion. Then, 3 weeks later she successfully started PD treatment again.

3. Patient 2

The patient had been a 54-year-old male with CKD stage 5 secondary to multiple myeloma (MM). He was on PD since November 2015. After 2 months on CAPD he started APD using Fresenius Sleep-Safe Cycler. His dialysis regimen was 12,0 liters of 1,5% glucose solution. He had well preserved residual renal function (RRF) with residual diuresis approximately 1,5 liters daily. His ultrafiltration rate ranges from 600 to 800ml daily. Moreover, his medical history included diabetes type 2, hypertension, psoriasis, hernia esophagi, peptic ulcer, and spinal column rupture (compression rupture Th5-Th8) related to MM. On admission to the hospital he presented mild abdominal pain and turbid dialysate. Physical examination revealed the following: his temperature was 37,5°C; his pulse rate was 78 beats/min; blood pressure was 120/70mmHg; respiration rate was 18 per minute; his abdomen was tender to palpation with positive Blumberg sign. Laboratory tests were as follows: WBC 8,280/mm^3, Hgb 7,8g/dl; platelets count 307.000; CRP 71,38mg/L; BUN 66,2mg/dl; serum creatinine 7,02mg/dl; serum albumin 3,1g/dl; total protein 5,3g/dl; total cholesterol 228mg/dl; dialysate leukocyte count 530/mm^3 (neutrophils/lymphocytes 78% vs 10%), serum calcium 1,77mmo/l; phosphorus 2,1mmo/l; sodium 139,1mmo/l; potassium 3,9mmo/l. Samples of peritoneal fluid, blood, and urine were inoculated. Growth of *S. suis* from peritoneal dialysis fluid was confirmed by our clinical microbiology laboratory. Blood culture and urine culture were negative. Current methods for serotyping a strain of *S. suis* are serology, PCR using specific primers (for cps genes) or whole-genome sequencing, and analysis of the cps genes, which were not available in the laboratory. The strain was identified using MALDI-TOF MS technique on MALDI Biotyper apparatus (Bruker) as described above. *S. suis* colonies were sensitive to penicillin G, ampicillin, cefotaxime, ceftriaxone, imipenem, and clindamycin, as described above. After 2 days of empiric intraperitoneal antibiotics administration (cefazoline+ceftazidime ip), we changed the treatment according to antibiogram results into ceftriaxone iv. We continued ceftriaxone iv 2,0g per day for 2 weeks. His clinical condition improved. There was no abdominal pain; peritoneal fluid was transparent. Control peritoneal fluid culture was negative. After 2 weeks of hospital treatment the patient was discharged. In his case we did not observe relapse of peritonitis.

4. Discussion

4.1. A. xylosoxidans PD Related Peritonitis. *A. xylosoxidans* is Gram negative, nonfermenting, aerobic, oxidase- and catalase-positive bacterium. Natural environments of *A. xylosoxidans* are soil and water. *A. xylosoxidans* is also a part of normal human flora. It can be encountered in dairy products. The clinical presentation of *A. xylosoxidans* infections is pneumonia, meningitis, urinary tract infection, endocarditis, bacteremia, and catheter related infections especially in immunocompromised patients. This bacterium is also detected in skin and gastrointestinal tract as normal human flora [4]. *A. xylosoxidans* infection in PD patients is very rare. According to literature data, 11 cases of *A. xylosoxidans* peritonitis have been described so far. These cases were reported mainly in diabetic kidney disease patients and primary glomerulonephritis (IgA nephropathy). Moreover, 2 cases of ESI caused by *A. xylosoxidans* were described. Jun-Li et al. reported first case of *A. xylosoxidans* related tunnel infection in a patient receiving PD. PD related peritonitis was also diagnosed in this patient. *A. xylosoxidans* related tunnel infection was confirmed in CT. The Tenckhoff catheter was removed and new one was inserted at the opposite site [5]. The risk factor for *A. xylosoxidans* infection is CKD per se according to its immunocompromised nature. Aqueous environment and glucose containing PD solution facilitate *A. xylosoxidans* infections. *A. xylosoxidans* colonies can form biofilm on PD catheters and therefore removal of infected catheters is the best method of treatment [5, 6]. In our patient, because of *A. xylosoxidans* relapsing peritonitis removal of PD catheter was performed. After she was transferred to hemodialysis, we continued antibiotic administration for the following 2 weeks. It is worth mentioning that *A. xylosoxidans* infections may occur in long-term hemodialysis patients especially in these having permanent catheters. Moreover, risk factors for *A. xylosoxidans* infections are poor socioeconomic status, contact with animals, poor personal hygiene, and contamination of catheters. In HD patients source of *A. xylosoxidans* infection comprises catheters presence, use of the heparin multidose vials, the dialysate itself, and hands and clothes of healthcare staff [7].

4.2. S. suis PD Related Peritonitis. Another peritonitis reported in our PD center was peritonitis caused by *Streptococcus suis*. This bacterium is common in pigs, piglets, and farm animals. It is also detected in ruminants, dogs, cats, deer, wild boars, and horses. Almost all pigs and farms worldwide are *S. suis* carriers. *S. suis* infection is common zoonosis especially in Southeast Asia. In Hong Kong *S. suis* meningitis is the most frequent bacterial meningitis in adults. There is an increasing evidence of *S. suis* infections in North America and Western countries. In France and United Kingdom *S. suis* infection is recognized as an industrial disease. *S. suis* may cause serious, even life threating diseases in humans. Meningitis and septicemia related to *S. suis* infection were first described in 1968 in Denmark [8]. Clinical presentation of *S. suis* infection is as follows: meningitis, pneumonia, arthritis, endophthalmitis, endocarditis, spontaneous bacterial peritonitis, skin lesions, bacteremia, and septic shock [3, 9]. Partial or complete deafness is an important complication of *S. suis* meningitis. The risk of this zoonosis is related to exposure to pigs (people at risk are farmers, veterinarians, and truck drivers who have direct contact with infected pigs) and pork-derived products (people handling fresh pork processing, people handling carcasses, people such as slaughterhouse workers, butchers, and people handling raw meat at home for cooking). *S. suis* infection is almost absent in children and is highly reported in men, with very high male to female ratio. It is generally considered as an occupational disease [8, 10, 11]. The main route of entry of *S. suis* is through contact of cutaneous lesions (on hands, arms) with contaminated animals, carcasses, or meat or oral route especially in Asian countries where infection has been reported after consumption of undercooked contaminated pork products. As wild boars are also carriers of *S. suis*, the cases of hunters that were infected while handling the carcasses were reported especially in France. In area of Barcelona in Spain, urban wild boars were considered to be a novel public health risk factor for nonhunters [12]. The real infection rate of *S. suis* remains unknown. Human microbiology diagnostic laboratories in Americas and European countries are not aware of this zoonosis and commonly misidentified *S. suis* as enterococci, *S. pneumoniae, S. bovis, S. viridans* group streptococci (*Streptococcus anginosus* and *Streptococcus vestibularis),* or *Listeria.* According to the available literature, serotype 2 ST1 is predominant in Europe. It does not present cross reactivity with other serotypes, in contrast to serotype 14, for example, [13]. The tested strain presented the closest similarity to the reference strain DSM 9682T, belonging to serotype 2, which was originally derived from the pig. Since the MS identifies microorganisms mainly on the basis of ribosomal proteins, in the epidemiological investigations of *S. suis* infections preferably serotyping and molecular methods should be used. MALDI-TOF MS presents 100% sensitivity and specificity for identifying but not serotyping of the most of the *Streptococcus* spp. [14] and enables discrimination between *S. suis* and *S. porcinus* and *S. dysgalactiae* subsp. *equisimilis*. In summary MALDI-TOF MS represents a rapid, accurate, and cost-saving method for routine identification of *S. suis* isolates from both human and animal origins [15].

Peritonitis caused by *S. suis* was previously described in literature but we did not find a description of *S. suis* peritonitis in PD patients. Spontaneous *S. suis* peritonitis was described in patient with alcoholic liver damage [16].

Another case of *S. suis* peritonitis was described in 45-year-old Thai male with acute kidney injury (AKI) stage 3 related to trauma and rhabdomyolysis [17]. Alcoholism, diabetes, malignancy, and contact with infected animals (especially pigs) are considered to be predisposing factors for *S. suis* peritonitis. Our patient was mean age immunocompromised male with MM and CKD. He declared that he did not have any contacts with animals especially pigs or wild animals. He was not occupationally handling meat; he had retired a few years ago. No one from his relatives occupationally was handling meat products. In the past he worked as a sales representative of chemical company. He denied consuming fresh, undercooked pork meat. He denied any serious cutaneous lesions as a route of infection. He was not a hunter. The course of infection in his case was mild and there was a good response for the treatment and no relapse. We suspect that there was a contact with infected animal or pork product used in cooking that patient did not realized, while he was spending his weekends in the rural area. The possible route of infection in his case was improper hand washing before connecting to the cycler which is quite common in PD patients. In our opinion this is the first description of *S. suis* peritonitis in PD patient.

5. Conclusions

Peritonitis caused by rare pathogens such as *A. xylosoxidans* and *S. suis* should always be taken into consideration in PD patients, especially in immunocompromised individuals with diabetic kidney disease, malignancies, or other serious underlying diseases. Specific environmental factors or some patients' habits may facilitate infections caused by described pathogens.

Ethical Approval

Approval for this publication was given by Local Bioethics Committee.

Authors' Contributions

Rafał Donderski, Agnieszka Mikucka, Magdalena Grajewska, Beata Sulikowska, Eugenia Gospodarek-Komkowska, and Jacek Manitius equally contributed to this paper. All authors have read the manuscript and agreed on publication.

References

[1] D. G. Struijk, "Peritoneal Dialysis Western Countries," *Kidney Diseases*, vol. 1, no. 3, pp. 157–164, 2015.

[2] E. Yabuuchi and A. Ohyama, "Achrobacter xylosoxidans n.sp. from human ear discharge," *Japanese Journal of Microbiology*, vol. 15, pp. 477–481, 1971.

[3] J. Dejace, P. Bagley, and E. Wood, "Streptococcus suis meningitis can require a prolonged treatment course," *International Journal of Infectious Diseases*, vol. 65, pp. 34–36, 2017.

[4] J. M. Duggan, S. J. Goldstein, C. E. Chenoweth, C. A. Kauffman, and S. F. Bradley, "Achromobacter xylosoxidans bacteremia: report of four cases and review of the literature," *Clinical Infectious Diseases*, vol. 23, no. 3, pp. 569–576, 1996.

[5] J.-L. Tsai and S.-F. Tsai, "Case report: The first case of Achromobacter xylosoxidans-related tunnel infection in a patient receiving peritoneal dialysis," *Medicine (United States)*, vol. 96, no. 16, Article ID e6654, 2017.

[6] M. T. Tsai, W. C. Yang, and C. C. Lin, "Continuous ambulatory peritoneal dialysis-related exit-site Infections caused by Achromobacter denitrificans and A. xylosoxidans," *Peritoneal Dialysis International*, vol. 32, no. 3, pp. 362-363, 2012.

[7] A. Segarra-Medrano, E. Jatem-Escalante, C. Carnicer-Cáceres et al., "Evolution of antibody titre against the M-type phospholipase A2 receptor and clinical response in idiopathic membranous nephropathy patients treated with tacrolimus," *Nefrología*, vol. 34, no. 4, pp. 491–497, 2014.

[8] H. Wertheim, H. Nghia, W. Taylor, and C. Schultsz, *Clinical Infectious Diseases*, vol. 48, no. 5, pp. 617–625, 2009.

[9] P. Zalas-Wiecek, A. Michalska, E. Grabczewska, A. Olczak, M. Pawłowska, and E. Gospodarek, "Human meningitis caused by Streptococcus suis," *Journal of Medical Microbiology*, vol. 62, no. 3, pp. 483–485, 2013.

[10] V. T. L. Huong, N. Ha, N. T. Huy et al., "Epidemiology, clinical manifestations, and outcomes of streptococcus suis infection in humans," *Emerging Infectious Diseases*, vol. 20, no. 7, pp. 1105–1114, 2014.

[11] J. Dutkiewicz, J. Sroka, V. Zając et al., "Streptococcus suis: a re-emerging pathogen associated with occupational exposure to pigs or pork products. Part I – Epidemiology," *Annals of Agricultural and Environmental Medicine*, vol. 24, no. 4, pp. 683–695, 2017.

[12] X. Fernández-Aguilar, M. Gottschalk, V. Aragon et al., " Urban Wild Boars and Risk for Zoonotic ," *Emerging Infectious Diseases*, vol. 24, no. 6, pp. 1083–1086, 2018.

[13] G. Goyette-Desjardins, J.-P. Auger, J. Xu, M. Segura, and M. Gottschalk, "Streptococcus suis, an important pig pathogen and emerging zoonotic agent-an update on the worldwide distribution based on serotyping and sequence typing," *Emerging Microbes and Infections*, vol. 3, article e45, pp. 1–20, 2014.

[14] M. Pérez-Sancho, A. I. Vela, T. García-Seco et al., "Usefulness of MALDI-TOF MS as a Diagnostic Tool for the Identification of Streptococcus Species Recovered from Clinical Specimens of Pigs," *PLoS ONE*, vol. 12, no. 1, p. e0170784, 2017.

[15] M. Pérez-Sancho, A. I. Vela, T. García-Seco, M. Gottschalk, L. Domínguez, and J. F. Fernández-Garayzábal, "Assessment of MALDI-TOF MS as Alternative Tool for Streptococcus suis Identification," *Frontiers in Public Health*, vol. 3, no. 202, 2015.

[16] R. Callejo, M. Prieto, F. Salamone, J.-P. Auger, G. Goyette-Desjardins, and M. Gottschalk, "Atypical streptococcus suis in man, Argentina, 2013," *Emerging Infectious Diseases*, vol. 20, no. 3, pp. 500–502, 2014.

[17] R.-K. Vilaichone, V. Mahachai, and P. Nunthapisud, "Streptococcus suis peritonitis: Case report," *Journal of the Medical Association of Thailand*, vol. 83, no. 10, pp. 1274–1277, 2000.

they present with symptoms of infectious mononucleosis or with fever and localized or disseminated lymphoproliferation involving the lymph nodes and extranodal sites like the liver, lungs, kidney, bone marrow, central nervous system, or small intestine [4]. Although PTLD has increased extranodal involvement when compared with lymphoma in the general population [5], cases involving extranodal masses in the testes have very sparse representation in current literature. We report an unusual finding of PTLD in a kidney transplant patient presenting as lymphoma of the right testis. We include a comparison of this form of PTLD with primary testicular lymphoma in the immunocompetent patient and review literature considering the role of EBV in carcinogenesis.

Posttransplant Lymphoproliferative Disorder Presenting as Testicular Lymphoma in a Kidney Transplant Recipient: A Case Report

Steve Omoruyi Obanor,[1,2] Michelle Gruttadauria,[3] Kayla Applebaum,[3] Mohammad Eskandari,[4] Michelle Lieberman Lubetzky,[1] and Stuart Greenstein[1]

[1]Montefiore Einstein Center for Transplantation, Montefiore Medical Center, Albert Einstein College of Medicine, Bronx, NY, USA
[2]Department of Internal Medicine, Maimonides Medical Center, Brooklyn, NY, USA
[3]Albert Einstein College of Medicine, Bronx, NY, USA
[4]Department of Pathology, Montefiore Medical Center, Albert Einstein College of Medicine, Bronx, NY, USA

Correspondence should be addressed to Stuart Greenstein; sgreenst@montefiore.org

Academic Editor: Władysław Sułowicz

Posttransplant lymphoproliferative disorder (PTLD) is a malignancy caused by the immunosuppression that occurs after transplantation. It is primarily a nodal lesion but frequently it involves extranodal masses. Treatment is usually by reducing immunosuppressive therapy. Testicular lymphoma as PTLD is notably rare in documented literature and there is limited evidence of definitive treatment guidelines. This manuscript describes a patient who developed diffuse large B-cell lymphoma of his right testis one year following kidney transplantation. A diagnosis of PTLD was made and treatment with rituximab, locoregional radiotherapy, and intrathecal methotrexate in addition to the standard reduction of immunosuppression resulted in complete remission until now. We submit this case along with literature review of similar cases in the past and a review of specific peculiarities of our case with emphasis on our treatment plan to further the understanding of this diversiform disease.

1. Introduction

Posttransplant lymphoproliferative disorder (PTLD) is a heterogeneous group of lesions that can develop in patients receiving chronic immunosuppression after solid organ transplantation [1]. The clear majority of these are proliferations of B-cell origin, triggered by Epstein-Barr virus (EBV) infection [2]; this can either be a primary infection after transplant in a seronegative recipient or reactivation of latent EBV infection in a seropositive recipient, the former posing higher risk of development of PTLD [3]. They present with symptoms of infectious mononucleosis or with fever and localized or disseminated lymphoproliferation involving the lymph nodes and extranodal sites like the liver, lungs, kidney, bone marrow, central nervous system, or small intestine [4]. Although PTLD has increased extranodal involvement when compared with lymphoma in the general population [5], cases

2. Materials and Methods: The Case Report

A 68-year-old Hispanic male (postrenal transplant) presented to our follow-up clinic in December 2013 with a 2-week history of painless right testicular swelling. He denied trauma. There was no associated history of fever, weight loss, anorexia, night sweats, or urinary symptoms.

His past medical history was significant for morbid obesity, diabetes, lone atrial fibrillation, and end-stage renal

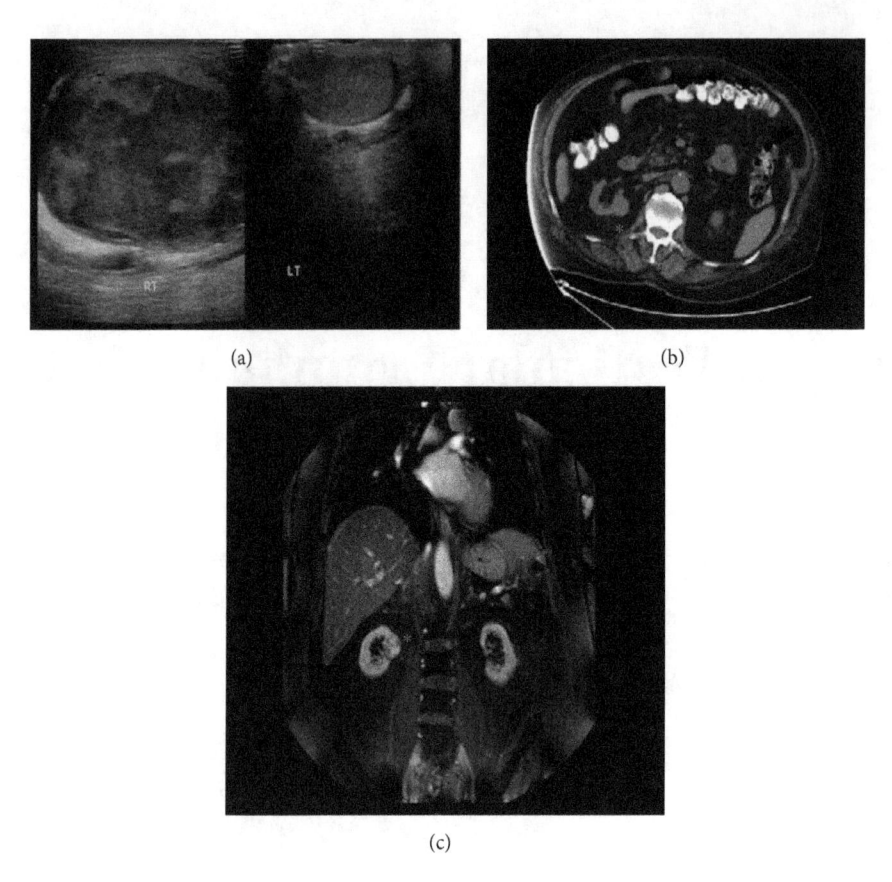

FIGURE 1: (a) Sonogram of both testes: sagittal view showing grossly enlarged right testis in comparison with the left. (b) T2-weighted MRI of the abdomen with contrast, transverse, and (c) sagittal views; renal cell carcinoma (red asterisk) noted on the right native kidney.

disease secondary to hypertensive nephrosclerosis for which he underwent a deceased donor renal transplant one year prior to presentation. He received a Public Health Service and Centers for Disease Control (PHS/CDC) high-risk kidney. EBV IgG and IgM and Cytomegalovirus (CMV) IgG and IgM of donor were negative. For the recipient, EBV IgG and CMV IgG were positive; however, EBV viral capsid antigen IgM, EBV DNA PCR, and CMV IgM were negative. Calculated Panel Reactive Antibody was 0. There were no donor-specific antigens (DSA). T&B cell flow crossmatches were negative. He received induction with basiliximab and maintenance immunosuppression with tacrolimus, mycophenolic acid, and prednisone. He had no episodes of graft rejection. He also had a history of Polyomavirus BK viremia, which necessitated a mycophenolate dose reduction (1000 mg twice a day (BID) to 500 mg BID). He was a former smoker but quit over 20 years ago and his mother is said to have had an unnamed cancer.

Initial management was with outpatient urology consult. Physical examination revealed an enlarged indurated right testicle with normal lie, firm-hard, nontender, nonfluctuant, and no regional or generalized lymphadenopathy. Left hemiscrotum was grossly normal. Blood and sonographic tests were ordered and he was asked to follow up in a month.

Serum tumor markers, alpha fetoprotein, beta human chorionic gonadotropin, prostate-specific antigen, and lactate dehydrogenase were all within normal limits. EBV and CMV serologies remained unchanged from pretransplant values. HIV was negative.

Doppler sonographic findings noted a markedly abnormal right testis, which was enlarged and nearly completely replaced by a zone or mass of heterogeneously decreased echogenicity and little if any internal vascular flow, suggestive of a subacute infarct or a hypovascular tumor (Figure 1(a)).

Prior to his next follow-up visit, however, he presented to the Emergency Department complaining of sudden sharp, nonradiating right testicular pain without fever or urinary symptoms. Noncontrast CT revealed an incidental, solitary, 2.3×2.1 cm, partially exophytic upper pole lesion on the right native kidney, suspicious for neoplasm; there was no abdominal or pelvic lymphadenopathy. Magnetic resonance imaging with contrast showed a small enhancing right renal nodule suspicious for cortical malignancy but there was no evidence of metastatic disease (Figures 1(b) and 1(c)). Mycophenolic acid was withheld due to concern for undetected malignancy.

In January 2014, he underwent a right total nephrectomy and right radical orchiectomy.

Pathological analysis established the diagnosis of renal cell carcinoma (RCC) and clear cell type (Fuhrman Nuclear grade 2). The lesion was 2.5 cm in its greatest dimension and unifocal and was limited to the kidney with all margins clear. Histological analysis of the right testis revealed a

(a) (b)

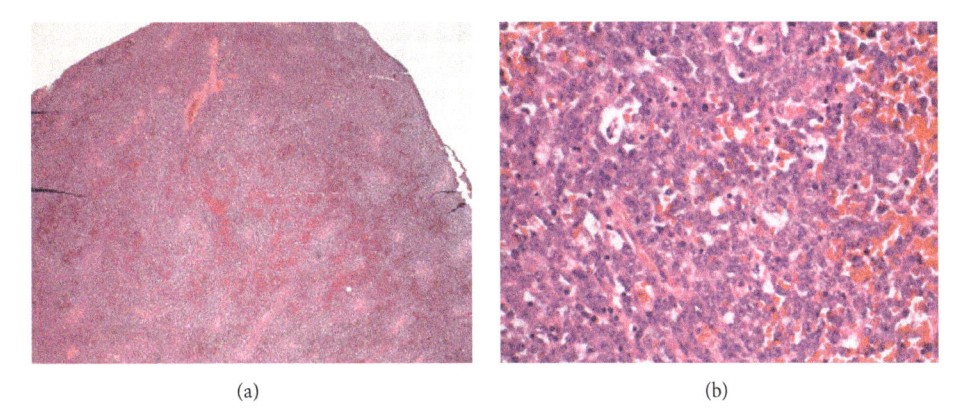

FIGURE 2: Section of the right testis stained with hematoxylin and eosin. (a) Low power (2x) shows diffuse infiltration of the testis by large neoplastic cells. There is geographic necrosis. (b) Higher magnification (40x) shows the large cells with irregular nuclei, vesicular chromatin, and prominent nucleoli. Occasional mitoses and apoptotic bodies present.

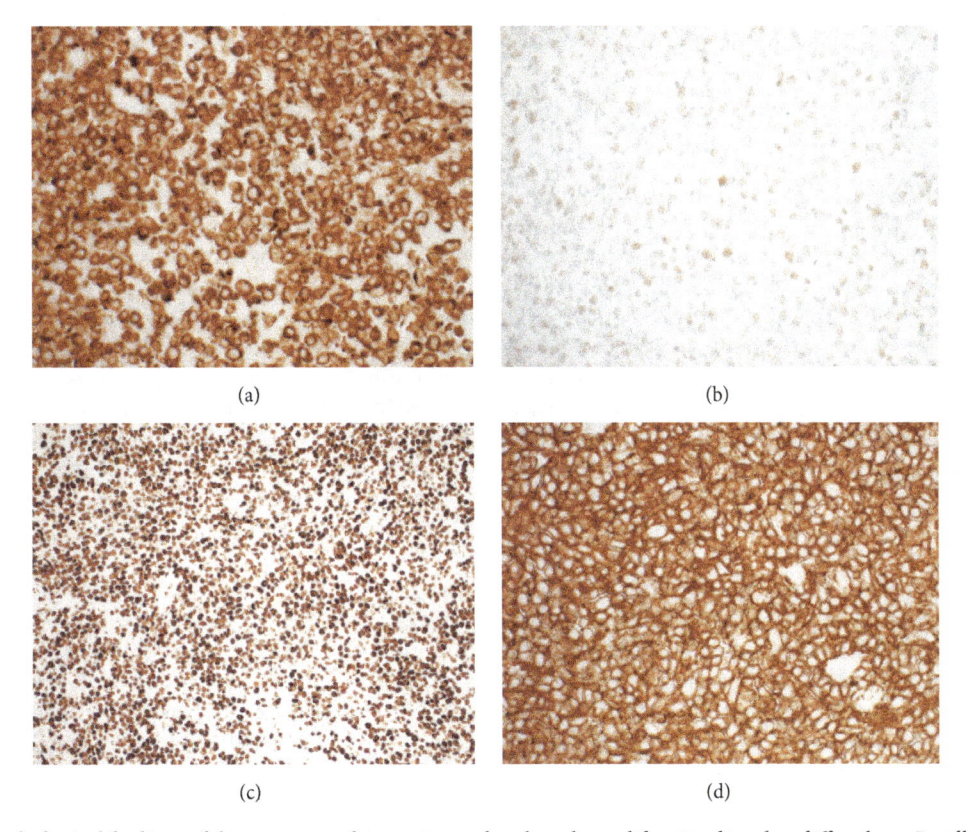

(a) (b)

(c) (d)

FIGURE 3: Histopathological findings of the monomorphic posttransplant lymphoproliferative disorder; diffuse large B-cell lymphoma of the right testis. Immunophenotyping, via immunohistochemistry, revealed neoplastic cells positive for Bcl-2 (a), Bcl-6 (b), Ki-67 (proliferation index > 90%) (c), and CD20 (d). Magnification for all panels: 40x.

monomorphic posttransplant lymphoproliferative disorder: diffuse large B-cell lymphoma (DLBCL) (Figure 2). Immunohistochemistry of the abnormal B-cells was positive for CD20, Bcl-2, Bcl-6, MUM1, Ki-67 (at least 90%), and EBV latent membrane protein 1 (EBV LMP-1) (Figure 3). The cells were negative for CD3, CD5, CD10, c-Myc, CD30, and HHV8. Fluorescent in situ hybridization and molecular studies were not performed.

Upon diagnosis of lymphoma, he had reduction of immunosuppression (mycophenolic acid was withheld) and was maintained on low-dose tacrolimus (0.5 mg q12 h) and prednisone (5 mg daily). Five days prior to diagnosis of lymphoma, the patient's tacrolimus level was 7 nanograms/mL. Cerebrospinal fluid (CSF) cytology, CSF flow cytometry, and CT guided bone marrow biopsy all showed no evidence of clonal B-cell expansion. PET/CT from base of skull to mid-thigh showed no evidence of metastatic disease which further characterized the disease as Stage IE.

Considering the rare nature of posttransplant testicular lymphoma, two oncologic opinions were sought. The initial recommendation was rituximab, cyclophosphamide, hydroxydaunorubicin, and prednisone (R-CHOP) regimen, in combination with intrathecal methotrexate and radiation to the contralateral testes. However, given his advanced age and immunosuppressed state, an alternative opinion to receive the above treatment without the CHOP regimen was recommended.

He went on to receive intrathecal methotrexate, 4 courses of rituximab, and radiation to the contralateral testes, which was completed in July 2014. Within 6 months, he achieved complete remission while maintaining excellent allograft function. His current creatinine is 1.2, although he has developed de novo DSA in the setting of reduced immunosuppression. He has no proteinuria and this is being followed closely as well as regular follow-up with oncology, with recurrence surveillance provided by regular PET/CT scans per oncology protocols.

3. Discussion

The incidence of PTLD in adult kidney transplant recipients ranges from 1 to 2.3% [6] and although immunosuppression, as can be seen after a transplant, puts the male patient at a 20 to 50 times greater risk of development of testicular neoplasm [7, 8], testicular lymphoma is still exceedingly rare in this population. A retrospective study analyzed malignant testicular neoplasms in immunocompromised (AIDS and posttransplant) patients over a period of 20 years. This study reviewed histopathology of testicular tumors, patient ages at presentation, disease stage at presentation, management schemes, type and incidence of adverse effect of therapy, and/or outcome after therapy. The tumors found were germ cell tumors (seminomas and nonseminomas, with equal prevalence) and lymphomas. However, no lymphomas were noted among posttransplant patients [9]. Prior to this case, only two solid organ recipients had been reported to develop testicular lymphoma after transplant: a 52-year-old with a primary occurrence of aggressive large cell CD45+ epididymal lymphoma seven years after transplant treated with reduction in immunosuppression and CHOP [10] and an 8-year-old heart transplant patient with CD20+, EBV+ polymorphic PTLD of the testicle six years after transplant treated with rituximab and autologous EBV-specific cytotoxic T lymphocytes [11].

Organ transplant recipients maintained on chronic immunosuppressive therapy have a heightened chance of developing de novo cancer within the first few years of transplantation [12]. However, on presentation with initial symptoms, our patient seemed to have a low risk of developing PTLD and presence of latent EBV infection as opposed to a primary one; the type of organ transplanted was the kidney, being the least likely to result in PTLD; induction therapy was by basiliximab as opposed to muromonab-CD3 (OKT3) or thymoglobulin; he had no prior rejection episodes and was neither CMV nor Hepatitis C Virus (HCV) positive. This stresses the need to have a high index of suspicion of PTLD. In addition to testicular lymphoma, he also developed a right renal cell carcinoma, an occurrence which can be attributed to his immunosuppressed state, morbid obesity, or even his family history of cancer. Several studies, however, have described the possible role of EBV in the etiopathogenesis of tumors after transplant. Lee et al. studied three children in whom smooth-muscle tumors developed at varying periods of time after transplant [13]. They found that a single form of EBV DNA was present in each tumor, defining them as neoplasia. Also, on analysis of EBV DNA in the tumors, features akin to those found in PTLD including unique EBV DNA episomes (EBV small RNA, EBER, and EBV nuclear antigen-2 (EBNA-2)) were noted. These unique episomes showed that they were present before the clonal population was derived, strongly supporting a causative role for EBV in the development of smooth-muscle tumors after transplantation. Shimakage et al. have several studies reporting the role of EBV in the pathogenesis of many human cancers. One of their studies [14] attempted to investigate EBV expression in renal cell carcinoma with the aim of inferring a causal relationship. Formalin-fixed paraffin-embedded tissue samples from nine patients with RCC and two patients with nephroblastoma were subjected to mRNA in situ hybridization and indirect immunofluorescence staining. Their results indicated that mRNA and proteins of EBV were expressed in all RCC and nephroblastoma tissues, suggesting an oncogenic and tumor progressive role of EBV in these conditions. This was in keeping with a prior study [15] on EBNA-2 transgenic mice, 90% of which developed kidney adenocarcinoma (immunohistochemistry demonstrated nuclear expression of EBNA-2 in hyperplastic tubular cells and tumor cells). Shimakage et al. also observed that EBV expression was more commonly present in papillary and clear cell RCC than chromophobe cell RCC (chromophobe cell RCC described to be less malignant than other RCC). Furthermore, EBV was expressed at higher rates in high-grade RCC than in low-grade RCC. These both suggested that EBV expression correlated with RCC malignancy. It is possible therefore to postulate that both neoplastic occurrences in our patient resulted as a consequence of EBV infection after transplant.

Primary testicular lymphoma in an immunocompetent patient is an aggressive form of extranodal lymphoma. Though rare, it is the most common testicular malignancy in men aged above 60 years (median age at diagnosis is 66 to 68 years). Our patient was 68 years old at presentation of symptoms and had atypical transplant serologic markers for PTLD. He was EBV IgG+ with an EBV− donor kidney. It was therefore paramount to distinguish his lymphoma as a PTLD in order to decide upon appropriate treatment. The presence of EBV LMP-1 (latent membrane protein 1) in the tissue sufficiently establishes this diagnosis. Serologic markers of EBV infection have also been used by some clinicians in making the diagnosis of PTLD, serum EBV DNA PCR (EBV DNAemia) being one of the most widely studied. Although EBV DNAemia has been suggested as a means of surveillance for suspected PTLD cases and monitoring established cases, several studies have shown its use to be debatable [16]. Initially thought to have 100% sensitivity and specificity, EBV

DNAemia has now been found to be relatively less sensitive though maintaining fairly high specificity for the detection of PTLD [17–19]. EBV DNA was negative in peripheral blood samples in our patient; possible reasons for this could be the fact that the PTLD was not driven by EBV or the effect of EBV infection on lymphoproliferation was localized [20]. Since our case showed EBV association histologically, the latter option is highly probable. Several studies show similar cases of localized PTLD failing to provoke a corresponding EBV DNAemia [20, 21]. One of such studies involves a case of isolated CNS lymphoma after allogenic hematopoietic stem cell transplant, in which EBV DNA load was elevated in the cerebrospinal fluid but was not detected in the peripheral blood [22]. In this case, it is important to note the special characteristics shared by both the CNS and the testes, as both are immune privileged sites, with tight junctions which isolate these cells from peripheral blood. This may play a role in negative EBV DNAemia seen in localized forms of PTLD.

The current international standard of care for primary testicular lymphoma irrespective of immune status is R-CHOP every 21 days with intrathecal methotrexate and locoregional radiation therapy [23]. In the international trial, intrathecal rather than systemic CNS prophylaxis was used as it is better tolerated by elderly patients than aggressive high-dose systemic prophylaxis [23]. There are no specific guidelines for testicular PTLD due to the rarity of its presentation. After consultations with 2 independent oncology services, we opted out of systemic chemotherapy, primarily because of the patient's advanced age and comorbidities. Local consensus studies also suggest that systemic chemotherapy is most useful in patients with monomorphic histology, a large mass lesion, fulminant PTLD, or evidence of graft rejection [24]. Furthermore, existing literature pertaining to the management of primary testicular lymphoma was reviewed, which found that adverse prognostic factors [25] include age above 70 years, advanced stage, presence of B symptoms, >1 extranodal site, involvement of extranodal sites other than testis, tumor diameter > 10 cm, elevated lactate dehydrogenase, elevated B2-microglobulin, hypoalbuminemia, and involvement of the left testes, all of which were negative in our patient. This also helped inform the decision for treatment without CHOP therapy. Estimated CNS involvement in primary testicular lymphoma has been reported in smaller series as up to 44% [25]. This risk has been noted, in a large retrospective study [26], to be higher in extranodal DLBCL as opposed to their nodal counterparts. Given CD20+ status of the lesion and the above considerations, treatment with rituximab, intrathecal methotrexate, and locoregional radiotherapy was agreed upon. Although this treatment course resulted in a positive outcome in this patient, strong conclusions cannot be made with this limited evidence of success and short follow-up period. It instead highlights the need for further investigation and discussion.

4. Conclusion

In summary, we report a unique manifestation of PTLD presenting as a testicular lymphoma, still a rare form of extranodal PTLD. Standard management of PTLD is usually with reduction of immunosuppression alone; however, given the aggressive nature of the lymphoma, we came up with a unique combination of surgical excision, reduction of immunosuppression, rituximab, intrathecal methotrexate, and radiotherapy. With this strategy, complete remission and a disease-free state until now were achieved.

Disclosure

Steve Omoruyi Obanor and Michelle Gruttadauria are co-first authors of the manuscript.

Authors' Contributions

Kayla Applebaum contributed to "Case Report" section and to review of the final manuscript. Mohammad Eskandari was responsible for the histopathology materials. Michelle Lieberman Lubetzky, patient's transplant nephrologist, was responsible for immunosuppressive treatment and outpatient follow-up and contributed to all chapters as well as review and correction of the manuscript. Stuart Greenstein, patient's transplant surgeon, was responsible for supervision of the patient during in-hospital and perioperative care as well as for obtaining imaging records and contributed to review and correction of the manuscript.

References

[1] T. Greiner, J. O. Armitage, and T. G. Gross, "Atypical lymphoproliferative diseases," *Hematology American Society of Hematology Education Program*, pp. 133–146, 2000.

[2] S. Gottschalk, C. M. Rooney, and H. E. Heslop, "Post-transplant lymphoproliferative disorders," *Annual Review of Medicine*, vol. 56, pp. 29–44, 2005.

[3] R. C. Walker, W. F. Marshall, J. G. Strickler et al., "Pretransplantation assessment of the risk of lymphoproliferative disorder," *Clinical Infectious Diseases*, vol. 20, no. 5, pp. 1346–1353, 1995.

[4] J. I. Cohen, "Epstein-Barr virus infection," *The New England Journal of Medicine*, vol. 343, no. 7, pp. 481–492, 2000.

[5] C. N. Kotton and J. A. Fishman, "Viral infection in the renal transplant recipient," *Journal of the American Society of Nephrology*, vol. 16, no. 6, pp. 1758–1774, 2005.

[6] A. L. Taylor, R. Marcus, and J. A. Bradley, "Post-transplant lymphoproliferative disorders (PTLD) after solid organ transplantation," *Critical Review in Oncology/Hematology*, vol. 56, no. 1, pp. 155–167, 2005.

[7] I. Penn, "Malignancy," *Surgical Clinics of North America*, vol. 74, article 1247, 1994.

[8] D. J. Kwan and F. C. Lowe, "Genitourinary manifestations of the acquired immunodeficiency syndrome," *Urology*, vol. 45, no. 1, pp. 13–27, 1995.

[9] I. Leibovitch, J. Baniel, R. G. Rowland, E. R. Smith Jr., J. K. Ludlow, and J. P. Donohue, "Malignant testicular neoplasms in immunosuppressed patients," *The Journal of Urology*, vol. 155, no. 6, pp. 1938–1942, 1996.

[10] R. Maniyur, K. Anant, S. Aneesh, E. Vinita, J. Manoj, and P. Rakesh, "Posttransplant epididymal lymphoma: An aggressive variant," *Transplantation*, vol. 75, no. 2, pp. 246-247, 2003.

[11] S. Basso, M. Zecca, L. Calafiore et al., "Successful treatment of a classic Hodgkin lymphoma-type post-transplant lymphoproliferative disorder with tailored chemotherapy and Epstein-Barr virus-specific cytotoxic T lymphocytes in a pediatric heart transplant recipient," *Pediatric Transplantation*, vol. 17, no. 7, pp. E168-E173, 2013.

[12] I. Penn, "Why do immunosuppressed patients develop cancer?" *Critical Reviews in Oncogenesis*, vol. 1, pp. 27-52, 1989.

[13] E. S. Lee, J. Locker, M. Nalesnik et al., "The association of Epstein-Barr virus with smooth-muscle tumors occurring after organ transplantation," *The New England Journal of Medicine*, vol. 332, no. 1, pp. 19-25, 1995.

[14] M. Shimakage, K. Kawahara, S. Harada, T. Sasagawa, T. Shinka, and T. Oka, "Expression of Epstein-Barr virus in renal cell carcinoma," *Oncology Reports*, vol. 18, no. 1, pp. 41-46, 2007.

[15] J. Törnell, S. Farzad, A. Espander-Jansson, G. Matejka, O. Isaksson, and L. Rymo, "Expression of Epstein-Barr nuclear antigen 2 in kidney tubule cells induces tumors in transgenic mice," *Oncogene*, vol. 12, no. 7, pp. 1521-1528, 1996.

[16] D. A. Axelrod, R. Holmes, S. E. Thomas, and J. C. Magee, "Limitations of EBV-PCR monitoring to detect EBV associated post-transplant lymphoproliferative disorder," *Pediatric Transplantation*, vol. 7, no. 3, pp. 223-227, 2003.

[17] M. H. Collins, K. T. Montone, A. M. Leahey et al., "Posttransplant lymphoproliferative disease in children," *Pediatric Transplantation*, vol. 5, no. 4, pp. 250-257, 2001.

[18] H.-J. Wagner, M. Wessel, W. Jabs et al., "Patients at risk for development of posttransplant lymphoproliferative disorder: Plasma versus peripheral blood mononuclear cells as material for quantification of Epstein-Barr viral load by using real-time quantitative polymerase chain reaction," *Transplantation*, vol. 72, no. 6, pp. 1012-1019, 2001.

[19] M. Green, J. Bueno, D. Rowe et al., "Predictive negative value of persistent low Epstein-Barr virus viral load after intestinal transplantation in children," *Transplantation*, vol. 70, no. 4, pp. 593-596, 2000.

[20] F. Baldanti, V. Rognoni, A. Cascina, T. Oggionni, C. Tinelli, and F. Meloni, "Post-transplant lymphoproliferative disorders and Epstein-Barr virus DNAemia in a cohort of lung transplant recipients," *Virology Journal*, vol. 8, article no. 421, 2011.

[21] B. M. Levenson, S. A. Ali, C. F. Timmons, N. Mittal, A. Muthukumar, and D. A. Payne, "Unusual case of Epstein-Barr virus DNA tissue positive: Blood negative in a patient with post-transplant lymphoproliferative disorder," *Pediatric Transplantation*, vol. 13, no. 1, pp. 134-138, 2009.

[22] H. Shimizu, T. Saitoh, H. Koya et al., "Discrepancy in EBV-DNA load between peripheral blood and cerebrospinal fluid in a patient with isolated CNS post-transplant lymphoproliferative disorder," *International Journal of Hematology*, vol. 94, no. 5, pp. 495-498, 2011.

[23] U. Vitolo, A. Chiapella, A. J. M. Ferreri et al., "First-line treatment for primary testicular diffuse large-b-cell lymphoma with rituximab-CHOP, CNS prophylaxis, and contralateral testis irradiation: Final results of an international phase II trial," *Journal of Clinical Oncology*, vol. 29, no. 20, pp. 2766-2772, 2011.

[24] National Guideline Clearinghouse (NGC), "Guideline summary: Evidence based clinical practice guideline for management of EBV-associated post-transplant lymphoproliferative disease (PTLD) in solid organ transplant. In: National Guideline Clearinghouse (NGC). Rockville (MD): Agency for Healthcare Research and Quality (AHRQ); 2012 Jan 01," https://www.guideline.gov.

[25] C. Y. Cheah, A. Wirth, and J. F. Seymour, "Primary testicular lymphoma," *Blood*, vol. 123, no. 4, pp. 486-493, 2014.

[26] E. Zucca, A. Conconi, T. I. Mughal et al., "Patterns of outcome and prognostic factors in primary large-cell lymphoma of the testis in a survey by the international extranodal lymphoma study group," *Journal of Clinical Oncology*, vol. 21, no. 1, pp. 20-27, 2003.

Mucin-1 Gene Mutation and the Kidney: The Link between Autosomal Dominant Tubulointerstitial Kidney Disease and Focal and Segmental Glomerulosclerosis

H. Trimarchi,[1] M. Paulero,[1] T. Rengel,[1] I. González-Hoyos,[1] M. Forrester,[1] F. Lombi,[1] V. Pomeranz,[1] R. Iriarte,[1] and A. Iotti[2]

[1]Nephrology Service, Hospital Británico de Buenos Aires, Buenos Aires, Argentina
[2]Pathology Service, Hospital Británico de Buenos Aires, Buenos Aires, Argentina

Correspondence should be addressed to H. Trimarchi; htrimarchi@hotmail.com

Academic Editor: John A. Sayer

Glomerular diseases are one of the most frequent causes of chronic kidney disease, focal and segmental glomerulosclerosis being one of the commonest glomerulopathies. However, the etiology of this glomerular entity, which merely depicts a morphologic pattern of disease, is often not established and, in most of the patients, remains unknown. Nephrologists tend to assume focal and segmental glomerulosclerosis as a definitive diagnosis. However, despite the increasing knowledge developed in the field, genetic causes of glomerular diseases are currently identified in fewer than 10% of chronic kidney disease subjects. Moreover, unexplained familial clustering among dialysis patients suggests that genetic causes may be underrecognized. Secondary focal and segmental glomerulosclerosis due to genetic mutations mainly located in the podocyte and slit diaphragm can occur from childbirth to adulthood with different clinical presentations, ranging from mild proteinuria and normal renal function to nephrotic syndrome and renal failure. However, this histopathological pattern can also be due to primary defects outside the glomerulus. The present report illustrates an adult case of secondary focal and segmental glomerulosclerosis with a dominant tubulointerstitial damage that led to the pursue of its cause at the tubular level. In this patient with an undiagnosed family history of adult kidney disease, a genetic study unraveled a mutation in the mucin-1 gene and a final diagnosis of adult dominant tubular kidney disease-MUC1 was made.

1. Introduction

Focal and segmental glomerulosclerosis (FSGS) is classified into primary and secondary causes [1]. While the former is mainly due to still unidentified controversial circulating permeability factors and presents clinically with severe nephrotic syndrome and a grim prognosis, the latter may be due to numerous widely dissimilar etiologies with completely different pathophysiological mechanisms [1, 2]. In general, secondary causes of focal and segmental glomerulosclerosis present with lower levels of proteinuria and a slow decline in kidney function. Regardless of the cause, the main concern that encompasses focal and segmental glomerulosclerosis is the fact that it refers just to a morphological pattern of disease [1]. Finally, in general nephrologists tend to accept FSGS as a definitive diagnosis and mainly focus on the management of the clinical markers of kidney disease progression, as proteinuria and hypertension. Rarely do nephrologists search for the genetic causes that may cause FSGS and assume it to be of glomerular origin when evident causes of its secondary essence have been discarded, as HIV infection, ureteralvesical reflux, obesity, pharmacological causes, hyperfiltration due to a reduction in the glomerular mass, cocaine abuse, and sickle cell disease, among others [1, 2]. Interestingly, the usually nonnephrotic range of proteinuria cannot differentiate between FSGS due to podocyte mutations from the other causes. In this regard, the clinical background, renal imaging, and certain histopathological features encountered in the kidney biopsy can guide or suggest a possible etiology. In this case report, the coexistence of glomerulosclerosis and relevant tubulointerstitial damage with mononuclear infiltration suggested an extraglomerular origin of FSGS.

Caucasian family, Italian origin

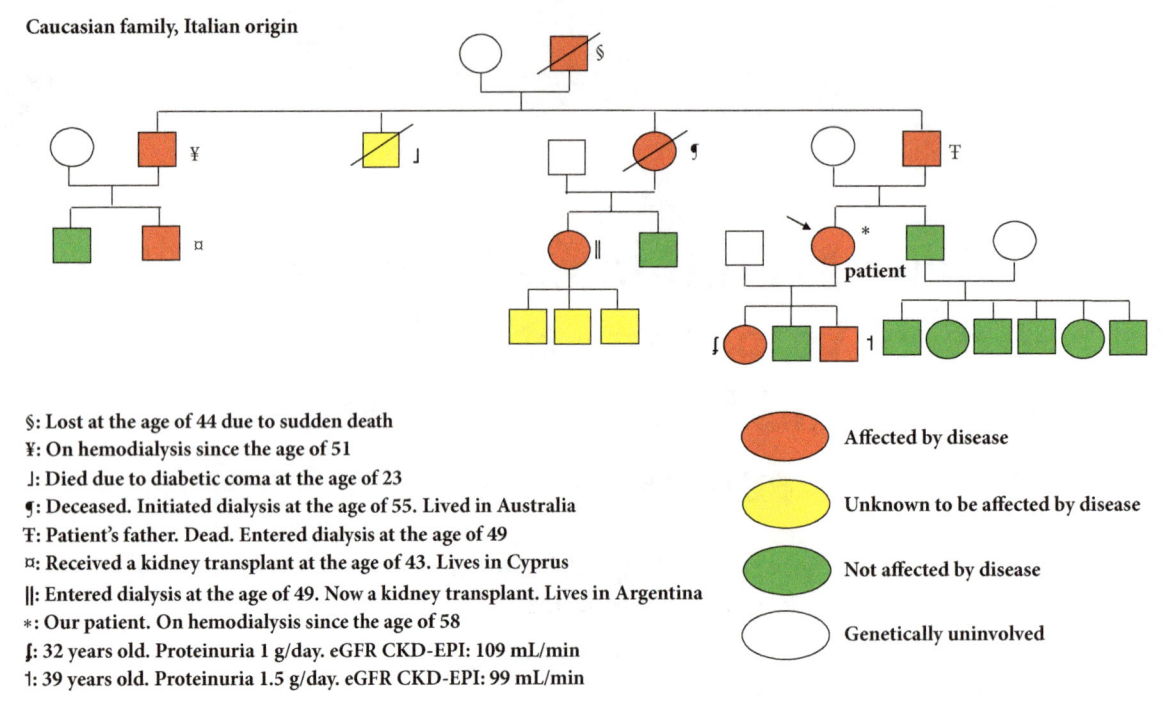

FIGURE 1: Family tree.

§: Lost at the age of 44 due to sudden death
¥: On hemodialysis since the age of 51
⌐: Died due to diabetic coma at the age of 23
¶: Deceased. Initiated dialysis at the age of 55. Lived in Australia
₮: Patient's father. Dead. Entered dialysis at the age of 49
¤: Received a kidney transplant at the age of 43. Lives in Cyprus
‖: Entered dialysis at the age of 49. Now a kidney transplant. Lives in Argentina
∗: Our patient. On hemodialysis since the age of 58
ʃ: 32 years old. Proteinuria 1 g/day. eGFR CKD-EPI: 109 mL/min
1: 39 years old. Proteinuria 1.5 g/day. eGFR CKD-EPI: 99 mL/min

- Affected by disease
- Unknown to be affected by disease
- Not affected by disease
- Genetically uninvolved

The unexpected diagnosis of a mutation in the mucin gene (MUC-1) was made and remarks how a tubular derangement can cause secondary glomerular damage as glomerulosclerosis, underscoring that FSGS is a pattern of disease.

2. Case Presentation

A 56-year-old female was referred to the nephrologist due to apparently chronic kidney disease (CKD), diagnosed on a routine laboratory check-up. The patient was asymptomatic, Past medical record was contributory for three normal pregnancies. There was no background of alcohol intake, tobacco consumption, drug abuse, or medication exposure. There was a family history of CKD (Figure 1). Physical examination was unremarkable. Abnormal blood tests were as follows: Haematocrit 37%; haemoglobin 11.9 g/dL; bicarbonate 21 mEq/L; urea 78 mg/dL (normal value 20-50 mg/dL); serum creatinine 2 mg/dL; uric acid 6.4 mg/dL; creatinine clearance 42 ml/min; proteinuria 0.2 g/day; urinary sodium excretion 188 mEq/day; urine pH: 6, urinary density 1015. Urinary sediment was unremarkable. HIV, HCV, and HBV were negative; C3, C4, and CH50 were within normal limits. ANA, p-ANCA, c-ANCA, antiglomerular basement membrane antibody, and antiphospholipid antibodies were reported as negative. Renal sonogram disclosed two kidneys, normal in shape- and size. A kidney biopsy was performed. Light microscopy disclosed 30 glomeruli: 6 completely obliterated, 8 presented peripheral sclerosis of the glomerular tuft with adhesions between parietal and visceral epithelial cells of Bowman's capsule, and 6 depicted mild mesangial expansion (Figure 2).

Tubular atrophy and interstitial fibrosis were 30%. Blood vessels showed mild intimal sclerosis in arterioles. Immunofluorescence was negative. Electron microscopy: diffuse effacement of podocyte foot processes existed with microvillous transformation. Basal membrane was normal. Tubules were normal. Pathology report was as follows: focal and segmental glomerulosclerosis with moderate interstitial fibrosis and tubular atrophy. Patient was started on enalapril 5 mg twice a day and simvastatin 10 mg/day and on appropriate diet.

She was lost to follow-up. Sixteen months later the patient returned to the nephrologist due to asthenia, fatigue, and cramps. Blood pressure was 110/70 mmHg. Significant blood test results were as follows: Haematocrit 32%; haemoglobin 9.2 g/dL; potassium 5.5 mEq/L; bicarbonate 19 mEq/L; serum calcium 9.5 mg/dL; serum phosphate 6.2 mg/dL; serum magnesium 2.2 mg/dL; urea 111 mg/dL; serum creatinine 3.78 mg/dL; uric acid 8.1 mg/dL; albumin 4.3 g/dL; creatinine clearance 21 ml/min; proteinuria 0.29 g/day; urinalysis was unremarkable. Urine pH was 7 and urinary density 1010. A renal magnetic resonance imaging was noncontributory. The patient was prescribed erythropoietin 2000 U every other day, enalapril 5 mg bid, calcium carbonate 2 g/day, sodium bicarbonate two tea spoons daily, and polystyrene calcium sulfonate. Six months later the patient was started on hemodialysis (creatinine clearance 12 mL/min). A genetic study disclosed the insertion of a cytosine nucleotide in the VNTR (Variable Number Tandem Repeats) region of the MUC-1 gene, consistent with a mutation of the mucin-1 gene previously reported [3]: cDNA NM_001204286.1, protein NP_001191215.1, SNaPshot. The diagnosis of ADTKD-MUC1 (Autosomal Dominant Tubulointerstitial Kidney Disease-Mucin-1) was finally made. The laboratory results of the

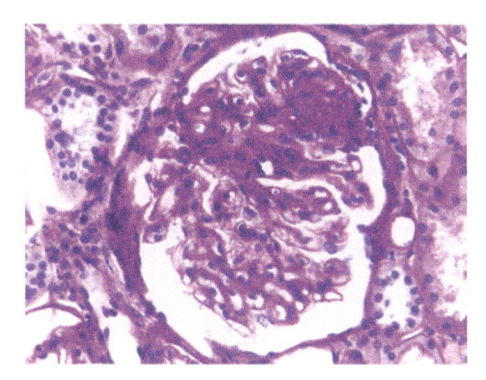

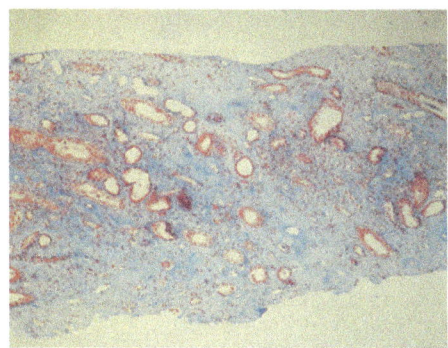

(a) Segmental sclerosis of glomerular capillaries PAS 400x

(b) Moderate to severe interstitial fibrosis. Mason Trichromic 200x

FIGURE 2

patient's daughter revealed mild proteinuria and normal kidney function (Figure 1). A kidney biopsy revealed mild tubulointerstitial disease and focal and segmental glomerulosclerosis in 2 out of 16 glomeruli. She was started on enalapril and nephroprotection and genetic counseling was given to her.

3. Discussion

Our patient presented with a long lasting undiagnosed family history of chronic kidney disease (CKD) while some of her relatives had progressed to end-stage kidney disease as adults. As the clinical case was assumed as idiopathic chronic kidney disease, the kidney biopsy was considered mandatory. Moreover, the family background showed a slow but progressive trend of the disease that urged to obtain tissue promptly, as the benefits of performing a biopsy with diagnostic purposes is lower at advanced stages of CKD. In our opinion, as long-term proteinuria was mild, a primary glomerulopathy appeared unlikely. However, the pathology report informed that FSGS dominated the glomerular architecture. This was accompanied by moderate interstitial fibrosis, tubular atrophy, and interstitial inflammation, which were in accordance with the glomerular level of compromise and also with the clinical picture. Therefore, a secondary cause of FSGS was pursued. The concomitant occurrence of FSGS in a case of ADTKD, as previously reported [4], could be a histological pattern of injury secondary to the common end result of many chronic kidney conditions, in a nonspecific manner, and not as a direct cause of FSGS by the MUC-1 mutation.

The family tree suggested an autosomal dominant pattern of inheritance. In addition, the middle-age adult onset on chronic kidney insufficiency and end-stage kidney disease was an important aspect to take into consideration. Noteworthily, hypertension was not present either at stage 3 of CKD (at the time of diagnosis) or when the patient entered dialysis. Finally, both a low-grade proteinuria plus the medullar histologic findings were indicating a genetic tubular cause was to be ruled out. In this regard, an autosomal dominant tubulointerstitial kidney disease was taken into consideration [4–6].

Autosomal dominant tubulointerstitial kidney disease is a rare entity and is subclassified on a genetic basis that encompasses four mutations in the genes encoding uromodulin (UMOD), hepatocyte nuclear factor 1-β (HNF 1B), renin (REN), and mucin-1 (MUC-1) [4]. This novel and practical classification replaces cumbersome and confusing previous ones and suggests straightforward diagnostic criteria. Most of the clinical and histologic findings are nonspecific. As remarked in the KDIGO guidelines, there is usually a known familial history of kidney disease, and some members may have not been diagnosed properly due to death even before CKD symptoms arise, as it was the case in our patient's father [4]. The average age of renal replacement therapy entrance is between 40 and 60 years, although this may depend on other variables as degree of penetrance of the mutation, hyperuricemia, and comorbidities [4–6]. Hypertension is typically absent in these subjects, while cysts are not predominant, although they can be more frequently encountered at advanced stages of these diseases, consequently not contributing to renal damage [4]. Due to their rarity, the prevalence and incidence of the different types of ADTKD remains unknown [4]. The main features although not exclusive of the four types are depicted in Table 1. Briefly, in ADTKD-UMOD, hyperuricemia and gout appear most frequently in adulthood and cysts are not frequent, but if present they tend to be cortical [4, 7, 8]. In ADTKD-REN, anemia (which resolves in puberty) and hypotension are present at childhood, while hyperuricemia and hyperkalemia are distinguishing features [4, 9]. In ADTKD-HNF1B, diabetes mellitus, pancreatic atrophy, and urogenital abnormalities are present, together with hypomagnesemia, hypokalemia, and liver function test abnormalities [10]. Finally, in ADTKD-MUC1, there are occasional cortical cysts and no other main characteristics [3, 4]. It may be presumed that the abnormal secreted mucin protein plugs in the distal tubule and causes an increase in the intraluminal pressure of the tubules, behaving as a postrenal cause of CKD. In this setting, this chronic situation impedes a normal clearance at the glomerular filtration barrier, leading to inflammation and glomerulosclerosis, as found in our patient (Figure 2). As

Table 1: Main findings of the different genetic subtypes of ADTKD.

	UMOD	MUC1	REN	HNF 1β
Clinical findings	Gout Occasional cortical cysts	Occasional cortical cysts	Hypotension Anemia	Diabetes mellitus Pancreatic atrophy Urogenital anomalies
Age at presentation	adulthood	adulthood	childhood	Early childhood
Laboratory findings	Hyperuricemia	No characteristic findings	Hyperuricemia Hyperkalemia	Hypomagnesemia Hypokalemia Elevated liver enzyme levels
Pathology findings	Tubulointerstitial damage. Secondary FSGS Intracellular UMOD deposits in Thick Ascending Henle's limbs	Tubulointerstitial damage. Secondary FSGS Intracellular accumulation of MUC1 in distal tubules	Tubulointerstitial damage. Secondary FSGS	

ADTKD, Adult dominant tubulointerstitial kidney disease; UMOD, uromodulin; MUC1, mucin-1; REN, renin; HNF 1β, Hepatocyte nuclear factor 1β; FSGS, focal and segmental glomerulosclerosis.

mentioned above, the interstitial inflammation and tubular atrophy tend to dominate the biopsy picture. In the case of ADTKD-MUC1, distal tubular intracellular accumulation of the abnormal codified peptide named mucin fs can be identified for research purposes [4]. Histologically, FSGS has been described as a nonspecific finding in kidney biopsies of patients with ADTKD [4, 8, 11] (Table 1).

Mucins are highly molecular heavily glycosylated transmembrane proteins classified as secretory or membrane-bound. MUC1 is a membrane-bound mucin with a high expression throughout the distal nephron and is involved in the protection and lubrication of the distal tubular lumen [12, 13]. In addition, as a transmembrane protein it is involved in many intracellular functions, particularly in signal transduction [12, 13]. Although genetic testing for UMOD, REN, and HNF1B mutations is well established, MUC1 genetic testing remains challenging [11]. Finally, there is no specific therapy for this disease. In ADTKD, diuretics should be used with caution or avoided, as they may aggravate hyperuricemia and volumen depletion [14]. Liberal water intake is recommended to compensate for possible urinary concentration defects. Nonsteroidal anti-inflammatory drugs should be avoided [4].

In conclusion, an initially diagnosed case of end-stage renal disease due to focal and segmental glomerulosclerosis with moderate tubulointerstitial compromise was later encountered to be secondary to a rare genetic mutation in mucin at the tubular level, known as ADTKD-MUC1.

References

[1] L. Zand, R. J. Glassock, A. S. de Vriese, S. Sethi, and F. C. Fervenza, "What are we missing in the clinical trials of Focal and Segmental Glomerulosclerosis?" *Nephrology Dialysis and Transplantationvol*, vol. 32, pp. 14–21, 2017.

[2] H. Trimarchi, "Primary focal and segmental glomerulosclerosis. Why are pieces of this puzzle still missing?" *European Medical Journal Nephrology*, vol. 3, no. 1, pp. 104–110, 2015.

[3] A. Kirby, A. Gnirke A, D. B. Jaffe et al., "Mutations causing medullary cystic kidney disease type 1 lie in a large VNTR in MUC1 missed by massively parallel sequencing," *Nature Genetics*, vol. 45, no. 3, pp. 299–303, 2013.

[4] K. U. Eckardt, S. L. Alper, C. Antignac et al., "Autosomal dominant tubulointerstitial kidney disease: diagnosis, classification, and management-A KDIGO consensus report," *Kidney International*, vol. 88, pp. 676–683, 2015.

[5] A. J. Bleyer and S. Kmoch, "Autosomal dominant tubulointerstitial kidney disease. of names and genes," *Kidney International*, vol. 86, pp. 459–461, 2014.

[6] A. J. Bleyer, S. Hart, and S. Kmoch, "Hereditary interstitial kidney disease," *Seminars in Nephrology*, vol. 30, no. 4, pp. 366–373, 2010.

[7] F. Scolari, G. Caridi, L. Rampoldi et al., "Uromodulin storage diseases: clinical aspects and mechanisms," *American Journal of Kidney Diseases*, vol. 44, no. 6, pp. 987–999, 2004.

[8] L. Rampoldi, F. Scolari, A. Amoroso et al., "The rediscovery of uromodulin (Tamm-Horsfall protein): from tubulointerstitial nephropathy to chronic kidney disease," *Kidney International*, vol. 80, no. 4, pp. 338–347, 2011.

[9] M. Zivna, H. Hulkova, M. Matignon et al., "Dominant renin gene mutations associated with early-onset hyperuricemia, anemia, and chronic kidney failure," *American Journal of Human Genetics*, vol. 85, no. 2, pp. 204–213, 2009.

[10] S. Faguer, S. Decramer, N. Chassaing et al., "Diagnosis, management, and prognosis of HNF1B nephropathy in adulthood," *Kidney International*, vol. 80, no. 7, pp. 768–776, 2011.

[11] X. M. Lens, J. F. Banet, P. Outeda, and V. Barrio-Lucía, "A novel pattern of mutation in uromodulin disorders: autosomal dominant medullary cystic kidney disease type 2, familial juvenile hyperuricemic nephropathy, and autosomal dominant glomerulocystic kidney disease," *American Journal of Kidney Diseases*, vol. 46, no. 1, pp. 52–57, 2005.

[12] K. Mehla and P. K. Singh, "A novel master metabolic regulator," *Biochemical Biophysical Acta*, vol. 1845, no. 2, pp. 126–135, 2014.

[13] P. J. Singh and M. A. Hollingsworth, "Cell surface-associaed mucins in signal transduction," *Trends in Cell Biology*, vol. 16, no. 9, pp. 467–479, 2006.

Successful Resuscitation of a Patient with Life-Threatening Metabolic Acidosis by Hemodialysis: A Case of Ethylene Glycol Intoxication

Ikuyo Narita,[1] Michiko Shimada,[1] Norio Nakamura,[2] Reiichi Murakami,[1] Takeshi Fujita,[1] Wakako Fukuda,[3] and Hirofumi Tomita[1]

[1]*Department of Cardiology and Nephrology, Hirosaki University Graduate School of Medicine, Hirosaki, Japan*
[2]*Community Medicine, Hirosaki University Graduate School of Medicine, Hirosaki, Japan*
[3]*Murakami Shinmachi Hospital, Aomori, Japan*

Correspondence should be addressed to Michiko Shimada; mshimada@hirosaki-u.ac.jp

Academic Editor: Yoshihide Fujigaki

Background. Ethylene glycol intoxication causes severe metabolic acidosis and acute kidney injury. Fomepizole has become available as its antidote. Nevertheless, a prompt diagnosis is not easy because patients are often unconscious. Here we present a case of ethylene glycol intoxication who successfully recovered with prompt hemodialysis. *Case Presentation.* A 52-year-old Japanese male was admitted to a local hospital due to suspected food poisoning. The patient presented with nausea and vomiting, but his condition rapidly deteriorated, with worsening conscious level, respiratory distress requiring mechanical ventilation, hypotension, and severe acute kidney injury. He was transferred to the university hospital; hemodialysis was initiated because of hyperkalemia and severe metabolic acidosis. On recovering consciousness, he admitted having ingested antifreeze solution. Thirty-seven days after admission, the patient was discharged without requiring HD. *Conclusions.* We reported a case of ethylene glycol intoxication who presented with a life-threatening metabolic acidosis. In a state of severe circulatory shock requiring catecholamines, hemodialysis should be avoided, and continuous hemodiafiltration may be a preferred approach. However, one should be aware of the possibility of intoxication by unknown causes, and hemodialysis could be life-saving with its superior ability to remove toxic materials in such cases.

1. Introduction

Ethylene glycol is used in commercially available products such as antifreeze solution, windshield, or cold-pack and is readily accessible in the household. It is odorless and has a sweet taste; therefore, accidental or suicidal ingestion may occur. Ethylene glycol poisoning is relatively uncommon, although it is an important cause of intoxication. In 2013, the American Association of Poison Control Centers Toxic Exposure Surveillance System reported 699 cases of ethylene glycol poisoning, resulting in 7 deaths, and this number should have been underestimated [1]. Ethylene glycol toxicity is related to the production of toxic metabolites by alcohol dehydrogenase (ADH) and aldehyde dehydrogenase that result in high anion gap metabolic acidosis (Figure 1). Calcium oxalate is produced from oxalates, and its precipitation in the renal tubules is one of the suggested causes of acute kidney injury. Therefore, the presence of calcium oxalate crystals in urinary sediment is an important clue for the diagnosis of ethylene glycol poisoning. Fomepizole, an inhibitor of ADH, is an antidote that prevents the production of toxic metabolites from ethylene glycol. Previously, ethanol infusion was widely used to inhibit ADH; however, the American Academy of Toxicology recommends treatment with fomepizole rather than ethanol, if available [2]. Fomepizole is used as an antidote for methanol intoxication as well. In the US, fomepizole was approved for the treatment of ethylene glycol intoxication in 1997, and in Japan, it was approved in 2015. However, it

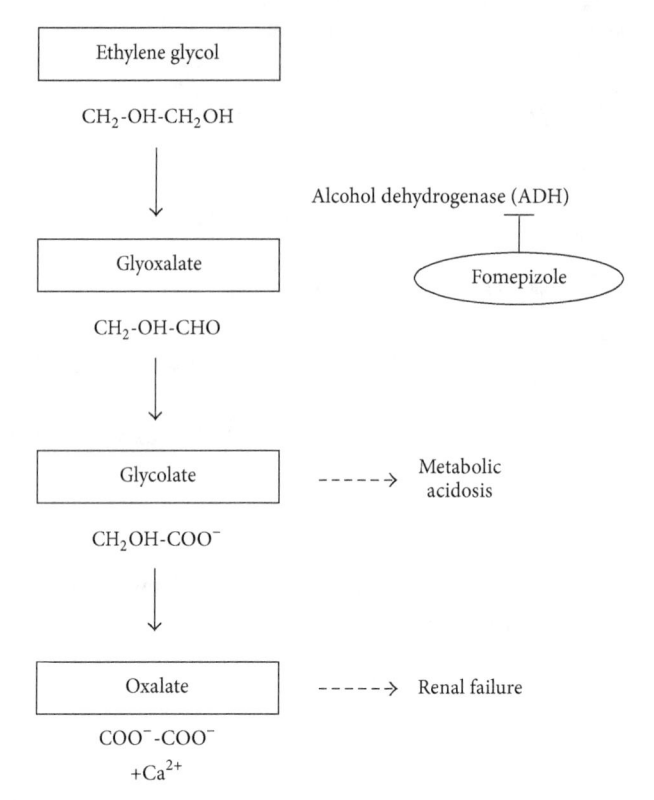

FIGURE 1: Metabolism of ethylene glycol and its mechanism of toxicity. Fomepizole acts as inhibitor of alcohol dehydrogenase and, therefore, prevents the formation of acidic ethylene glycol metabolites.

is not always easy to diagnose ethylene glycol intoxication because patients are often unconscious or small children [3] or have a cognitive impairment [4], and the use of fomepizole is limited to cases in which there is some clue of ethylene glycol ingestion.

Here we present a case of a life-threatening metabolic acidosis and acute kidney injury due to ethylene glycol intoxication who successfully recovered with prompt hemodialysis.

2. Case Presentation

A 52-year-old Japanese male was admitted to the gastroenterology department of a local hospital with suspected food poisoning. He presented with nausea and vomiting and had to be transported via an ambulance because he was unable to walk. On admission, he was awake, and his blood pressure and renal function were normal. During the next 24 hours (h), his condition rapidly deteriorated, with worsening conscious level, respiratory distress requiring mechanical ventilation, decreased blood pressure, and severe acute kidney injury. Thus, he was transferred to the university hospital. Laboratory data in the first hospital were shown in Table 1. He developed anuria and his initial arterial blood gas analysis showed a high anion gap metabolic acidosis, with the following results: pH, 6.92; pCO2, 20.6 mmHg; pO2, 538 mmHg; bicarbonate, 4.1 mmol/L; base excess, −30.3 mmol/L; anion gap, 15.9 mmol/L; and lactate, 21 mmol/L, under mechanical ventilation. Physical examination showed that his body temperature was 38.9°C, blood pressure was 80/50 mmHg, and pulse rate was regular at 106 beats/min. No remarkable findings were observed in his chest and abdomen, but his legs showed cyanosis. Laboratory tests revealed an increased white blood cell count of 36800/μL. Serum creatinine (Cr) levels were elevated at 3.27 mg/dL, and potassium levels were 7.0 mEq/L. In order to improve hyperkalemia and severe metabolic acidosis, hemodialysis (HD) was initiated within 1 h on arrival. HD was performed under norepinephrine infusion for 4 h and followed by continuous hemodiafiltration (CHDF). Metabolic acidosis was dramatically improved, and on day 2 of admission his respiratory condition improved and he was extubated. On recovering consciousness, he said that he ingested antifreeze solution 6 to 12 h before the admission to the first hospital because it was sweet. He denied having committed suicide. We also referred him to the psychiatrist, and mental illness was denied. He denied simultaneous ethanol ingestion. Thus we suspected that his illness was caused by ethylene glycol intoxication. Anuric phase was persistent for the next 7 days; therefore, he had been on CHDF during his stay in the ICU. On day 9, he was shifted from ICU to the general ward, and intermittent HD was initiated three times a week for 4 h. HD was discontinued on day 26 of admission because his Cr levels had decreased to 2.3 mg/dL and urine volume had increased. The patient was discharged on day 37 of admission. Later, serum ethylene glycol level on admission to our hospital turned out to be 15 mg/dL. In 3 months, his Cr levels returned to normal.

TABLE 1: Laboratory data in the first hospital.

Parameters	Day −1		Day 1	
	1 am	4 pm	9 pm	4 am
RBC ($\times 10^4$ /μL)	544	639	590	544
Hb (g/dL)	16.7	17	19.6	16.6
WBC (/μL)	8,570	22,350	34,770	87,860
Plt ($\times 10^4$/μL)	25.3	30.3	34.3	34.1
TP (g/dl)	7.8	10.3	9.0	7.8
Alb (g/dl)	5.1	6.7	5.8	5.0
LDH (IU/L)	176	347	254	386
BUN (mg/dl)	13.9	11.8	17.2	29.8
Cr (mg/dl)	0.69	0.94	1.38	3.1
eGFR (mL/min/1.73 m^2)	91.2	65.1	42.7	17.6
Na (mEq/L)	142	144	141	145
K (mEq/L)	5.1	6.2	6.0	7.0
Cl (mEq/L)	107	117	115	115
Ca (mg/dl)	10.3	11.3	10.4	9.4
CRP (mg/dl)	<0.3	<0.3	<0.3	0.5
Arterial pH		7.07	7.0	6.8
PaO$_2$ (mmHg)		138	209	211
PaCO$_2$ (mmHg)		10	16	21
Bicarbonate (mmol/L)		2.8	7.8	6.2
Base excess (mmol/L)		−24	−25	−28

3. Discussion

In this case, the patient was initially suspected as having food poisoning, but none of his family members who had the same meal had any digestive symptoms. Then, his condition rapidly deteriorated, and his doctor made an emergency call to a nephrologist in the university hospital, early in the morning. Food poisoning and acute kidney injury suggested the possibility of hemolytic uremic syndrome, but hemolytic anemia or low platelet count was not observed. At this time, the patient was transferred via an ambulance, and due to his life-threatening conditions, he was directly admitted to the ICU. His blood gas analysis revealed a high anion gap and severe metabolic acidosis, and his serum potassium level was 7.0 mEq/L. At this point, neither we nor his family was aware of the possibility that he had ingested ethylene glycol. On recovering consciousness, he admitted having ingested antifreeze solution because it was sweet. Usually, hemodialysis is avoided in cases with deteriorating vital signs with severe hypotension [5], and continuous hemodiafiltration may be preferred. However, fortunately, in this case, hemodialysis was selected because of patient's high potassium levels, and it was more efficient in removing ethylene glycol and its toxic metabolites.

It has been reported that clinically evident toxicity is usually seen with serum ethylene glycol levels of >20 mg/dL. A dose of >30 mg/dL is potentially lethal and that of 1.4 mL/kg is assumed to be lethal [6]. The patient stated that he ingested only a cap of antifreeze, and his ethylene glycol level (15 mg/dL) was below the toxic dose on arrival to our hospital, which was 48 to 72 h since ingestion. Considering that half-life of ethylene glycol is 3 to 9 h, the blood level at the time of admission to the first hospital should have been higher, possibly lethal level. It is possible that he did not remember the exact ingested amount. However, this case suggests that a relatively small amount of ethylene glycol can cause a life-threatening intoxication. At most facilities, the analysis of serum ethylene glycol levels requires several days. Thus, the general condition and the level of metabolic acidosis should be preferentially considered for therapeutic decisions. It has been suggested that hemodialysis is required despite the use of fomepizole in the event of metabolic acidosis with pH < 7.25, acute kidney injury or electrolyte imbalances that do not respond to conventional therapy, and deteriorating vital signs [5].

Previous case reports showed that the initial assessment took several hours, and 4 h after admission, either fomepizole [3] or hemodialysis [7] was initiated, and both cases were survived. In this case, we initiated hemodialysis within 1 h on arrival, and we assume that the prompt initiation of hemodialysis was an important factor in his survival.

4. Conclusions

We reported a case of ethylene glycol poisoning who presented with a life-threatening metabolic acidosis. In a state of severe circulatory shock requiring catecholamines, hemodialysis should be avoided, and continuous hemodiafiltration may be preferred. However, one should be aware of the possibility of intoxication by unknown causes, and hemodialysis can be life-saving with its superior ability to remove toxic materials.

Abbreviations

ADH: Alcohol dehydrogenase
Cr: Creatinine
HD: Hemodialysis
CHDF: Continuous hemodiafiltration
ICU: Intensive care unit.

Authors' Contributions

Ikuyo Narita, Michiko Shimada, and Wakako Fukuda prepared the manuscript and performed the literature search. Hirofumi Tomita revised the manuscript. Ikuyo Narita, Michiko Shimada, Norio Nakamura, Takeshi Fujita, Reiichi Murakami, and Hirofumi Tomita treated the patient. All authors have read and approved the final manuscript.

References

[1] J. B. Mowry, D. A. Spyker, L. R. Cantilena Jr., N. McMillan, and M. Ford, "2013 annual report of the American Association of Poison Control Centers' National Poison Data System (NPDS): 31st annual report," *Clinical Toxicology*, vol. 52, no. 10, pp. 1032–1283, 2014.

[2] D. G. Barceloux, E. P. Krenzelok, K. Olson, W. Watson, and H. Miller, "American academy of clinical toxicology practice guidelines on the treatment of ethylene glycol poisoning. Ad Hoc committee," *Journal of Toxicology—Clinical Toxicology*, vol. 37, no. 5, pp. 537–560, 1999.

[3] G. Hann, D. Duncan, G. Sudhir, P. West, and D. Sohi, "Antifreeze on a freezing morning: ethylene glycol poisoning in a 2-year-old," *BMJ Case Reports*, 2012.

[4] T. Fujita, N. Nakamura, H. Hitomi, and K. Okumura, "Risk of sweet 'ethylene glycol' consumption," *Internal Medicine*, vol. 52, no. 3, p. 409, 2013.

[5] G. Bayliss, "Dialysis in the poisoned patient," *Hemodialysis International*, vol. 14, no. 2, pp. 158–167, 2010.

[6] B. Mégarbane, "Treatment of patients with ethylene glycol or methanol poisoning: Focus on fomepizole," *Open Access Emergency Medicine*, vol. 2, pp. 67–75, 2010.

[7] D. P. Davis, K. J. Bramwell, R. S. Hamilton, and S. R. Williams, "Ethylene glycol poisoning: case report of a record-high level and a review," *Journal of Emergency Medicine*, vol. 15, no. 5, pp. 653–667, 1997.

Bartonella Endocarditis Mimicking Crescentic Glomerulonephritis with PR3-ANCA Positivity

Joseph Vercellone,[1] Lisa Cohen,[1] Saima Mansuri,[1] Ping L. Zhang,[2] and Paul S. Kellerman[1]

[1]Department of Internal Medicine, Oakland University William Beaumont School of Medicine, Royal Oak, MI, USA
[2]Department of Pathology, Oakland University William Beaumont School of Medicine, Royal Oak, MI, USA

Correspondence should be addressed to Joseph Vercellone; joseph.vercellone@beaumont.org

Academic Editor: Kouichi Hirayama

Bartonella henselae is a fastidious organism that causes cat scratch disease, commonly associated with fever and lymphadenopathy but, in rare instances, also results in culture-negative infectious endocarditis. We describe a patient who presented with flank pain, splenic infarct, and acute kidney injury with an active urinary sediment, initially suspicious for vasculitis, which was subsequently diagnosed as *B. henselae* endocarditis. *Bartonella* endocarditis may present with a crescentic glomerulonephritis (GN) and elevated PR3-ANCA antibody titers, mimicking ANCA-associated GN, with 54 cases reported in the literature. Unique to our case in this series is a positive PR3-ANCA antibody despite a negative IIF-ANCA. Thus, the presentation of *Bartonella* can mimic ANCA-associated GN, and renal biopsy showing immune complex deposition is critical for diagnosis and appropriate treatment.

1. Introduction

Bartonella henselae is a fastidious organism commonly known for causing cat scratch disease. Cat scratch disease had been described over 50 years ago, but the first causal evidence of disease was not documented until 1983 [1]. Cat scratch disease typically presents with cutaneous lesions at the site of infection that progresses to lymphadenopathy and fever approximately two weeks after exposure to the bacteria. Visceral organ involvement, albeit unusual, typically involves the liver and spleen with marked hepato- and splenomegaly. Rarely, *B. henselae* results in culture-negative endocarditis, an illness that can be difficult to diagnose and a challenge to treat effectively and in a timely manner. Herein, we present a case of *B. henselae* with endocarditis, in a previous healthy male, causing crescentic glomerulonephritis with PR3-ANCA positivity mimicking an ANCA-associated vasculitis.

2. Case Report

A 47-year-old male with a past history of nephrolithiasis, irritable bowel syndrome, and mild depression presented to the emergency center with two weeks of flank pain and four days of cola-colored urine. He described a throbbing, stabbing pain in his left flank that persisted and progressively worsened, which was associated with dark urine, nausea, unmeasured fever, chills, and a 10-lb weight loss. He denied dysuria or urinary hesitancy.

On physical exam, vital signs showed a temperature of 37.2°C, blood pressure of 121/55 mmHg, pulse of 95 bpm, and respirations at 20 breaths per minute while saturating at 94% on room air. He was alert and oriented x 3, but in moderate distress from his left-sided flank pain. There was no cervical, axillary, or femoral lymphadenopathy present. On auscultation, he was noted to have bilateral, basilar crackles without rhonchi or wheezing. Cardiac exam showed a regular rate and rhythm, with a 2/6 systolic, crescendo-decrescendo murmur heard best over the left sternal border. There was severe, left CVA tenderness on exam, but his abdomen was soft, nondistended, and nontender. Extremities showed no edema, and skin exam showed no evidence of petechiae or rashes.

Initial laboratory data showed a WBC of 3.8 bil/L, Hgb of 7.7 g/dL, platelet count of 89 bil/L, sodium of 138 mmol/L,

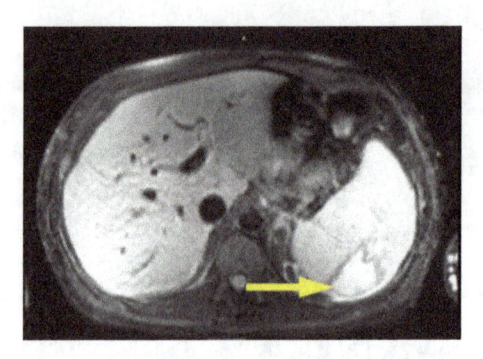

FIGURE 1: CT scan showing large splenic infarct.

potassium of 4.4 mmol/L, chloride of 114 mmol/L, CO2 21 of mmol/L, calcium of 7.4 mg/dL, phosphorus of 3.0 mg/dL, BUN of 19 mg/dL, creatinine of 2.36 mg/dL, and glucose of 97 mg/DL. Urinalysis showed 3+ blood, 1+ protein, > 50 RBC/HPF, 0-5 WBC/HPF, and RBC casts.

Abdominal ultrasound showed a 12.6 cm right kidney, 12.4 cm left kidney with no hydronephrosis, and a spleen with wedge-shaped areas suggestive of infarct. An MRI showed splenomegaly of 17.9 cm and a wedge-shaped infarct (Figure 1)

Further blood test results showed a haptoglobin of 159 mg/DL, LDH of 272 U/L, fibrinogen of 248 mg/dL, an elevated CRP of 4.9 mg/dL, ESR of 25 mm/hr, C3 of 94 mg/dL, C4 of 23 mg/dL, negative antibodies to hepatitis A, B, and C, and negative ANA, ASO, and anticardiolipin antibodies. ANCA testing was negative using an indirect immunefluorescent assay (IIF) with a positive lab test considered for results greater than 1:20. Myeloperoxidase antibody (MPO-ANCA) was negative, but proteinase-3 (PR3-ANCA) antibody titer was elevated at 160 units, using an enzyme-linked immunosorbent assay (ELISA) with a positive result greater than 21 units. Blood cultures were negative and remained so after 5 days.

A renal biopsy was performed. Light microscopy (Figure 2, left) showed focal proliferative injury with two non-necrotic crescents. Immunofluorescence was positive for IgM, IgA, C3, and C1q located predominantly along the glomerular capillary loops and rarely in the mesangial areas. Electron microscopy (Figure 2, right) showed segmental foot process fusion with mesangial and subendothelial immune deposits with no subepithelial deposits, consistent with an immune complex GN.

Concerned with the heart murmur and renal biopsy results, a transthoracic echocardiogram was performed and was negative for valvular vegetations. A subsequent transesophageal echocardiogram showed a bicuspid aortic valve with a vegetation. Culture-negative endocarditis was diagnosed and valve replacement performed with pathology showing necrosis, neutrophils, and *B. henselae* on tissue culture and specialized stains.

The patient received 6 weeks of antibiotic therapy with doxycycline and rifampin and clinically improved with decrease in flank pain. Urinalysis also improved showing 4-10 RBC/HPF, 0-5 WBC/HPF, and no visible casts. Creatinine decreased to 1.4 mg/dL, and ESR and CRP normalized within 2 months to 3 mm/hr and <0.4 mg/dL respectively. Repeat proteinase-3 antibodies remained elevated at 121-163 units despite antibiotic therapy.

3. Discussion

Initial testing for ANCA-associated vasculitis typically uses IIF-ANCA. The specificity of ANCA testing is very high, with a very low false negative rate, but measurement of PR3-ANCA or MPO-ANCA antibodies with a positive IIF-ANCA improves sensitivity by ruling out false positive tests.

Positive tests for IIF-ANCA, PR3-ANCA, and MPO-ANCA antibodies may be found in patients with subacute bacterial endocarditis. Common organisms include Viridans streptococci, Staphylococcus aureus, and other staph species. The association of infectious endocarditis with these antibodies has led to postulated causal mechanisms for vasculitis. Unmethylated CpG is a constituent of bacterial DNA and has been shown to stimulate ANCA production in B cells of ANCA-associated vasculitis patients. Staph aureus tsst-1 superantigen nasal carriage carries a high rate of relapse in granulomatous polyangiitis patients. Diseases with barrier dysfunction to microbes, such as inflammatory bowel disease, show increased incidence of ANCA positivity. Neutrophil extracellular traps (NETs), which play a role in extracellular killing of microbes, may also release ANCA-associated antigens [2].

On the other hand, a retrospective review of patients with IIF-ANCA-negative, positive MPO-ANCA, or PR3-ANCA antibody testing such as that found in this case, showed that only 1 of 38 of these patients actually developed ANCA-associated vasculitis. There is evidence for cross-reactivity in the assays, as PR3-ANCA-positive antibodies have also been found in nonvasculitic inflammatory conditions such as rheumatoid arthritis, inflammatory bowel disease, and SLE [3]. Most relevant to our case, in contrast to ANCA-associated vasculitis, endocarditis-associated ANCAs typically show immune complex deposits in the kidney and resolution of kidney disease with treatment of the infection. Thus, although there is argument for bacterial endocarditis antigens being causal for renal vasculitis, current evidence favors ANCA antibody production as a nonpathologic result of bacterial endocarditis.

We present a case of culture-negative endocarditis and acute kidney injury due to glomerulonephritis, due to *Bartonella henselae* cardiac valve infection. Culture-negative infectious endocarditis is estimated to comprise 3-48% of all endocarditis cases. A literature search revealed 54 cases of *Bartonella*-induced infective endocarditis associated with glomerulonephritis reported in 14 publications, with 77% of cases presenting with serologic positivity of either IIF-ANCA, PR3-ANCA, or both. Unique to our case is a high titer positive PR3-ANCA antibody with a negative IIF-ANCA (Figure 3). A review of glomerular light-microscopy findings associated with the aforementioned 54 cases of *Bartonella*-induced infective endocarditis demonstrated similar findings of focal proliferative injury with both necrotic and

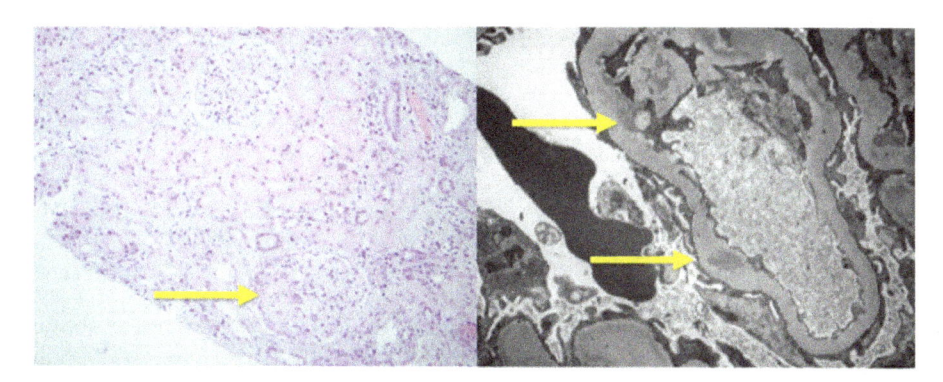

Figure 2: Light microscopy (left) of kidney showing focal proliferation with cellular crescent and electron microscopy (right) showing focal foot process fusion and subendothelial deposits.

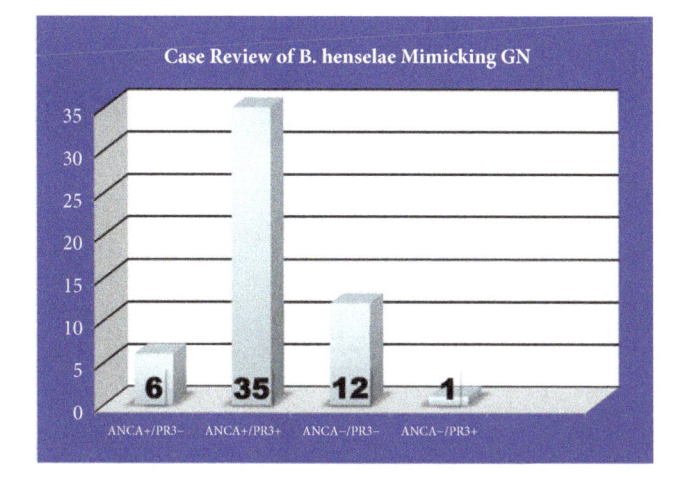

Figure 3: Case review [4–17].

nonnecrotic crescents in both ANCA-positive and ANCA-negative cases [4–17]. Of the cases describing pathology in more detail, all but one showed positive immunofluorescence indicative of immune complex disease.

In summary, this case highlights how *Bartonella henselae* endocarditis may present with a crescentic and proliferative GN and elevated PR3-ANCA antibodies, thus mimicking an ANCA-associated GN. Because *Bartonella* is fastidious and often does not grow in blood cultures, as opposed to more typical endocarditis microbes such as Staphylococcus aureus and Viridans streptococci, clinical symptoms and lab results may lead to an incorrect diagnoses of ANCA vasculitis. An incorrect diagnosis may expose patients to immunosuppressive regimens potentially hazardous to patients with bacterial endocarditis. Thus, a kidney biopsy showing immune complex deposition is critical to establishing appropriate therapy.

Disclosure

This research was presented in poster format at the American Society of Nephrology's (ASN) Kidney Week 2017 in New Orleans, Louisiana, on November 1, 2017.

References

[1] D. Wear, A. Margileth, T. Hadfield, G. Fischer, C. Schlagel, and F. King, "Cat scratch disease: a bacterial infection," *Science*, vol. 221, no. 4618, pp. 1403–1405, 1983.

[2] E. Csernok, P. Lamprecht, and W. L. Gross, "Clinical and immunological features of drug-induced and infection-induced proteinase 3-antineutrophil cytoplasmic antibodies and myeloperoxidase-antineutrophil cytoplasmic antibodies and vasculitis," *Current Opinion in Rheumatology*, vol. 22, no. 1, pp. 43–48, 2010.

[3] D. A. Rao, K. Wei, J. F. Merola et al., "The significance of MPO-ANCA and PR3-ANCA without immunoflorescent ANCA found by routine clinical testing," *Journal of Rheumatology*, vol. 42, no. 5, pp. 847–852, 2015.

[4] E. Aslangul, C. Goulvestre, Z. Mallat, and J.-L. Mainardi, "Human Bartonella infective endocarditis is associated with high frequency of antiproteinase 3 antibodies," *The Journal of Rheumatology*, vol. 41, no. 2, pp. 408–410, 2014.

[5] S. V. H. Heijmeijer, D. Wilmes, S. Aydin, C. Clerckx, and L. Labriola, "Necrotizing ANCA-positive glomerulonephritis secondary to culture-negative endocarditis," *Case Reports in Nephrology and Dialysis*, vol. 2015, Article ID 649763, 5 pages, 2015.

[6] H. Liapis, *Necrotizing glomerulonephritis caused by Bartonella henselae endocarditis. CIN2007*, 2007, http://www.uninet.edu/CIN2007.

[7] A. Mahr, F. Batteux, S. Tubiana et al., "Prevalence of Antineutrophil Cytoplasmic Antibodies in Infective Endocarditis," *Arthritis & Rheumatology*, vol. 66, no. 6, pp. 1672–1677, 2014.

[8] T. F. Olsen and S. U. A. Gill, "Bartonella Endocarditis Imitating Anca-Associated Vasculitis," *Journal of Cardiology Clinical Research*, p. 1054, 2016.

[9] S. Paudyal, D. T. Kleven, and A. M. Oliver, "Bartonella Henselae endocarditis mimicking ANCA associated vasculitis," *Case Reports in Internal Medicine*, vol. 3, no. 2, 2016.

[10] J. E. Raybould, A. L. Raybould, M. K. Morales et al., "Bartonella Endocarditis and Pauci-Immune Glomerulonephritis: A Case Report and Review of the Literature," *Infectious Diseases in Clinical Practice*, vol. 24, no. 5, pp. 254–260, 2016.

[11] C. Salvado, A. Mekinian, P. Rouvier, P. Poignard, I. Pham, and O. Fain, "Rapidly progressive crescentic glomerulonephritis and aneurism with antineutrophil cytoplasmic antibody: *Bartonella henselae* endocarditis," *La Presse Médicale*, vol. 42, no. 6, pp. 1060-1061, 2013.

[12] S. H. Shah, C. Grahame-Clarke, and C. N. Ross, "Touch not the cat bot a glove: ANCA-positive pauci-immune necrotizing glomerulonephritis secondary to *Bartonella henselae*," *Clinical Kidney Journal*, vol. 7, no. 2, pp. 179–181, 2014.

[13] H. Sugiyama, M. Sahara, Y. Imai et al., "Infective endocarditis by *Bartonella quintana* masquerading as antineutrophil cytoplasmic antibody-associated small vessel vasculitis," *Cardiology*, vol. 114, no. 3, pp. 208–211, 2009.

[14] L. S. G. Teoh, H. H. Hart, M. C. Soh et al., "Bartonella henselae aortic valve endocarditis mimicking systemic vasculitis," *BMJ Case Reports*, 2010.

[15] R. M. van Tooren, R. van Leusen, and F. H. Bosch, "Culture negative endocarditis combined with glomerulonephritis caused by *Bartonella* species in two immunocompetent adults," *The Netherlands Journal of Medicine*, vol. 59, no. 5, pp. 218–224, 2001.

[16] H. R. Vikram, A. K. Bacani, P. A. DeValeria, S. A. Cunningham, and F. R. Cockerill III, "Bivalvular *Bartonella henselae* prosthetic valve endocarditis," *Journal of Clinical Microbiology*, vol. 45, no. 12, pp. 4081–4084, 2007.

[17] C.-M. Ying, D.-T. Yao, H.-H. Ding, and C.-D. Yang, "Infective endocarditis with antineutrophil cytoplasmic antibody: report of 13 cases and literature review," *PLoS ONE*, vol. 9, no. 2, pp. 1–6, 2014.

Nephrologists Hate the Dialysis Catheters: A Systemic Review of Dialysis Catheter Associated Infective Endocarditis

Kalyana C. Janga,[1] Ankur Sinha,[2] Sheldon Greenberg,[1] and Kavita Sharma[3]

[1]*Department of Nephrology, Maimonides Medical Center, Brooklyn, NY, USA*
[2]*Department of Internal Medicine, Maimonides Medical Center, Brooklyn, NY, USA*
[3]*Department of Infectious Diseases, Maimonides Medical Center, Brooklyn, NY, USA*

Correspondence should be addressed to Ankur Sinha; ANsinha@maimonidesmed.org

Academic Editor: Władysław Sułowicz

A 53-year-old Egyptian female with end stage renal disease, one month after start of hemodialysis via an internal jugular catheter, presented with fever and shortness of breath. She developed desquamating vesiculobullous lesions, widespread on her body. She was in profound septic shock and broad spectrum antibiotics were started with appropriate fluid replenishment. An echocardiogram revealed bulky leaflets of the mitral valve with a highly mobile vegetation about 2.3 cm long attached to the anterior leaflet. CT scan of the chest, abdomen, and pelvis showed bilateral pleural effusions in the chest, with triangular opacities in the lungs suggestive of infarcts. There was splenomegaly with triangular hypodensities consistent with splenic infarcts. Blood cultures repeatedly grew *Candida albicans*. Despite parenteral antifungal therapy, the patient deteriorated over the course of 5 days. She died due to a subsequent cardiac arrest. Systemic review of literature revealed that the rate of infection varies amongst the various types of accesses, and it is well documented that AV fistulas have a much less rate of infection in comparison to temporary catheters. All dialysis units should strive to make a multidisciplinary effort to have a referral process early on, for access creation, and to avoid catheters associated morbidity.

1. Introduction

End stage renal disease (ESRD) is rampant in the population today. As per the data reported in the US renal data reporting system by the national institutes of health (NIH), the number of patients being treated by hemodialysis is at a record high [1]. They reported 678,383 prevalent cases of ESRD, and the number continues to rise by about 21000 cases per year. The onus falls on the nephrologists to provide safe and good quality dialysis, while the patients wait for their transplant. This includes getting appropriate vascular access for performing the procedure.

Infective endocarditis is an infection of the endocardial layer of the heart. Patients receiving chronic hemodialysis are at an increased risk of infective endocarditis [2] and the disease course is protracted with significant mortality and morbidity [3]. It is a well known fact that temporary vascular access in the form of central lines and dialysis catheters further increase the risk of life threatening bacteremia and in turn infective endocarditis.

We report a case of severe endocarditis with marked complications associated with a temporary vascular access in a patient recently commenced on dialysis. We aim to shed light on the pitfalls of continuing dialysis on such forms of vascular accesses and to review the diagnosis and management of infective endocarditis in similar cases.

2. Case Presentation

A 53-year-old Egyptian female with past medical history of hypertension with nephropathy leading to end stage renal disease, one month after the start of hemodialysis, presented with fever and shortness of breath at an Egyptian hospital. Blood cultures grew *Staphylococcus aureus* and the sepsis was treated aggressively with piperacillin with tazobactam

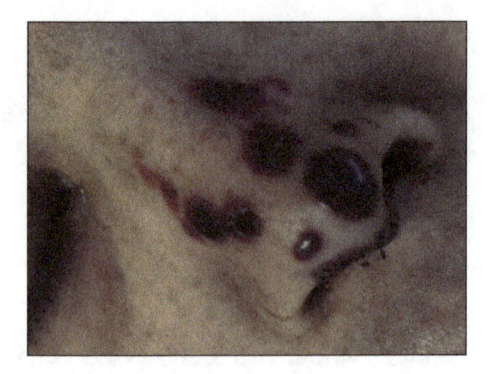

FIGURE 1: Image depicting severe end arteriolar embolic phenomenon to the nose.

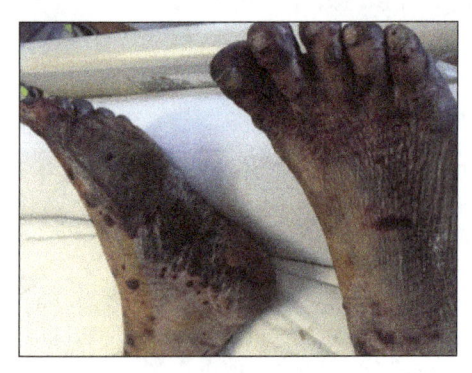

FIGURE 2: Image depicting desquamating vesiculobullous lesions of the feet.

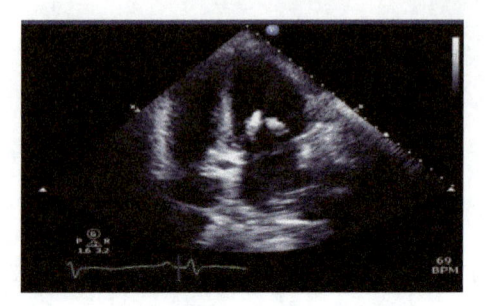

FIGURE 3: Image depicting a transthoracic echo cardiogram, depicting vegetation and severe mitral regurgitation.

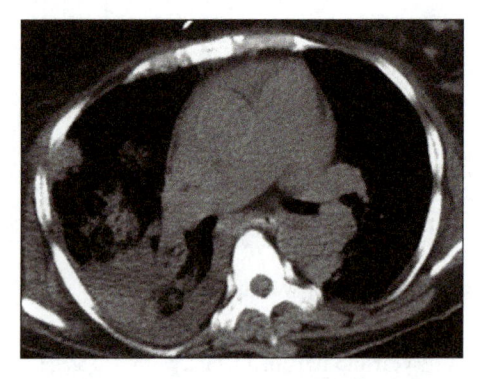

FIGURE 4: CT scan of the chest, depicting wedge shaped large pulmonary infarct.

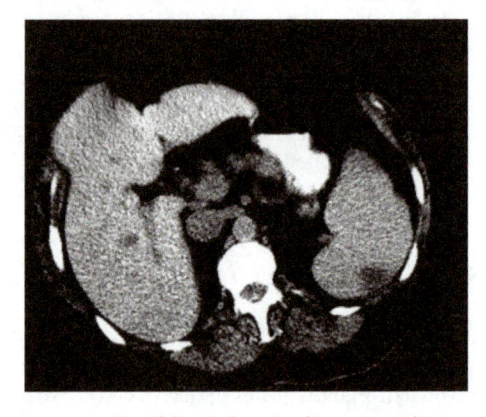

FIGURE 5: CT scan of the abdomen, depicting splenic infarct.

and Imipenem. She was transported from Egypt for further treatment in the United States.

On presentation at the referral center the patient was found to be in septic shock.

Her blood pressure on admission was 73/41 mm of mercury, with a heart rate of 120 beats per minute and a respiratory rate of 22 breaths per minute. Her white cell count on admission was 9,400 cells/μL; the differential count included 97.9% neutrophils with 2% lymphocytes. C-reactive protein on admission was 4.7 mg/dL. She was hypotensive and tachycardic. She had vesiculobullous lesions on the nose (Figure 1), forearms, and the feet (Figure 2). Some of the lesions desquamated to leave ulcers. She had a previously placed left sided internal jugular central line for hemodialysis. This central line was immediately removed on presentation and a fresh dialysis catheter was placed. Blood cultures grew *Candida albicans* on day 1 and continued to grow in all blood culture bottles consistently, during her stay. Appropriate investigations for infective endocarditis were performed.

A transthoracic echocardiogram revealed bulky leaflets of the mitral valve with a highly mobile vegetation about 2.3 cm long attached to the anterior leaflet (Figure 3). This vegetation was prolapsing into the left atrium and was causing moderate mitral regurgitation. Computed tomogram (CT) scan of the chest, abdomen, and pelvis was also performed. It showed bilateral pleural effusions in the chest, with triangular opacities in the lungs suggestive of infarcts (Figure 4). There was mild splenomegaly with triangular hypodensities consistent with splenic infarcts (Figure 5). A CT scan of the abdomen and pelvis was found to appropriately visualize the renal system; there were atrophic kidneys bilaterally, with no evidence of stones. The bladder was collapsed on the scan.

Despite initiating parenteral antifungal therapy, the patient deteriorated over the course of 5 days. Her disease progressed to cause multiple organ failure and she was placed on palliative care due to grave prognosis and to honor the family's wishes. She died due to a cardiac arrest.

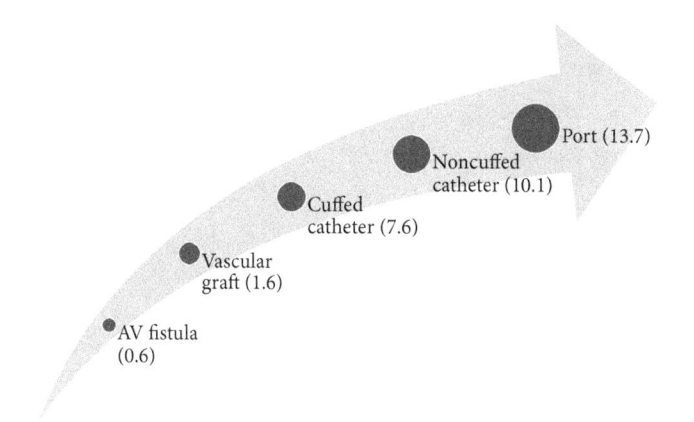

FIGURE 6: Depicting vascular access infection rate by type of vascular access.

3. Discussion

3.1. Microbiology. The center for disease control and prevention (CDC) issued a dialysis surveillance report with data for participating centers the United States. This report utilized the CDC's national health safety network (NHSN) for reporting facts about patients receiving hemodialysis. This network involved reporting of adverse events associated with dialysis and analyzing the data. Out of the 599 bacterial isolates from the 532 positive blood cultures following an adverse event, 77% (461 isolates) were associated with central lines. Although common skin contaminants took a major chunk of these isolates (44.3%), *Staphylococcus aureus* also represented major causation (19.7%). It is also concerning to note that there is a stark difference in the rate of bacteremia in temporary lines in comparison to patients with a graft or arteriovenous fistula (138 isolates comprising of 17%) [4]. 42% of all reported isolates of Staphylococcus aureus were MRSA.

It is interesting to note that fungal infections leading to endocarditis, similar to our patient, comprised of a mere 1.7% in Central line associated infections and 2.9% in fistula or graft associated infections.

3.2. Predisposing Factors. Strom et al. reported a 16.9% relative risk of IE in hemodialysis patients in comparison to the general population [5]. One of the most important factors is the propensity of having bacteremia in patients needing HD. These frequent episodes of bacteremia can be attributed to repeated IV access through vascular catheters, grafts, and fistulas [6]. The rate of infection varies amongst the various types of access, and it is well documented that AV fistulas have a much lower rate of infection in comparison to temporary catheters. Figure 6 depicts the rate of vascular access infection as per a report by the CDC [7]. This theory is confirmed by the fact that rate of endocarditis is less in patients getting peritoneal dialysis in comparison to general population [8]. While the patients with peritoneal dialysis have lower rates of infection than hemodialysis their rates of infective endocarditis are still higher than general population [3].

There is literature suggesting salvage of central lines if it is technically unfeasible to remove the lines. The suggested measures include antibiotic lock therapy with varying concentrations of solutions like antibiotics [9], ethanol [10], and nitroglycerin [10]. The consensus is to remove the infected line unless an extenuating circumstance prevents removing the line.

Some practices have been suggested to decrease the rate of infections associated with central lines; these include use of chlorhexidine impregnated dressings, catheter care with chlorhexidine solution, and dressing changes every 5–7 days. Catheter hubs and ports should be cleaned with either 70% alcohol or chlorhexidine [11].

Patients with ESRD have an increased incidence of heart valve disease. The valve disorders are secondary to calcification leading to regurgitation or stenosis [12]. The onset of valve disease in HD patients is earlier by 10–20 years in comparison to general population. This has been attributed to abnormal calcium and phosphorus metabolism, secondary to hyperparathyroidism [13].

ESRD results in an impaired immune status. This is multifactorial and includes a defect in antigen presenting cells. This leads to reduced stimulation of T Lymphocytes. This has been well documented and was originally observed due to decreased response to hepatitis vaccine in patients with ESRD [14]. T cell activation is hampered in patient with ESRD, and there is a predisposition of T Helper Cell 1 (TH1) pattern instead of T Helper 2 (TH2) pattern. This leads to a decrease in amount of antibody production [15]. There is a decrease in the number of circulating monocytes on starting HD. This is secondary to their activation on coming in contact with the dialyzing membrane and a state of chronic inflammation [16], although it is yet to be proven if this has any effect on the decreased immune response. Figure 7 depicts the pathophysiology of impaired immune function in renal failure.

3.3. Diagnosis. The diagnosis of infective endocarditis is specifically challenging in patients on HD. Duke's criterion is most trusted for predicting and diagnosing infective endocarditis, but applying the criterion to patient with ESRD on HD is tricky. Duke's criteria have major and minor criteria; one of the key major criteria is two positive blood cultures with an organism consistent with infective endocarditis, in the absence of a focus of infection. The frequent presence of a plausible source of infection, in the form of central lines, or ports can often make it difficult to differentiate between endocarditis and an uncomplicated line infection [17]. Similarly, fever is a minor criterion in Duke's Criteria. Patients with ESRD have a flattened immune response, and they do not mount fevers as effectively as the general population [2].

Thus echocardiography in the presence of a high suspicion of endocarditis in a patient with HD can be life-saving. Like any other patient with suspected infective endocarditis the initial imaging modality is a transthoracic echocardiogram, followed by a transesophageal echocardiogram if the image quality is questionable. Another indication of a

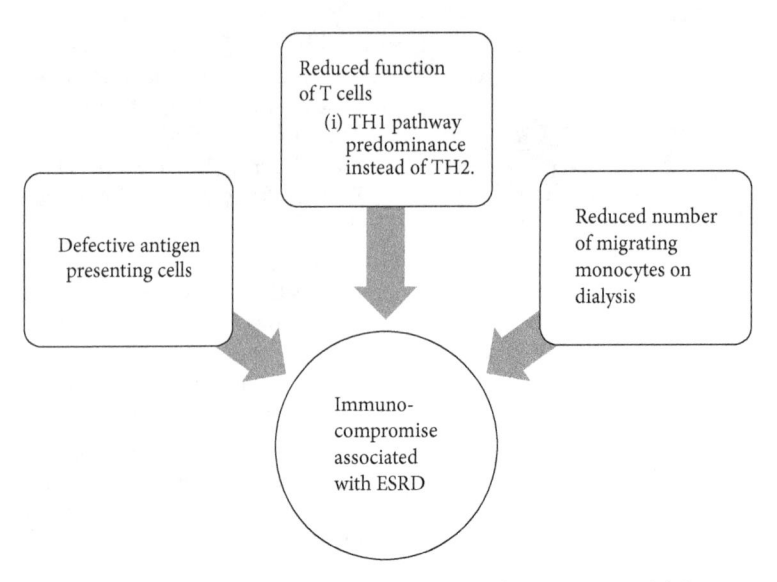

Figure 7: Pathophysiology of impeded immune function in renal failure.

Table 1: High suspicion features mandating TTE in patients with HD and suspected IE.

High suspicion features for infective endocarditis mandating transesophageal echocardiogram after a TTE
(i) Patients with HD catheters
(ii) New onset congestive heart failure
(iii) Stigmata of endocarditis
(iv) HD related hypotension in a previously hypertensive patient
(v) Prior or repeated episodes of IE
(vi) Prior valvular surgery
(vii) Typical organisms for IE
(viii) Relapsing bacteremia after antibiotic discontinuation, regardless of causative pathogen

Gaetano et al., European heart journal (2007) 28, 2307–2312 doi:10.1093/eurheartj/ehm278.

transesophageal echocardiogram would be high suspicion even after a transthoracic study negates the diagnosis. Gaetano et al. published some high suspicion features mandating transesophageal study; these features are depicted in figure. They recommend a mandatory TEE with a TTE if any of these features are present (Table 1).

3.4. Treatment. The treatment of IE involves prompt diagnosis with the start of empiric therapy. After blood cultures have isolated an organism, a more directed approach can be followed. Table 2 depicts the appropriate therapy for empiric as well as organism specific therapy as per published guidelines for American family physicians.

Special consideration should be made in patients with ESRD and vancomycin should be avoided for methicillin susceptible *S. aureus* as it has lower bactericidal action in comparison to oxacillin or cefazolin. It also contributes to selection of S aureus strains with reduced sensitivity to glycopeptides and vancomycin resistant enterococci [18]. Vancomycin remains the first choice for MRSA infections. Due to the rising rate of *S. aureus* strains with increased minimal inhibitory concentration of vancomycin, drugs like daptomycin and linezolid should be considered [19].

Candida endocarditis is a rare entity in native valves, and the risk of having a fungal infection causing endocarditis rises in the immunocompromised, IV drug abusers, and in patients with indwelling foreign bodies like pacemakers, catheters, or prosthetic joints [20]. Current treatment regime as per the infectious disease society of America (IDSA) is valve replacement with initial antifungal treatment with amphotericin B with or without flucytosine followed by long term suppression with fluconazole [21]. Patients who are poor surgical candidates should be placed in chronic lifelong suppression with fluconazole 400–800 mg (6–12 mg/kg) [18].

3.5. Surgical Management. Operative intervention should be considered in all individuals with the criterion mentioned in Table 3. Special consideration should be made to the clinical situation of the patient, and the likelihood of surviving the surgery on a case-to-case basis should be made. The main aim of surgery should be to eradicate infection and improve patient survival.

Mitral valve insufficiency precedes the development of heart failure and early intervention is recommended to improve survival. Antibiotic therapy alone does not lead to an improvement of mitral insufficiency [22]. The chances of a vegetation embolizing to distal circulation depend directly on the vegetation size. The chances of having an embolic phenomenon are as high as 70% in vegetation larger than 15 mm, in comparison to 27% in patients with size less than 15 mm. Similarly the mobile vegetation is much more likely to cause an embolism [23].

In case of a suspected embolic stroke, MRI scan of the brain is considered the most sensitive test for neurological imaging. Stroke can be seen in as much as 80% patients who

TABLE 2: Depicting the suggested treatment regime for infective endocarditis in the general population as per guidelines published in American Family Physician.

	Treatment regimen for Infectious endocarditis in general population
Empiric therapy	(i) Vancomycin or ampicillin/sulbactam with an aminoglycoside (ii) Add rifampin in patients with prosthetic valves
Penicillin susceptible *viridans* Streptococcus or *Streptococcus bovis* (*S. bovis*)	(i) Penicillin G or ceftriaxone for 4 weeks Or (ii) Penicillin G plus gentamycin for 2 weeks Or (iii) Ceftriaxone plus gentamycin for 2 weeks Or (iv) Vancomycin for 4 weeks
Relatively penicillin resistant *viridans* Streptococcus or *S. bovis*	(i) Penicillin G or ceftriaxone for 4 weeks, plus gentamycin for 2 weeks Or (ii) Vancomycin for 4 weeks
Penicillin-resistant *viridans* Streptococcus or *S. bovis*	(i) Ampicillin plus gentamycin for 4–6 weeks Or (ii) Penicillin G plus gentamycin for 4–6 weeks Or (iii) Vancomycin for 6 weeks
Oxacillin- susceptible staphylococci	(i) Nafcillin or oxacillin for 6 weeks, plus gentamycin for 3–5 days (optional) Or (ii) Cefazolin for 6 weeks plus gentamycin for 3–5 days (optional)
Oxacillin-resistant staphylococci	(i) Vancomycin for 6 weeks

TABLE 3: Indication of surgical management of Mitral valve IE.

Indications for surgery in native valve endocarditis of mitral valve
(i) Moderate to severe or severe mitral regurgitation with or without heart failure
(ii) Vegetation size measuring more than 10 mm
(iii) Mobile vegetation
(iv) Paravalvular abscess
(v) Evidence of a single embolic phenomenon including stroke
(vi) Failure of antibiotic therapy
(vii) Infection with a fungal organism

[22].

have a left sided IE, on MRI scan. This MRI scan should be preceded by a noncontrast CT scan of the head to rule out bleeding; this may be secondary to a mycotic aneurysm and should warrant immediate neurosurgical evaluation. Patients with an active intracranial bleed are poor candidates for surgery [24, 25].

Splenic infarction is frequent in left sided IE and should not delay surgery. A CT scan of the abdomen and pelvis should be performed to rule out a splenic abscess. The missed diagnosis of a splenic abscess has grave consequences as it may cause infections of the new valve [26]. Table 4 summarizes the preoperative investigations for surgical approach.

The surgery should be timed as early as possible to avoid significant morbidity and improve survival. The main motive remains to avoid embolic phenomenon. There is limited data on the outcomes of valve surgery following infective endocarditis. A single center retrospective study noted that survival rates following surgery are acceptable with 30 day mortality at 8.5% and cumulative late mortality of 25.6% [27]. There is limited literature to comment on outcomes of valve surgery in cases with concurrent ESRD with IE.

4. Conclusion

Advances in medicine, public health, and economic developments have added an extra decade of life to the average human lifespan. Hemodialysis vascular access for initiation of hemodialysis has become crucial. Catheters are still common form of vascular access used for dialysis initiation due to late placement of AVF before dialysis, primary AVF failure, urgent initiation following acute kidney injury, unexpected decline in glomerular filtration rate, medical insurance issues, Surgeon shortage, and a lack of predialysis nephrology care. All dialysis units should take a multidisciplinary approach and have a referral process early on for access creation and avoid catheters and associated mortality. Patients who are not candidates for fistulas and grafts, as well as peritoneal dialysis, should be involved in a detailed goal of care discussion. The aim should be improving maximal care while compromising least on the quality of life.

TABLE 4: Suggested preop workup for surgical candidates.

	Suggested preoperative work-up prior to considering surgery
Initial CT head	(i) Embolic stroke (ii) Mycotic aneurysm (iii) Intracranial bleed
MRI Brain	(i) More sensitive for neuroradiological diagnosis
CT chest, abdomen and pelvis	(i) Pulmonary Infarcts (ii) Splenic and Hepatic Infarcts (iii) Splenic abscess contraindicating surgery
Transesophageal echocardiography	(i) More sensitive than TTE in visualization of vegetation (ii) Paravalvular Abscess

[22].

Acknowledgments

The authors acknowledge the sincere contribution of the Department of Nephrology and Internal Medicine.

References

[1] NIH and U.S. Renal Data System, *USRDS 2016 Annual Data Report*, 2016.

[2] S. Maraj, L. E. Jacobs, S.-C. Kung et al., "Epidemiology and outcome of infective endocarditis in hemodialysis patients," *The American Journal of the Medical Sciences*, vol. 324, no. 5, pp. 254–260, 2002.

[3] K. C. Abbott and L. Y. Agodoa, "Hospitalizations for bacterial endocarditis after initiation of chronic dialysis in the United States," *Nephron*, vol. 91, no. 2, pp. 203–209, 2002.

[4] R. M. Klevens, J. R. Edwards, M. L. Andrus et al., "Dialysis surveillance report: National Healthcare Safety Network (NHSN)—data summary for 2006 R," *Seminars in Dialysis*, vol. 21, no. 1, pp. 24–28, 2008.

[5] B. L. Strom, E. Abrutyn, J. A. Berlin et al., "Risk factors for infective endocarditis: oral hygiene and nondental exposures," *Circulation*, vol. 102, no. 23, pp. 2842–2848, 2000.

[6] N. R. Powe, B. Jaar, S. L. Furth, J. Hermann, and W. Briggs, "Septicemia in dialysis patients: incidence, risk factors, and prognosis," *Kidney International*, vol. 55, no. 3, pp. 1081–1090, 1999.

[7] R. M. Klevens, J. I. Tokars, and M. Andrus, "Electronic reporting of infections associated with hemodialysis," *Nephrology News & Issues*, vol. 19, no. 7, pp. 37–43, 2005.

[8] J. Fernández-Cean, A. Alvarez, S. Burguez, G. Baldovinos, P. Larre-Borges, and M. Cha, "Infective endocarditis in chronic haemodialysis: two treatment strategies," *Nephrology Dialysis Transplantation*, vol. 17, no. 12, pp. 2226–2230, 2002.

[9] I. Raad, A.-M. Chaftari, R. Zakhour et al., "Successful salvage of central venous catheters in patients with catheter-related or central line-associated bloodstream infections by using a catheter lock solution consisting of minocycline, EDTA, and 25% ethanol," *Antimicrobial Agents and Chemotherapy*, vol. 60, no. 6, pp. 3426–3432, 2016.

[10] R. A. Reitzel, J. Rosenblatt, C. Hirsh-Ginsberg et al., "In vitro assessment of the antimicrobial efficacy of optimized nitroglycerin-citrate-ethanol as a nonantibiotic, antimicrobial catheter lock solution for prevention of central line-associated bloodstream infections," *Antimicrobial Agents and Chemotherapy*, vol. 60, no. 9, pp. 5175–5181, 2016.

[11] Z. Han, S. Y. Liang, and J. Marschall, "Current strategies for the prevention and management of central line-associated bloodstream infections," *Infection and Drug Resistance*, vol. 3, pp. 147–163, 2010.

[12] E. Umana, W. Ahmed, and M. A. Alpert, "Valvular and perivalvular abnormalities in end-stage renal disease," *American Journal of the Medical Sciences*, vol. 325, no. 4, pp. 237–242, 2003.

[13] E. C. Madu, I. A. D'Cruz, B. Wall, N. Mansour, and S. Shearin, "Transesophageal echocardiographic spectrum of calcific mitral abnormalities in patients with end-stage renal disease," *Echocardiography*, vol. 17, no. 1, pp. 29–35, 2000.

[14] H. Kohler, W. Arnold, G. Renschin et al., "Active hepatitis B vaccination of dialysis patients and medical staV," *Kidney International*, vol. 25, pp. 124–128, 1984.

[15] M. Girndt, U. Sester, M. Sester, H. Kaul, and H. Kohler, "Impaired cellular immune function in patients with end-stage renal failure," *Nephrology Dialysis Transplantation*, vol. 14, no. 12, pp. 2807–2810, 1999.

[16] M. Girndt, H. Kaul, U. Sester et al., "Selective sequestration of cytokine producing mononuclear cells during hemodialysis treatment," *Journal of the American Society of Nephrology*, vol. 8, article 236, 1997.

[17] D. L. Robinson, V. G. Fowler, D. J. Sexton, R. G. Corey, and P. J. Conlon, "Bacterial endocarditis in hemodialysis patients," *American Journal of Kidney Diseases*, vol. 30, no. 4, pp. 521–524, 1997.

[18] T. L. Smith, M. L. Pearson, K. R. Wilcox et al., "Emergence of vancomycin resistance in Staphylococcus aureus," *The New England Journal of Medicine*, vol. 340, no. 7, pp. 493–501, 1999.

[19] M. Drees and H. Boucher, "New agents for *Staphylococcus aureus* endocarditis," *Current Opinion in Infectious Diseases*, vol. 19, no. 6, pp. 544–550, 2006.

[20] L. C. Pierrotti and L. M. Baddour, "Fungal endocarditis, 1995-2000," *Chest*, vol. 122, no. 1, pp. 302–310, 2002.

[21] P. G. Pappas, C. A. Kauffman, D. Andes et al., "Clinical practice guidelines for the management of candidiasis: 2009 update by the Infectious Diseases Society of America," *Clinical Infectious Diseases*, vol. 48, no. 5, pp. 503–535, 2009.

[22] C. F. Evans and J. S. Gammie, "Surgical management of mitral valve infective endocarditis," *Seminars in Thoracic and Cardiovascular Surgery*, vol. 23, no. 3, pp. 232–240, 2011.

[23] G. Di Salvo, G. Habib, V. Pergola et al., "Echocardiography predicts embolic events in infective endocarditis," *Journal of the American College of Cardiology*, vol. 37, no. 4, pp. 1069–1076, 2001.

[24] H. A. Cooper, E. C. Thompson, R. Laureno et al., "Subclinical brain embolization in left-sided infective endocarditis: results from the evaluation by MRI of the brains of patients with left-sided intracardiac solid masses (EMBOLISM) pilot study," *Circulation*, vol. 120, no. 7, pp. 585–591, 2009.

[25] P. J. Peters, T. Harrison, and J. L. Lennox, "A dangerous dilemma: management of infectious intracranial aneurysms complicating endocarditis," *Lancet Infectious Diseases*, vol. 6, no. 11, pp. 742–748, 2006.

[26] S. L. Robinson, J. M. Saxe, C. E. Lucas et al., "Splenic abscess associated with endocarditis," *Surgery*, vol. 112, no. 4, pp. 781–787, 1992.

[27] K. Spiliopoulos, G. Giamouzis, A. Haschemi et al., "Surgical management of infective endocarditis: early and long-term mortality analysis. single- center experience and brief literature review," *Hellenic Journal of Cardiology*, vol. 55, no. 6, pp. 462–474, 2014.

Renal Tubular Acidosis and Hypokalemic Paralysis as a First Presentation of Primary Sjögren's Syndrome

Arun Sedhain,[1] Kiran Acharya,[2] Alok Sharma,[3] Amir Khan,[2] and Shital Adhikari[4]

[1]Nephrology Unit, Department of Medicine, Chitwan Medical College, Bharatpur, Chitwan, Nepal
[2]Department of Medicine, Chitwan Medical College, Bharatpur, Chitwan, Nepal
[3]Department of Renal Pathology & Electron Microscopy, National Reference Laboratory, Dr. Lal Pathlabs Ltd, New Delhi, India
[4]Pulmonology and Critical Care Unit, Department of Medicine, Chitwan Medical College, Bharatpur, Chitwan, Nepal

Correspondence should be addressed to Arun Sedhain; arunsedhain@gmail.com

Academic Editor: Władysław Sułowicz

Sjögren's syndrome is an autoimmune disease with multisystem involvement and varying clinical presentation. We report the clinical course and outcome of a case who presented with repeated episodes of hypokalemia mimicking hypokalemic periodic paralysis and metabolic acidosis, which was later diagnosed as distal renal tubular acidosis secondary to primary Sjögren's syndrome. A 50-year-old lady, who was previously diagnosed as hypokalemic periodic paralysis, presented with generalized weakness and fatigue. She was found to have severe hypokalemia with normal anion-gap metabolic acidosis consistent with distal renal tubular acidosis. Subsequent evaluation revealed Sjögren's syndrome as the cause of her problems. Kidney biopsy done to evaluate significant proteinuria revealed nonproliferative morphology with patchy acute tubular injury and significant chronic interstitial nephritis. The patient responded well to potassium supplementation and oral prednisolone. Presentation of this case highlights the necessity of close vigilance while managing a case of repeated hypokalemia, which could be one of the rare clinical manifestations of Sjögren's syndrome.

1. Introduction

Sjögren's syndrome (SS) is a slowly progressing autoimmune disease characterized by lymphocytic infiltration of the exocrine glands, mainly the lacrimal and salivary glands, resulting in impaired secretory function. The disease has an estimated prevalence of 0.3 to 1 per 1000 persons and a peak incidence at approximately 50 years of age with female-to-male predominance of 9:1 [1].

Renal involvement is seen in 5% of patients with SS, with the most common of which being chronic interstitial nephritis [2–4]. Renal tubular acidosis (RTA) occurs in up to 25% of patients with the disease [5], most of which are usually asymptomatic. We report a case requiring multiple hospital admissions with a clinical diagnosis of hypokalemic periodic paralysis previously presented to us with severe hypokalemia associated with metabolic acidosis, which was later diagnosed to be secondary to Sjögren's syndrome.

2. Case Report

A 50-year-old woman presented to the Emergency Department (ED) of Chitwan Medical College, Bharatpur, Chitwan, Nepal, with the history of weakness of both lower limbs for two days that was preceded by muscle cramps of three days' duration. Her weakness was insidious in onset and gradually progressive in nature affecting the upper limbs by next day with no history of altered sensorium, seizure, and bladder or bowel involvement. Her past medical history was positive for repeated hospital admissions following episodes of weakness and fatigue associated with hypokalemia for the past three years, which was managed in the line of hypokalemic periodic paralysis that responded well to supplemental potassium alone. She also had similar problems episodically for the past three years requiring repeated hospital admissions. The lady also had a history of drooping of her bilateral eyelids, foreign body sensation in the eyes, dry mouth, and recurrent

TABLE 1: Laboratory and biochemical parameters at presentation.

Test	Result
Hb	10.0 (g/dl)
WBC	5600 (per mm^3)
Platelets	298,000 (per mm3)
ESR	67 (mm/1st hour)
Serum Na$^+$	148 (mEq/L)
Serum K$^+$	1.6 (mEq/L)
Serum Urea	29 (mg/dL)
Serum Creatinine	1.0 (mg/dL)
Random blood sugar	130 (mg/dL)
Serum Magnesium	2.5 (mg/dL)
Serum Calcium	8.36 (mg/dL)
Serum pH	7.20
pCO$_2$	18.8 (mmHg)
HCO$_3$	7.1 (mEq/L)
pO$_2$	89 (mmHg)
Serum Chloride	130 (mmol/L)
Anion Gap	11.9 (mmol/L)
Serum Vitamin 25(OH) D	6.40 (ng/ml)
Parathyroid hormone	145 (pg/ml)
TSH	8.74 (mIU/ml)
Urine pH	5.0
Urine K$^+$	34.6
HIV, HBsAg, Anti-HCV	Negative

Hb: hemoglobin, ESR: erythrocyte sedimentation rate, RBS: random blood sugar, TSH: thyroid stimulating hormone. Serum anion gap = Na − (Cl + HCO3).

muscular weakness for the past three years. She denied history of vomiting and intake of diuretics, alcohol, or laxatives. Previous medical records revealed negative results for antibody against acetylcholine receptor that ruled out myasthenia gravis.

On physical examination, vital signs were within normal limit and higher mental functions were intact. Her oral cavity was dry and there was no lymphadenopathy. Motor power was 3/5 on the lower limbs and 4/5 on the upper limb affecting both proximal and distal group of muscles. Deep tendon reflexes were diminished bilaterally. There was no sensory deficit and cranial nerve examination was unremarkable. Cardiovascular, respiratory, gastrointestinal, and thyroid examination findings were normal.

She was found to have hypokalemia (documented serum K+ of 1.6 meq/L; normal range 3.5-5.5 meq/L) (Table 1). ECG showed a sinus bradycardia with global T wave inversion and the presence of subtle U wave.

In the Emergency Department, the patient was started on intravenous potassium supplementation at the rate of 20 meq/hour via central line and was admitted to the intensive care unit (ICU), where treatment was continued and serial monitoring of potassium level was done. Consecutive serum potassium levels at 6th, 12th, and 48th hour after initiation of treatment were 1.75 mmol/L, 2.1 mmol/L, and 3.7 mmol/L, respectively. Intravenous magnesium supplementation and injection sodium bicarbonate were also given. After 12 hours of treatment, her clinical condition improved significantly with normalization of the muscle power.

With the urinary pH of 5.0, negative urine culture, no history of diuretic usage, vomiting, and diarrhea, and the arterial blood gas (ABG) showing hyperchloremic normal anion-gap metabolic acidosis in a patient with severe hypokalemia (serum potassium 1.7 mmol/L), the diagnosis of distal renal tubular acidosis (DRTA) was made. With the history of xerostomia and xerophthalmia without any secondary causes for them, SS was suspected, which was later confirmed by the significantly raised titers of anti-Ro/SSA and/or anti-La/SSB antibodies and positive Schirmer test (4.8 mm in 5 minutes) as per the latest classification criteria [6].

She was started on oral prednisolone at 1 mg/kg/day after which ptosis showed partial recovery in the first 7 days. She was discharged with the same dose of prednisolone and was advised for regular follow-up in nephrology clinic.

The patient attended the nephrology clinic after 7 days with palpable purpuric rashes in both of the lower limbs associated with minimal pedal edema (Figure 1). She was reevaluated and skin biopsy was suggested, but she refused it. She was found to have normal hemogram and bleeding profile and negative perinuclear antineutrophil cytoplasmic antibodies (P-ANCA), antineutrophil cytoplasmic antibodies (C-ANCA), and cryoglobulins. Urine examination showed 2+ albumin without associated hematuria and 24-hour urinary protein was 1600 mg, for which she underwent kidney biopsy. Light microscopy showed nonproliferative glomerular morphology (Figure 2) with patchy acute tubular injury and multifocal chronic interstitial inflammation (Figure 3). Direct immunofluorescent examination revealed no significant glomerular immune deposits. Transmission electron microscopy revealed relatively well-preserved visceral epithelial cell foot processes (Figure 4) and no evidence of glomerular or extraglomerular electron dense deposits. Endothelial tubuloreticular inclusions were not seen. Proximal tubular epithelial cells did not reveal abnormal inclusions or giant mitochondria.

The patient is on regular follow-up for the last eight months and the oral steroids is getting tapered gradually. She is doing well with improvement in proteinuria, resolution of acidosis, and hypokalemic episodes.

3. Discussion

Our patient presented with the complaints of muscle weakness secondary to severe hypokalemia (serum K+ 1.6 meq/L). On further evaluation in our center, she had normal anion-gap hyperchloremic metabolic acidosis (HCMA). Despite lack of a more comprehensive evaluation, the biochemical findings of renal potassium loss in association with HCMA were supportive of the diagnosis of distal renal tubular acidosis (RTA) in our patient. Further history obtained from the patient revealed that she had a history of foreign body sensation in the eyes and dry mouth for the past three years, which prompted us to evaluate for the possibility of Sjögren's syndrome as the root cause of her recurrent clinical problems.

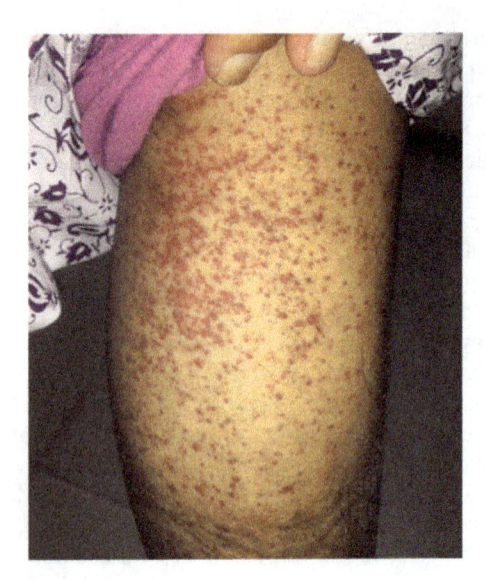

FIGURE 1: Palpable purpura on the lower limb.

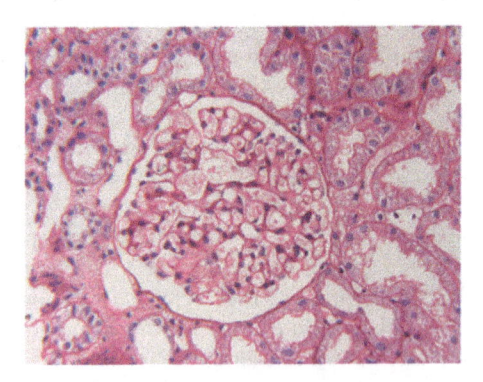

FIGURE 2: Photomicrograph from renal biopsy showing an unremarkable appearing glomerulus (PAS X 200).

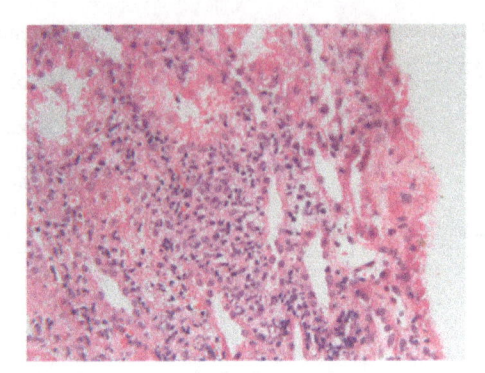

FIGURE 3: Photomicrograph showing dense chronic lymphoplasmacytic interstitial inflammation (H&E X 160).

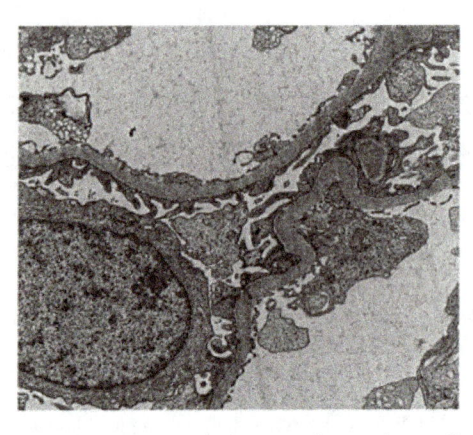

FIGURE 4: Electron micrograph showing glomerular capillaries with well-preserved foot processes of visceral epithelial cells (uranyl acetate and lead citrate X 3000).

Significantly raised titers of anti-Ro/SSA and anti-La/SSB antibodies and positive Schirmer test confirmed Sjögren's syndrome. She later developed significant proteinuria, for which kidney biopsy was done showing nonproliferative morphology with patchy acute tubular injury and focal chronic interstitial inflammation. She was started with oral prednisolone and was kept on regular follow-ups with significant clinical improvements.

Sjögren's syndrome is a systemic autoimmune disorder characterized by a unique set of signs and symptoms predominantly caused by a cell-mediated autoimmunity against exocrine glands [7]. Systemic manifestations occur in approximately 30 to 40% of the patients with primary Sjögren's syndrome [2]. Lymphocytic infiltration can cause interstitial nephritis, autoimmune primary biliary cholangitis, and obstructive bronchiolitis. Immune complex deposition can result in palpable purpura, cryoglobulinemia-associated glomerulonephritis, interstitial pneumonitis, and peripheral neuropathy [8].

The most common affected nonexocrine organ in Sjögren's syndrome is kidney with the prevalence ranging between 2 and 67% [9, 10]. Most common form of renal involvement in Sjögren's syndrome is interstitial nephritis followed by distal renal tubular acidosis (dRTA), nephrogenic diabetes insipidus, and different forms of glomerular diseases, of which membranoproliferative glomerulonephritis (MPGN) and membranous nephropathy (MN) are the most common [3, 4]. Although dRTA is common in Sjögren's syndrome, it is usually asymptomatic and in most cases it remains undetected. Hypokalemia is the most common electrolyte abnormality in patients with dRTA. The causes of hypokalemia include decreased distal tubular Na+ delivery, secondary hyperaldosteronism, defective H+-K+ ATPase, and bicarbonaturia. Hypokalemic paralysis seen in SS is rare and may sometimes mimic hypokalemic periodic paralysis (HPP). However, there are case reports of single presentation of severe hypokalemic paralysis, which was later confirmed as Sjögren's syndrome [11].

A diagnosis of primary Sjögren's syndrome is often considered based on the classic symptoms of mouth and eye dryness, fatigue, and pain [2]. However, systemic complications sometimes provide the first clue to the disease as seen in our case, in which the presenting complaint was muscle weakness secondary to severe hypokalemia and metabolic acidosis. Anti-SSA antibodies (antibodies against Sjögren's syndrome–related antigen A) are present in two-thirds of patients and should be assessed in all suspected cases of primary Sjögren's syndrome. Biopsy of minor salivary glands is typically recommended for establishing a diagnosis of primary Sjögren's syndrome in the absence of anti-SSA antibodies. Schirmer's test to assess the ocular dryness is a useful examination. A recent set of classification criteria for SS were published by the ACR/EULAR in 2016 [6] and the score of ≥4 is required for the diagnosis.

Management of primary SS is symptomatic. In the acute setting, when the patient presents with hypokalemia, the priority will be to reverse the severe hypokalemia with intravenous potassium supplementation, followed by correction of the underlying acidosis. Long-term use of potassium supplementation might be required for majority of the patients. Use of muscarinic agonists (pilocarpine hydrochloride and cevimeline hydrochloride) is recommended for the treatment of oral dryness and, to a lesser extent, ocular dryness [12]. Neuropathic pain in patients with primary Sjögren's syndrome is typically treated with gabapentin, pregabalin, or duloxetine. Although no immunomodulatory drug has proved to be efficacious in primary SS, combination of corticosteroids and other immunosuppressive drugs has been reported to slow the progression of renal damage in Sjögren's syndrome [13]. Agents that are commonly used include hydroxychloroquine, prednisone, methotrexate, mycophenolate sodium, azathioprine, and cyclosporine. Few biologic agents have been rigorously studied in primary SS, and none have shown significant efficacy in multiple studies [14, 15]. The heterogeneity in the etiopathogenesis and clinical manifestation of the disease, in conjunction with a variable response to clinical therapeutics, warrants a more individualized approach to achieve improved long-term outcomes in patients with primary SS.

Our patient had repeated episodes of hypokalemia and metabolic acidosis in the past, which responded symptomatically to potassium supplementation alone. Thus, she was labelled as a case of hypokalemic periodic paralysis but detailed workup for the etiopathogenesis of her problem was missed.

4. Conclusion

Although Sjögren's syndrome might have a varying clinical presentation, presentation of a person with renal symptoms in the form of hypokalemia as the first symptom might create the confusion to reach the diagnosis. This case highlights the importance of high index of suspicion for possibility of Sjögren's syndrome, especially in the middle-aged females, who present with hypokalemia and metabolic acidosis.

References

[1] B. Qin, J. Wang, Z. Yang et al., "Epidemiology of primary Sjögren's syndrome: a systematic review and meta-analysis," *Annals of Rheumatic Diseases*, vol. 74, pp. 1983–1989, 2015.

[2] S. Retamozo, P. Brito-Zerón, M. Zeher et al., "Epidemiologic subsets drive a differentiated clinical and immunological presentation of primary Sjögren syndrome: Analysis of 9302 patients from the Big Data International Sjögren Cohort," *Arthritis Rheumatol*, vol. 69, supplement 10, pp. 876–877, 2017.

[3] D. Kidder, E. Rutherford, D. Kipgen, S. Fleming, C. Geddes, and G. A. Stewart, "Kidney biopsy findings in primary Sjögren syndrome," *Nephrology Dialysis Transplantation*, vol. 30, no. 8, pp. 1363–1369, 2015.

[4] S. Maripuri, J. P. Grande, T. G. Osborn et al., "Renal involvement in primary sjögren's syndrome: a clinicopathologic study," *Clinical Journal of the American Society of Nephrology*, vol. 4, no. 9, pp. 1423–1431, 2009.

[5] J. M. Poux, P. Peyronnet, Y. Le Meur et al., "Hypokalemic quadriplegia and respiratory arrest revealing primary Sjögren's syndrome," *Clinical Nephrology*, vol. 37, no. 4, pp. 189–191, 1992.

[6] C. H. Shiboski, S. C. Shiboski, R. Seror et al., "2016 American College of Rheumatology/European League Against Rheumatism classification criteria for primary Sjögren's syndrome: A consensus and data-driven methodology involving three international patient cohorts," *Annals of the Rheumatic Diseases*, vol. 69, no. 1, pp. 35–45, 2017.

[7] R. I. Fox, "Sjögren's syndrome," *The Lancet*, vol. 366, no. 9482, pp. 321–331, 2005.

[8] X. Mariette and L. A. Criswell, "Primary sjögren's syndrome," *New England Journal of Medicine*, vol. 378, no. 10, pp. 931–939, 2018.

[9] M. Pertovaara, M. Korpela, and A. Pasternack, "Factors predictive of renal involvement in patients with primary Sjögren's syndrome," *Clinical Nephrology*, vol. 56, no. 1, pp. 10–18, 2001.

[10] N. Bossini, S. Savoldi, F. Franceschini et al., "Clinical and morphological features of kidney involvement in primary Sjögren's syndrome," *Nephrology Dialysis Transplantation*, vol. 16, no. 12, pp. 2328–2336, 2001.

[11] B. Aygen, F. E. Dursun, A. Dogukan et al., "Hypokalemic quadriparesis associated with renal tubular acidosis in a patient with Sjögren's syndrome," *Clinical Nephrology*, vol. 69, pp. 306–309, 2008.

[12] M. Ramos-Casals, A. G. Tzioufas, J. H. Stone, A. Sisó, and X. Bosch, "Treatment of primary Sjögren syndrome: A systematic review," *Journal of the American Medical Association*, vol. 304, no. 4, pp. 452–460, 2010.

[13] H. Ren, W. M. Wang, and X. N. Chen, "Renal involvement and follow-up of 130 patients with primary Sjögren's syndrome," *The Journal of Rheumatology*, vol. 35, no. 2, pp. 278–284, 2008.

[14] X. Mariette, P. Ravaud, S. Steinfeld et al., "Inefficacy of Infliximab in Primary Sjögren's Syndrome: Results of the Randomized, Controlled Trial of Remicade in Primary Sjögren's Syndrome (TRIPSS)," *Arthritis & Rheumatology*, vol. 50, no. 4, pp. 1270–1276, 2004.

[15] V. Sankar, M. T. Brennan, M. R. Kok et al., "Etanercept in Sjögren's syndrome: A twelve-week randomized, double-blind, placebo-controlled pilot clinical trial," *Arthritis & Rheumatism*, vol. 50, no. 7, pp. 2240–2245, 2004.

Early Renal Involvement in a Girl with Classic Fabry Disease

Fernando Perretta,[1,2] Norberto Antongiovanni,[2,3] and Sebastián Jaurretche[2,4,5]

[1]Servicio de Terapia Intensiva del Hospital Dr. Enrique Erill de Escobar, Provincia de Buenos Aires, Argentina
[2]GINEF Argentina (Grupo de Investigación Nefrológica en la Enfermedad de Fabry), Buenos Aires, Argentina
[3]Centro de Infusión y Estudio de Enfermedades Lisosomales del Instituto de Nefrología Clínica Pergamino, Provincia de Buenos Aires, Argentina
[4]Centro de Neurociencias Los Manantiales, Grupo Gamma Rosario, Provincia de Santa Fe, Argentina
[5]Cátedra de Biofísica y Fisiología, Instituto Universitario Italiano de Rosario, Provincia de Santa Fe, Argentina

Correspondence should be addressed to Fernando Perretta; fjperretta@hotmail.com

Academic Editor: Hiro Matsukura

Fabry disease is an X-linked lysosomal storage disorder resulting from the deficiency or absence of the enzyme alpha galactosidase A; this defect leads to the systemic accumulation of globotriaosylceramide and its metabolites. Organic involvement in men is well known, but in women it is controversial, mainly due to the random X-chromosome inactivation in each of their cells (Lyon hypothesis). This would explain why women (heterozygotes) present a wide variability in the severity of their phenotype. The manifestations are multisystemic and begin in early childhood, reaching a severe compromise in adulthood. Typical acroparesthesia in hands and feet, gastrointestinal symptoms, angiokeratomas, dyshidrosis, hearing loss, arrhythmias, hypertrophic cardiomyopathy, cerebrovascular accidents, and renal failure can be observed. Nephropathy is one of the major complications of Fabry disease. Glomerular and vascular changes are present before progression to overt proteinuria and decreased glomerular filtration rate, even in pediatric patients. A case of incipient renal involvement in a girl with classic Fabry disease is reported.

1. Introduction

Fabry disease (FD) is caused by the lysosomal accumulation of complex glycosphingolipids, mainly globotriaosylceramide (Gb3) and its metabolites [1]. This deposit triggers physiopathogenic pathways in the vascular endothelium and cells of different tissues (cardiac, renal, and nervous among others) that lead to cell death, with progression to fibrosis and irreversible organic damage [2, 3]. The storage of Gb3 is due to the deficient or null activity of α-galactosidase A (α-galA, EC 3.2.1.22). The GLA gene, which encodes α-galA, is located on the X-chromosome (Xq22.1), whereby practically all men carrying a genetic mutation (hemizygous) develop the disease, while women (heterozygotes) exhibit a wide variability in the severity of their phenotype, mainly due to the random X-chromosomes inactivation in each of their cells (Lyon hypothesis) [4]. The symptoms intensity will depend mostly on the residual activity of the α-galA enzyme.

FD manifestations are multisystemic and begin in childhood, reaching severe impairment in the third or fourth decade of life. The main signs and symptoms of the disease are acroparesthesia in hands and feet, gastrointestinal disorders, angiokeratomas, dyshidrosis, intolerance to exercise and heat, hearing loss, arrhythmias, hypertrophic cardiomyopathy, cerebrovascular accidents, and renal failure [5, 6].

FD is panethnic and, given its low incidence, there is no accurate information regarding its prevalence, ranging from 1 : 40,000 men to 1 : 117,000 live births [7, 8]. Due to the great phenotypic and symptoms variability, it is difficult to perform a precise diagnosis, which is reached in adult ages when the organic involvement is already installed.

Thanks to systematic studies of FD detection in dialysis centers, it has been possible to advance in the determination of the prevalence in the dialysis population. It is 0.33% in men, showing that screening is a useful strategy in patients with chronic kidney damage [9].

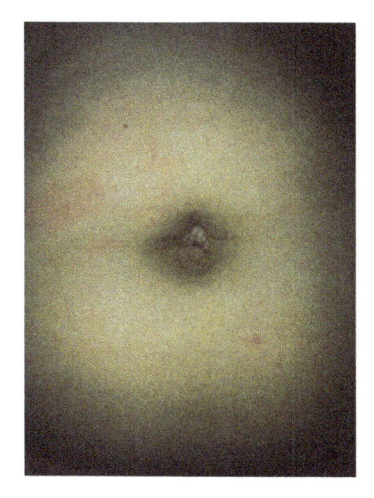

FIGURE 1: Periumbilical angiokeratomas.

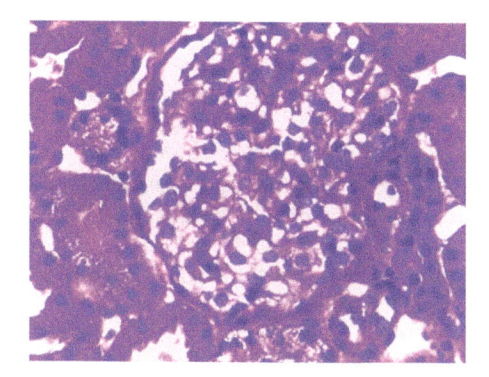

FIGURE 2: Light microscopy. PAS ×630.

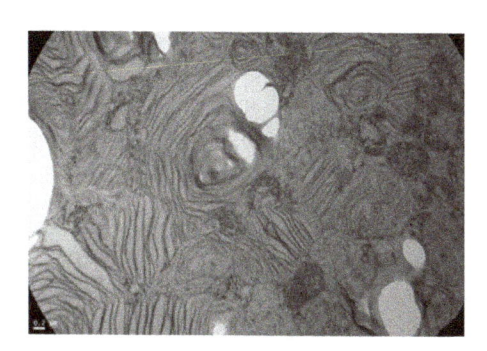

FIGURE 3: Electron microscopy ×25.000.

Once the diagnosis has been made, it is possible to work on the family screening, which will allow the identification of affected relatives, thus detecting patients at an earlier age [10].

In the last years there has been progress in understanding the pathophysiology of tissue damage in FD, mainly in early organ involvement due to the accumulation of Gb3, where it was observed that asymptomatic pediatric patients already present tissue alterations [11]. This report describes incipient renal involvement in a pediatric patient with classic FD.

2. Case Presentation

A 9-year-old female patient was diagnosed with FD by family screening at 5 years of age, mutation c.1244T>C (p.L415P) in heterozygous status, alpha galactosidase in dried blood spot on filter paper of 1.5 umol/l/h (reference value ≥ 4.0).

It is a patient with normal physical and neurological development according to age. On examination, the following is found: preserved vital signs with normal blood pressure, weight 52 kg, height 151 cm, rare bronchospasms, mild acroparesthesias with good response to carbamazepine 200 mg/day, and few periumbilical angiokeratomas (Figure 1).

Complementary Studies. Laboratory findings are as follows: creatinine of 0.34 mg/dl (estimated glomerular filtration rate by Schwartz formula of 183 ml/min), albuminuria of 2.7 ug/min (reference value from 0 to 15), and proteinuria of 30 mg/24 hours (reference value < 150), with blood Lyso-Gb3 of 69.9 nmol/l (reference value < 1.2), normal electrocardiogram for their age, Doppler echocardiography with physiologic tricuspid and pulmonary regurgitation, normal brain magnetic resonance imaging, ophthalmological examination with slit lamp showing cornea verticillata in both eyes, and normal abdominal and renal ultrasound.

Although the patient did not present clinical data of nephropathy (albuminuria/proteinuria), due to the presence of glomerular hyperfiltration associated with peripheral neuropathy and an elevated blood Lyso-Gb3, a renal biopsy was performed. Light microscopy: after staining with hematoxylin and eosin, periodic acid-Schiff, Masson's trichrome, and silver-methenamine (Jones stain), glomeruli were observed with some degree of podocyte vacuolization that occupies on average 30% of the podocytes. Tubules: some distal tubules with clarification and microvacuolization of the cytoplasm. Interstitium and vessels were without alterations (Figure 2). Electron microscopy: glomeruli showed microvacuolization in one-micron sections (Fogo classification score 2), with mild clarification in the cytoplasm of proximal and distal tubules and Interstitium and vessels without alterations. Typical myeloid or zebra bodies were observed in the cytoplasm of several podocytes, confirming the diagnosis of FD (Figure 3). After a multidisciplinary evaluation, it was decided to start enzyme replacement therapy (ERT) with agalsidase beta at doses of 1 mg/kg body weight every 2 weeks by intravenous infusion.

3. Discussion

Gb3 deposits have been found in placental tissue, suggesting that the storage is already present at birth [12]. However, children are not symptomatic in the first years of life [13]. Patients generally present at an earlier age symptoms that manifest the progressive function loss of small nerve fibers of the peripheral somatic and autonomic nervous systems [13]. Early symptoms may include chronic neuropathic pain and/or acute attacks of pain ("Fabry crisis"); absence or decrease in sweating; tinnitus; intolerance to cold, heat, or exercise; gastrointestinal disorders (e.g., diarrhea, nausea, vomiting, postprandial bloating, and pain); and difficulty gaining weight. In addition, skin lesions (angiokeratomas), corneal and lenticular opacities, and the presence of mild proteinuria (in adolescent males) are among the first manifestations [14]. These symptoms generally cause morbidity despite the absence of major organ dysfunction, limiting the child's physical, school, and social performances. It has been reported that the symptoms can occur in early childhood, before the age of 5 years [15].

Screening is a valid tool to detect patients with FD, and performing a detailed pedigree, as in this case, can help to identify them at an earlier age before organic damage occurs [10].

Nephropathy is one of the major complications of FD [10]. Renal biopsies demonstrate Gb3 accumulation in tubular, glomerular, and endothelial cells, even in pediatric patients without albuminuria or decreased glomerular filtration rate [16, 17]. At present the only tool to detect early involvement is the kidney biopsy, but its routine indication is controversial because of the potential risks of the procedure. Percutaneous renal biopsy is safe in all ages when performed by experienced physicians; reduced estimated GFR and smaller center size are associated with an increased risk of major complications [18]. For this reason, the interest in the last years has focused on the study of noninvasive biomarkers able to detect early kidney damage. Lyso-Gb3 has been associated with neuropathic pain and with prealbuminuric histological changes, as in this case. Plasma measurement of Lyso-Gb3 is valuable for confirming the diagnosis of FD, particularly in heterozygous women, and its values correlate with disease severity [19]. A pilot study about the identification of urinary podocytes as a potential biomarker of glomerular damage, in primary and secondary glomerulopathies, was performed in Argentina [20]. Fabry disease is associated with increased podocyte loss; the direct associations found between podocyturia and proteinuria and the inverse association found between podocyturia and glomerular filtration rate in male patients indicate that there are important correlations between podocyturia and severity of Fabry nephropathy [21]. However, new biomarkers are needed to help in the stratification and quantification of renal damage in patients with FD to replace kidney biopsies.

In the present report, we describe renal histological involvement in a pediatric patient with classic FD and nonspecific signs and symptoms, prior to urinary protein loss (albuminuria/proteinuria). The kidney biopsy describes a score 2 of the Fogo et al. classification [16]; moderate podocyte vacuolization. This finding confirms what Tøndel et al. published in 2008; glomerular and vascular changes are present before progression to overt proteinuria and decreased glomerular filtration rate [11]. It has also been described that podocyte foot process effacement is an early marker of nephropathy in young classic Fabry patients without albuminuria. For this reason, renal biopsies may be essential in the early diagnosis of FD nephropathy and also in the evaluation of ERT response [17]. In this patient, we highlight the renal hyperfiltration values that can be interpreted as a glomerular compensation sign, despite the limitation that they were estimated by formula, but not measured.

In this case report, kidney biopsy provided useful information for the diagnosis of FD nephropathy, confirming the clinical suspicion. The lack of noninvasive biomarkers that correlate with the degree of tissue damage determines that, despite the controversies, a kidney biopsy is a necessary intervention in certain patients, even at pediatric ages.

Since 2001, FD has had a specific treatment with ERT, which has also demonstrated safety and efficacy [22]. It has been described that early histological renal lesions have a good response to ERT when it begins early. The clearance of Gb3 and the improvement of these lesions have been confirmed in serial kidney biopsies of pediatric patients treated with ERT and have a dose-dependent correlation [11, 17], and reaccumulation was observed after the decrease of the indicated dose [23].

To conclude, we emphasize the importance of suspecting FD and its exhaustive study. The kidney biopsy is an important tool in the assessment of renal involvement and can lead to the early initiation of ERT, which will change the natural history of this disease.

References

[1] C. De Duve, "Exploring cells with a centrifuge," *Science*, vol. 189, no. 4198, pp. 186–194, 1975.

[2] R. J. Desnick, Y. A. Ioannou, and C. M. Eng, "Alpha-galactosidase a deficiency: fabry disease," in *The Metabolic And Molecular Basis of Inherited Disease*, C. R. Scriver, A. L. Beaudet, W. S. Sly, and D. Valle, Eds., pp. 2741–2784, McGraw-Hill, New York, 7th edition, 1995.

[3] S. Park, J. A. Kim, K. Y. Joo et al., "Globotriaosylceramide leads to KCa3.1 channel dysfunction: a new insight into endothelial dysfunction in fabry disease," *Cardiovascular Research*, vol. 89, no. 2, pp. 290–299, 2011.

[4] R. J. Desnick, K. Y. Allen, S. J. Desnick, and etal., "Fabrys disease: enzymatic diagnosis of hemizygotes and heterozygotes: alpha-galactosidase activities in plasma, serum, urine, and leukocytes," *Journal of Laboratory and Clinical Medicine*, vol. 81, pp. 157–171, 1973.

[5] R. J. Desnick, R. Brady, J. Barranger et al., "Fabry disease, an under-recognized multisystemic disorder: expert recommendations for diagnosis, management, and enzyme replacement therapy," *Annals of Internal Medicine*, vol. 138, no. 4, pp. 338–346, 2003.

[6] A. Mehta, R. Ricci, U. Widmer et al., "Fabry disease defined: baseline clinical manifestations of 366 patients in the fabry outcome survey," *European Journal of Clinical Investigation*, vol. 34, no. 3, pp. 236–242, 2004.

[7] R. J. Desnick, Y. A. Ioannou, and C. M. Eng, "Alpha-Galactosidase a deficiency: fabry disease," in *The Metabolic And Molecular Basis of Inherited Disease*, C. R. Scriver, A. L. Beaudet, W. S. Sly, and D. Valle, Eds., pp. 3733–3774, McGraw-Hill, New York, 8th edition, 2001.

[8] P. J. Meikle, J. J. Hopwood, A. E. Clague, and W. F. Carey, "Prevalence of lysosomal storage disorders," *Journal of the American Medical Association*, vol. 281, no. 3, pp. 249–254, 1999.

[9] G. E. Linthorst, M. G. Bouwman, F. A. Wijburg, and etal., "Screening for Fabry disease in high-risk populations: a systematic review," *Journal of Medical Genetics*, vol. 47, no. 4, pp. 217–222, 2010.

[10] S. Jaurretche, N. Antongiovanni, and F. Perretta, "Prevalence of chronic kidney disease in fabry disease patients: multicenter cross sectional study in Argentina," *Molecular Genetics and Metabolism Reports*, vol. 12, pp. 41–43, 2017.

[11] C. Tøndel, L. Bostad, A. Hirth, and E. Svarstad, "Renal biopsy findings in children and adolescents with fabry disease and minimal albuminuria," *American Journal of Kidney Diseases*, vol. 51, no. 5, pp. 767–776, 2008.

[12] A. C. Vedder, A. Strijland, M. A. vd Bergh Weerman, S. Florquin, J. M. F. G. Aerts, and C. E. M. Hollak, "Manifestations of Fabry disease in placental tissue," *Journal of Inherited Metabolic Disease*, vol. 29, no. 1, pp. 106–111, 2006.

[13] D. P. Germain, "Fabry disease," *Orphanet Journal of Rare Diseases*, vol. 5, 2010.

[14] R. J. Desnick and R. O. Brady, "Fabry disease in childhood," *Journal of Pediatrics*, vol. 144, no. 5, pp. S20–S26, 2004.

[15] D. A. Laney, D. S. Peck, A. M. Atherton et al., "Fabry disease in infancy and early childhood: a systematic literature review," *Genetics in Medicine*, vol. 17, no. 5, pp. 323–330, 2015.

[16] A. B. Fogo, L. Bostad, E. Svarstad et al., "Scoring system for renal pathology in Fabry disease: report of the international study group of fabry nephropathy (ISGFN)," *Nephrology Dialysis Transplantation*, vol. 25, no. 7, pp. 2168–2177, 2010.

[17] C. Tøndel, T. Kanai, K. K. Larsen et al., "Foot process effacement is an early marker of nephropathy in young classic fabry patients without albuminuria," *Nephron*, vol. 129, no. 1, pp. 16–21, 2015.

[18] C. Tøndel, B. E. Vikse, L. Bostad, and E. Svarstad, "Safety and complications of percutaneous kidney biopsies in 715 children and 8573 adults in Norway 1988–2010," *Clinical Journal of the American Society of Nephrology*, vol. 7, no. 10, pp. 1591–1597, 2012.

[19] S. M. Rombach, N. Dekker, M. G. Bouwman, and etal., "Plasma globotriaosylsphingosine: diagnostic value and relation to clinical manifestations of Fabry disease," *Biochimica et Biophysica Acta - Molecular Basis of Disease*, vol. 1802, no. 9, pp. 741–748, 2010.

[20] H. Trimarchi, R. Canzonieri, A. Muryan, and etal., "La identificación de podocitos urinarios. La utilidad potencial de un biomarcador novedoso de daño gomerular en las glomerulopatías primarias y secundarias. Un estudio piloto," *Revista Nefrología Argentina*, vol. 14, no. 1, 2016.

[21] B. Fall, C. R. Scott, M. Mauer et al., "Urinary podocyte loss is increased in patients with fabry disease and correlates with clinical severity of fabry nephropathy," *PLoS ONE*, vol. 11, no. 12, Article ID e0168346, 2016.

[22] W. R. Wilcox, M. Banikazemi, N. Guffon et al., "Long-term safety and efficacy of enzyme replacement therapy for Fabry disease," *American Journal of Human Genetics*, vol. 75, no. 1, pp. 65–74, 2004.

[23] R. Skrunes, E. Svarstad, K. Kampevold Larsen, S. Leh, and C. Tøndel, "Reaccumulation of globotriaosylceramide in podocytes after agalsidase dose reduction in young Fabry patients," *Nephrology Dialysis Transplantation*, vol. 32, no. 5, pp. 807–813, 2017.

Ureteropelvic Junction Obstruction and Parathyroid Adenoma: Coincidence or Link?

Salah Termos,[1] Majd AlKabbani,[1] Tim Ulinski,[2] Sami Sanjad,[3] Henri Kotobi,[2] Francois Chalard,[2] and Bilal Aoun[2,3]

[1]Hepatobiliary and Transplant Unit, Department of Surgery, Al-Amiri Hospital, Kuwait City, Kuwait
[2]Pediatric Nephrology, Armand Trousseau Hospital, APHP, Paris, France
[3]Division of Pediatric Nephrology, Department of Pediatrics, American University of Beirut, Beirut, Lebanon

Correspondence should be addressed to Salah Termos; salahtermos@gmail.com

Academic Editor: Salih Kavukcu

Congenital ureteropelvic junction obstruction (UPJO) is the most common cause of upper urinary tract obstruction in children. It is generally diagnosed in the routine work-up during antenatal period and is characterized by spontaneous recovery. It can be associated with urolithiasis; hence further investigation should be carried out. We report the case of a 15-year-old boy, who is known to have right UPJO, presented with right renal colic and discovered to have bilateral kidney stones. Further studies showed primary hyperparathyroidism and genetic analysis revealed a CDC73 mutation (initially HRPT2). We believe that association of UPJO and PHPT is a rare coincidence that can be linked. Careful work-up of children with UPJO and urolithiasis is recommended to exclude an underlying metabolic disease. Surgical correction can be evitable as treatment of the primary cause can lead to complete dissolution of kidney stones and improvement of the medical condition.

1. Introduction

Ureteropelvic junction obstruction (UPJO) has a reported incidence of 1 in 500 live births [1], more commonly in males than females and more frequently found on the left side. It can be congenital or acquired, but congenital cases are more common. It is considered the most common cause of antenatally detected hydronephrosis [2, 3].

Management of UPJO depends on symptoms and split renal function and it includes conservative management with observation and follow-up or surgical intervention. UPJO can lead to urolithiasis due to obstruction and urinary stasis; however, metabolic causes of urolithiasis should be investigated and ruled out [4–6]. We describe an unusual case of UPJO associated with PHTP and kidney stones.

2. Case Presentation

In our manuscript, we report the case of a 15-year-old boy with a longstanding history of unilateral ureteropelvic junction obstruction who was presented for right flank pain of three-month duration. The patient had been followed up for his right UPJO since birth, as he was diagnosed prenatally to have hydronephrosis. An early ultrasound imaging of the kidney was done at the age of three months and revealed a right renal pelvis dilatation of 15 mm (anteroposterior diameter) with normal kidney parenchyma. Later at the age of three years, a follow-up ultrasound noted an increased dilatation of the right pelvis up to 20 mm. Further studies were carried out; a MAG-3 scintigraphy was performed and showed a good contrast evacuation (10% residual radioactivity, 20 minutes after furosemide injection) and symmetric kidney function (45% for the right kidney and 55% for the left). Furthermore, the child was followed regularly with renal ultrasound that revealed a stationary course of pelvic dilation within 15–20 mm without any clinical manifestation.

At the age of 15 years, the patient presented to our institution for right flank pain, without urinary symptoms. Renal ultrasound showed bilateral kidney stones (8 to 9 mm). A CT-scan of the abdomen showed a moderately dilated right pelvis of 19 mm containing three stones, in addition to two stones in a nondilated left renal pelvis

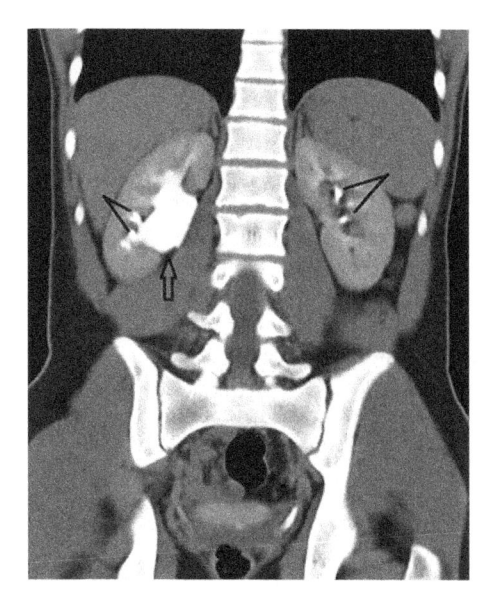

FIGURE 1: CT-scan of the abdomen and pelvis demonstrating moderately dilated right renal pelvis of 19 mm (headed arrow) and bilateral renal stones (dashes).

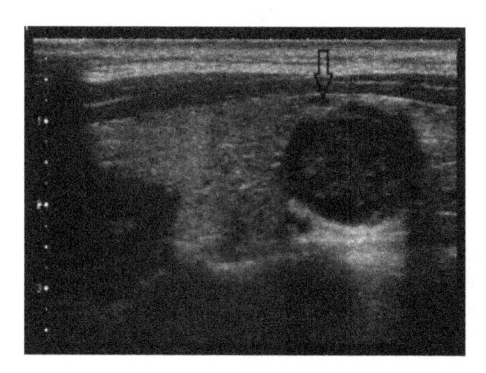

FIGURE 2: Ultrasound neck showing a well-defined hypoechoic parathyroid adenoma (arrow).

(Figure 1). There was also a lytic lesion in the right iliac bone.

Blood investigation showed a normal serum creatinine level of 60 μmol/L, elevated calcium level of 3.16 mmol/L (N = 2.20–2.50), and moderately decreased phosphorus level of 0.85 mmol/L (N = 0.97–1.81). Parathyroid hormone (PTH) was checked and revealed elevated level of 305 ng/L (N = 8–49). Moreover, the patient had a neck ultrasound showing multiple parathyroid adenomas (Figure 2) responsible for hyperparathyroidism leading to hypercalcemia and secondary bone lesions. The urine calcium level was also elevated with calcium/creatinine ratio of 1.6 mmol/mmol (N = 0.16–0.50). Genetic counseling found a mutation in CDC73 (HRPT2).

The patient had a parathyroidectomy that led to normalization of the calcium level within 72 hours (2.6 mmol/L). PTH level decreased to its normal value (45 ng/L) after one week of the surgery. His renal colic attacks became less frequent. Follow-up renal ultrasound three months later noted a decrease in the number of kidney stones and complete spontaneous disappearance of stones at the end of the first year.

MAG-3 scintigraphy revealed a rapid contrast evacuation with normal kidney function. Patient was not operated on for the UPJO and renal ultrasound on one-year follow-up showed normal findings.

3. Discussion

Congenital ureteropelvic junction obstruction is the most common cause of upper urinary tract obstruction in children. By definition, the diagnosis of UPJO signifies functionally impaired transport of urine from the renal pelvis into the ureter. Because the increased renal pelvic pressure from obstruction may lead to progressive renal injury and impairment, correct diagnosis is clinically important. The impairment may be primary or secondary in nature. This, along with the chronicity and severity of the condition, dictates the course of management [7, 8].

Routine antenatal ultrasonography readily recognizes the presence of hydronephrosis and this has led to earlier detection of UPJO [9]. Although the majority of cases are discovered in the neonatal period, many are still diagnosed later in life manifested with hematuria, kidney stones, or abdominal discomfort. The outcome usually is either improvement in the dilatation after birth or worsening with time which eventually may require surgical intervention [10].

Nuclear medicine scanning may be used to quantitatively assess the differential renal function. It has become a primary study for defining ureteropelvic junction obstruction (UPJO) and establishing the decision for surgery [11]. In our case, MAG3 noted bilateral rapid evacuation without abnormal findings giving us some advantage to avoid surgery for the right UPJO and safely monitor the period after parathyroidectomy until the complete dissolution of all kidney stones.

Parathyroid adenoma, which is responsible for primary hyperparathyroidism (PHPT) rarely, occurs in children with an estimated incidence of 2–5 cases per 100,000 of population. PHPT is most often sporadic but may also be seen with hyperplasia of the glands in patients with multiple endocrine neoplasia (MEN) I. Most of the patients with PHPT present with bone diseases mainly fractures or rickets [12, 13]. Although primary hyperparathyroidism is rare in children, presence of urolithiasis or any symptoms suggestive of urolithiasis such as hematuria in this age group should trigger the investigation and exclusion of parathyroid abnormalities [14], taking into account the fact that 50% of patients who are younger than 30 years and diagnosed with primary hyperparathyroidism have urolithiasis [15]. In addition, another study has concluded that 6% of children with urolithiasis had primary hyperparathyroidism [16].

In a view of UPJO and concurrent renal calculi in pediatrics patients, a long-term follow-up study has found that an identifiable metabolic etiology was found in the majority of cases and it suggested that the presence of metabolic abnormality significantly predisposes to recurrent nonstruvite renal lithiasis in such cases [17]. Patients with congenital UPJO and associated nephrolithiasis are found to have higher rate of metabolic abnormalities compared to those with nephrolithiasis not associated with UPJO. This finding supports the fact that urinary stasis alone cannot explain stone formation in patients with UPJO, prompting the need for further metabolic screening and investigations in cases of UPJO and nephrolithiasis [18]. The role of metabolic risk factors in the formation of renal calculi should be investigated, even in the picture of congenital UPJO; and the point of abnormal urinary biochemistry adding a role in the high incidence of nephrolithiasis in children with urinary tract anomalies should prompt a screening of urinary and serum biochemistry in these patients [19].

The incidence of renal calculi in patients with ureteropelvic junction obstruction (UPJO) is nearly 20% [17]. Soylu et al. suggest that it may be due to pelvic dilatation and urine stasis [20]. Our patient remained asymptomatic with his UPJO for a period of fourteen years, before manifesting with a right flank pain due to kidney stones that aggravated the underlying pelvic dilation. The presence of nephrolithiasis directed us towards metabolic work-up that later revealed hypercalcemia which was caused by a parathyroid adenoma leading to PHPT.

A linkage between hyperparathyroidism-jaw tumor syndrome (HPT-JT), which is linked to a chromosomal mutation in HRPT2, and renal diseases was published in a previous study, where two families with HPT-JT syndrome were followed and found to have adult renal hamartomas and cystic kidney disease as prominent features; and this possibly represented a new phenotypic variant of the HPT-JT syndrome. In one of the families, renal lesions were even more prominent, as five out of six individuals had renal lesions, while hyperparathyroidism was found in four individuals and jaw tumor was found in two individuals only [21]. What is interesting about our case is that symptomatic kidney stones led to the diagnosis of PHPT which was secondary to a mutation in CDC73 (HRPT2). PHPT can potentially be the only or the main cause of kidney stones since our patient had bilateral kidney stones despite having only unilateral right dilated pelvis. However, it is possible that UPJO is a second triggering factor that accelerated the formation of kidney stones and other related symptoms.

We believe that association of UPJO and PHPT is a rare coincidence that can be linked as a congenital anomaly and genetic mutation, role to be more investigated. Careful work-up of children with ureteropelvic junction obstruction who develop unilateral or bilateral urolithiasis is recommended to exclude a concomitant metabolic disease. Presence of kidney stones in UPJO is not always an indication for surgery mainly in the absence of renal function impairment. Treatment of the primary cause and close monitoring can lead to complete dissolution of kidney stones.

References

[1] S. A. Koff and K. H. Mutabagani, "Anomalies of the kidney," in *Adult and Pediatric Urology*, J. Y. Gillenwater, J. T. Grayhack, S. S. Howards, and M. E. Mitchell, Eds., p. 2129, Lippincott Williams and Wilkins, Philadelphia, Pa, USA, 4th edition, 2002.

[2] L. Morin, M. Cendron, T. M. Crombleholme, S. H. Garmel, G. T. Klauber, and M. E. D'Alton, "Minimal hydronephrosis in the fetus: Clinical significance and implications for management," *The Journal of Urology*, vol. 155, no. 6, pp. 2047–2049, 1996.

[3] H. P. Duong, A. Piepsz, F. Collier et al., "Predicting the clinical outcome of antenatally detected unilateral pelviureteric junction stenosis," *Urology*, vol. 82, no. 3, pp. 691–696, 2013.

[4] J. E. Heinlen, C. S. Manatt, B. C. Bright, B. P. Kropp, J. B. Campbell, and D. Frimberger, "Operative Versus Nonoperative Management of Ureteropelvic Junction Obstruction in Children," *Urology*, vol. 73, no. 3, pp. 521–525, 2009.

[5] S. A. Koff, "Postnatal management of antenatal hydronephrosis using an observational approach," *Urology*, vol. 55, no. 5, pp. 609–611, 2000.

[6] S. Josephson and A. P. Dickson, "Antenatally detected pelviureteric junction obstruction: Concerns about conservative management (multiple letters)," *BJU International*, vol. 85, no. 7, p. 973, 2000.

[7] Gomella L. G., *The 5-Minute Urology Consult*, Lippincott Williams & Wilkins, Philadelphia, Pa, USA, 2000.

[8] S. Halachmi and G. Pillar, "Congenital urological anomalies diagnosed in adulthood - Management considerations," *Journal of Pediatric Urology*, vol. 4, no. 1, pp. 2–7, 2008.

[9] D. B. Liu, W. R. Armstrong, and M. Maizels, "Hydronephrosis: Prenatal and Postnatal Evaluation and Management," *Clinics in Perinatology*, vol. 41, no. 3, pp. 661–678, 2014.

[10] N. Aksu, O. Yavaşcan, M. Kangin et al., "Postnatal management of infants with antenatally detected hydronephrosis," *Pediatric Nephrology*, vol. 20, no. 9, pp. 1253–1259, 2005.

[11] P. O. Kiratli, D. Orhan, G. K. Gedik, and S. Tekgul, "Relation between radionuclide imaging and pathologic findings of ureteropelvic junction obstruction in neonatal hydronephrosis," *Scandinavian Journal of Urology*, vol. 42, no. 3, pp. 249–256, 2008.

[12] J. S. Lee, B. H. Lau, M. L. Yeh, and C. C. Lee, "Urolithiasis and primary parathyroid adenoma: report of one case," *Acta Paediatr Taiwan*, vol. 44, pp. 372–374, 2003.

[13] R. W. Gasser, "Clinical aspects of primary hyperparathyroidism: Clinical manifestations, diagnosis, and therapy," *Wiener Medizinische Wochenschrift*, vol. 163, no. 17-18, pp. 397–402, 2013.

[14] Y. Ohata, T. Yamamoto, Y. Kitai et al., "A case of primary hyperparathyroidism in childhood found by a chance hematuria," *Clinical Pediatric Endocrinology*, vol. 16, no. 1, pp. 11–16, 2007.

[15] K. Cupisti, A. Raffel, C. Dotzenrath, M. Krausch, H.-D. Röher, and K.-M. Schulte, "Primary hyperparathyroidism in the young age group: Particularities of diagnostic and therapeutic schemes," *World Journal of Surgery*, vol. 28, no. 11, pp. 1153–1156, 2004.

[16] R. S. Malek and P. P. Kelalis, "Urologic Manifestations of Hyperparathyroidism in Childhood," *The Journal of Urology*, vol. 115, no. 6, pp. 717–719, 1976.

[17] D. A. Husmann, D. S. Milliner, and J. W. Segura, "Ureteropelvic junction obstruction with concurrent renal pelvic calculi in the pediatric patient: A long-term followup," *The Journal of Urology*, vol. 156, no. 2, pp. 741–743, 1996.

[18] S. F. Matin and S. B. Streem, "Metabolic risk factors in patients with ureteropelvic junction obstruction and renal calculi," *The Journal of Urology*, vol. 163, no. 6, pp. 1676–1678, 2000.

[19] A. Tekin, S. Tekgul, N. Atsu, A. Ergen, and S. Kendi, "Ureteropelvic junction obstruction and coexisting renal calculi in children: Role of metabolic abnormalities," *Urology*, vol. 57, no. 3, pp. 542–545, 2001.

[20] A. Soylu, Y. M. Uğraş, A. Güneş, and C. Baydinç, "Bilateral kidney stones with ureteropelvic junction obstruction," *Nature Clinical Practice Urology*, vol. 2, no. 7, pp. 351–354, 2005.

[21] B. T. Teh, F. Farnebo, U. Kristoffersson et al., "Autosomal dominant primary hyperparathyroidism and jaw tumor syndrome associated with renal hamartomas and cystic kidney disease: linkage to 1q21-q32 and loss of the wild type allele in renal hamartomas," *The Journal of Clinical Endocrinology & Metabolism*, vol. 81, no. 12, pp. 4204–4211, 1996.

Permissions

All chapters in this book were first published in CRN, by Hindawi Publishing Corporation; hereby published with permission under the Creative Commons Attribution License or equivalent. Every chapter published in this book has been scrutinized by our experts. Their significance has been extensively debated. The topics covered herein carry significant findings which will fuel the growth of the discipline. They may even be implemented as practical applications or may be referred to as a beginning point for another development.

The contributors of this book come from diverse backgrounds, making this book a truly international effort. This book will bring forth new frontiers with its revolutionizing research information and detailed analysis of the nascent developments around the world.

We would like to thank all the contributing authors for lending their expertise to make the book truly unique. They have played a crucial role in the development of this book. Without their invaluable contributions this book wouldn't have been possible. They have made vital efforts to compile up to date information on the varied aspects of this subject to make this book a valuable addition to the collection of many professionals and students.

This book was conceptualized with the vision of imparting up-to-date information and advanced data in this field. To ensure the same, a matchless editorial board was set up. Every individual on the board went through rigorous rounds of assessment to prove their worth. After which they invested a large part of their time researching and compiling the most relevant data for our readers.

The editorial board has been involved in producing this book since its inception. They have spent rigorous hours researching and exploring the diverse topics which have resulted in the successful publishing of this book. They have passed on their knowledge of decades through this book. To expedite this challenging task, the publisher supported the team at every step. A small team of assistant editors was also appointed to further simplify the editing procedure and attain best results for the readers.

Apart from the editorial board, the designing team has also invested a significant amount of their time in understanding the subject and creating the most relevant covers. They scrutinized every image to scout for the most suitable representation of the subject and create an appropriate cover for the book.

The publishing team has been an ardent support to the editorial, designing and production team. Their endless efforts to recruit the best for this project, has resulted in the accomplishment of this book. They are a veteran in the field of academics and their pool of knowledge is as vast as their experience in printing. Their expertise and guidance has proved useful at every step. Their uncompromising quality standards have made this book an exceptional effort. Their encouragement from time to time has been an inspiration for everyone.

The publisher and the editorial board hope that this book will prove to be a valuable piece of knowledge for researchers, students, practitioners and scholars across the globe.

List of Contributors

Homare Shimohata, Kentaro Ohgi, Hiroshi Maruyama, Yasunori Miyamoto, Mamiko Takayashu, Kouichi Hirayama and Masaki Kobayashi
Department of Nephrology, Tokyo Medical University Ibaraki Medical Center, Ibaraki, Japan

Michael Babigumira, Sherry Werner and Wajeh Qunibi
Division of Nephrology, University of Texas Health Science Center at San Antonio, 7703 Floyd Curl Drive, MSC 7882, San Antonio, TX 78229, USA

Benjamin Huang
San Antonio Uniformed Services Health Education Consortium, San Antonio, TX, USA

Klaus Stahl, Anke Schwarz, A. D. Wagner, Hermann Haller and Mario Schiffer
Department of Nephrology, Hannover Medical School, Carl-Neuberg-Strasse 1, 30625 Hannover, Germany

Michelle Duong
Department of Hospital Pharmacy, Hannover Medical School, Carl-Neuberg-Strasse 1, 30625 Hannover, Germany

Roland Jacobs
Department of Clinical Immunology and Rheumatology, Hannover Medical School, Hannover, Germany

Ahmet Karakurt
Department of Cardiology, Faculty of Medicine, Kafkas University, Kars, Turkey

Arnaud Devresse and Nada Kanaan
Division of Nephrology, Cliniques Universitaires Saint-Luc, Université Catholique de Louvain, Brussels, Belgium

Martine de Meyer
Division of Abdominal Surgery and Transplantation, Cliniques Universitaires Saint-Luc, Université Catholique de Louvain, Brussels, Belgium

Selda Aydin
Division of Pathology, Cliniques Universitaires Saint-Luc, Université Catholique de Louvain, Brussels, Belgium

Karin Dahan
Division of Nephrology, Cliniques Universitaires Saint-Luc, Université Catholique de Louvain, Brussels, Belgium
Division of Human Genetics, Cliniques Universitaires Saint-Luc, Université Catholique de Louvain, Brussels, Belgium
Center of Human Genetics, Institut de Pathologie et de Génétique, Gosselies, Belgium

H. Trimarchi, M. Paulero, M. Forrester, F. Lombi, V. Pomeranz, R. Iriarte, T. Rengel and I. Gonzalez-Hoyos
Nephrology, Hospital Británico de Buenos Aires, Buenos Aires, Argentina

R. Canzonieri, A. Schiel, A. Stern and A. Muryan
Biochemistry, Hospital Británico de Buenos Aires, Buenos Aires, Argentina

A. Iotti and E. Zotta
Pathology Services, Hospital Británico de Buenos Aires, Buenos Aires, Argentina

C. Costales-Collaguazo
IFIBIO Houssay-UBA CONICET, Facultad de Medicina, Universidad de Buenos Aires, Argentina

Dimitrios Patoulias, Theodoros Michailidis and Petros Keryttopoulos
Department of Internal Medicine, General Hospital of Veria, Veria, Greece

Thomas Papatolios and Rafael Papadopoulos,
Department of Nephrology, General Hospital of Veria, Veria, Greece

Vipuj Shah and Mary Hammes
Department of Medicine, Section of Nephrology, University of Chicago, Chicago, IL, USA

Rakesh Navuluri
Department of Interventional Radiology, University of Chicago, Chicago, IL, USA

Yolanda Becker
Department of Transplant Surgery, University of Chicago, Chicago, IL, USA

Chia Wei Teoh
Division of Nephrology, The Hospital for Sick Children, Toronto, ON, Canada
Department of Paediatric Nephrology and Transplantation, The Children's University Hospital, Temple Street, Dublin 1, Ireland
Department of Paediatrics, University of Toronto, Toronto, ON, Canada

Kathleen Mary Gorman, Niamh Marie Dolan, Michael Riordan and Atif Awan
Department of Paediatric Nephrology and Transplantation, The Children's University Hospital, Temple Street, Dublin 1, Ireland

Bryan Lynch
Department of Neurology, The Children's University Hospital, Temple Street, Dublin 1, Ireland

Timothy H. J. Goodship
Institute of Genetic Medicine, Newcastle University, International Centre for Life, Central Parkway, Newcastle upon Tyne, UK

Mary Waldron
Department of Paediatric Nephrology, Our Lady's Children's Hospital, Crumlin, Dublin 12., Ireland

Gunilla Einecke, Nils Hanke, Hermann Haller and Anke Schwarz
Department of Nephrology and Hypertension, Hannover Medical School, Hannover, Germany

Jan Hinrich Bräsen
Department of Pathology, Hannover Medical School, Hannover, Germany

Vimal Master Sankar Raj, Diana Warnecke, and Sarah Elhadi
Department of Pediatric Nephrology, University of Illinois College of Medicine at Peoria, Peoria, IL, USA

Julia Roberts
Department of Pediatrics, University of Illinois College of Medicine at Peoria, Peoria, IL, USA

Fabio Solis-Jimenez
Internal Medicine Service, General Hospital of Mexico "Dr. Eduardo Liceaga", Mexico City, Mexico

Hector Hinojosa-Heredia and Luis García-Covarrubias
Transplant Service, General Hospital of Mexico "Dr. Eduardo Liceaga", Mexico City, Mexico

Virgilia Soto-Abraham
Pathological Anatomy Service, General Hospital of Mexico "Dr. Eduardo Liceaga", Mexico City, Mexico

Rafael Valdez-Ortiz
Nephrology Service, General Hospital of Mexico "Dr. Eduardo Liceaga", Mexico City, Mexico

Meral Hassan Abualjadayel and Maysaa Adnan Banjari,
King Abdulaziz University, Jeddah, Saudi Arabia

Osama Y. Safdar and Sherif El Desoky
Center of Excellence in Pediatric Nephrology, King Abdulaziz University, Jeddah, Saudi Arabia

Ghadeer A. Mokhtar
Pathology Department, King Abdulaziz University, Jeddah, Saudi Arabia

Raed A. Azhar
Urology Department, King Abdulaziz University, Jeddah, Saudi Arabia

Dennis Narcisse
University of Tennessee College of Medicine, Memphis, TN, USA

Manyoo Agarwal and Aneel Kumar
Department of Internal Medicine, University of Tennessee Health Science Center, Memphis, TN, USA

Joshua M. Inglis
Department of General Medicine, Royal Adelaide Hospital, Adelaide, SA, Australia

George Passaris
Department of Renal Medicine, Flinders Medical Centre, Adelaide, SA, Australia

Jeffrey A. Barbara, Rajiv Juneja, Caroline Milton and Jordan Y. Z. Li
Department of Renal Medicine, Flinders Medical Centre, Adelaide, SA, Australia
School of Medicine, Flinders University, Adelaide, SA, Australia

Thaofiq Ijaiya, Sandhya Manohar and Kameswari Lakshmi
Department of Medicine, Montefiore New Rochelle Hospital, Albert Einstein College of Medicine, New Rochelle, NY, USA

List of Contributors

Rishi Raj and Aasems Jacob
University of Kentucky, Lexington, KY 40536, USA

Ajay Venkatanarayan, Mohankumar Doraiswamy and Manjula Ashok
Monmouth Medical Center, Long Branch, NJ 07740, USA

Phuong-Chi Pham, Pavani Reddy, Shaker Qaqish and Ashvin Kamath
Olive View-UCLA Medical Center, Division of Nephrology and Hypertension, Sylmar, CA 91342, USA

Johana Rodriguez, David Bolos and Martina Zalom
Olive View-UCLAMedical Center,Division of Hematology and Oncology, Sylmar, CA 91342, USA

Phuong-Thu Pham
Ronald Reagan UCLA Medical Center, Kidney Transplant, Los Angeles, CA 90095, USA

Maite Hurtado Uriarte
Nephrologist, University Hospital San Rafael, RTS Baxter, Bogota, Colombia

Carolina Larrarte
Nephrologist, University Hospital Militar, RTS Baxter, Bogota, Colombia

Laura Bravo Rey
Medical student, Javeriana University, Bogota, Colombia

Kevin T. Barton
Division of Pediatric Nephrology, Washington University in St. Louis School of Medicine, St. Louis, MO, USA

Aadil Kakajiwala
Division of Pediatric Nephrology, Washington University in St. Louis School of Medicine, St. Louis, MO, USA
Divisions of Nephrology, The Children's Hospital of Philadelphia, Philadelphia, PA, USA
Perelman School of Medicine,The University of Pennsylvania, Philadelphia, PA, USA

Elisha Rampolla and Christine Breen
Divisions of Nephrology, The Children's Hospital of Philadelphia, Philadelphia, PA, USA

Madhura Pradhan
Divisions of Nephrology, The Children's Hospital of Philadelphia, Philadelphia, PA, USA
Perelman School of Medicine, The University of Pennsylvania, Philadelphia, PA, USA

Ryan Jalleh and Richard Le Leu
Central and Northern Adelaide Renal and Transplantation Service, Royal Adelaide Hospital, Adelaide, South Australia, Australia

Gopal Basu and Shilpanjali Jesudason
Central and Northern Adelaide Renal and Transplantation Service, Royal Adelaide Hospital, Adelaide, South Australia, Australia
Department of Medicine, University of Adelaide, South Australia, Australia

Natacha Rodrigues, Fernando Caeiro, Alice Santana and Teresa Mendes
Hemodialysis Unit Diaverum Cruz Vermelha Portuguesa, Lisbon, Portugal

Leonor Lopes
Department of Dermatology, Centro Hospitalar Lisboa Norte, Lisbon, Portugal

Donlawat Saengpanit and Pongpratch Puapatanakul
Division of Nephrology, Department of Medicine, Faculty of Medicine, Chulalongkorn University, Bangkok, Thailand

Piyaporn Towannang
CAPD Excellent Center, King Chulalongkorn Memorial Hospital, Bangkok, Thailand

Talerngsak Kanjanabuch
Division of Nephrology, Department of Medicine, Faculty of Medicine, Chulalongkorn University, Bangkok, Thailand
CAPD Excellent Center, King Chulalongkorn Memorial Hospital, Bangkok, Thailand
Kidney and Metabolic Research Unit, Department of Medicine, Faculty of Medicine, Chulalongkorn University, Bangkok, Thailand

Chikayuki Morimoto, Risa Iino, Kei Taniguchi, Yosuke Kawamorita, Shinichiro Asakawa, Daigo Toyoki, Shinako Miyano, Wataru Fujii, Tatsuru Ota, Shigeru Shibata and Shunya Uchida
Department of Internal Medicine, Teikyo University School of Medicine, Itabashi-ku, Tokyo, Japan

Yoshihide Fujigaki
Department of Internal Medicine, Teikyo University School of Medicine, Itabashi-ku, Tokyo, Japan
Central Laboratory, Teikyo University School of Medicine, Itabashi-ku, Tokyo, Japan

Rishi Kora
Mount Carmel West Hospital, Columbus, OH, USA

Sergey V. Brodsky, Tibor Nadasdy and Anjali A. Satoskar
Ohio State UniversityWexner Medical Center, Columbus, OH, USA

Dean Agra
Columbus Nephrology, Columbus, OH, USA

Muhammad Siddique Khurram, Ahmed Alrajjal, Warda Ibrar, Jacob Edens, Umer Sheikh, Ameer Hamza and Hong Qu
St. John Hospital andMedical Center,Detroit,MI, USA

Caprice Cadacio, Ruchika Bhasin, Anita Kamarzarian and Phuong-Chi Pham
Olive View-UCLA Medical Center, 14445 Olive View Drive, 2B-182, Sylmar, CA 91342, USA

Phuong-Thu Pham
Ronald Reagan UCLA Medical Center, 200 Medical Plaza, Los Angeles, CA 90095, USA

Mazen Toushan Hassan D. Kanaan, Limin Yu, Mitual B. Amin and Ping L. Zhang,
Division of Anatomic Pathology, Department of Pathology, Beaumont Health, Royal Oak, MI, USA

Ashka Atodaria, Stephen D. Lynch and Mamon Tahhan
Department of Internal Medicine, Beaumont Health, Royal Oak, MI, USA

Paul S. Kellerman and Abhishek Swami
Division of Nephrology, Department of Internal Medicine, Beaumont Health, Royal Oak, MI, USA

Ronak A. Patel, Hayden P. Baker and Sara B. Smith
College of Medicine, University of Illinois at Chicago, Chicago, IL, USA

Nobuo Tsuboi, Naoko Nakaosa, Kotaro Haruhara, Go Kanzaki, Kentaro Koike, Akihiro Shimizu, Akira Fukui, Hideo Okonogi, Yoichi Miyazaki, Tetsuya Kawamura, Makoto Ogura and Takashi Yokoo
Division of Nephrology and Hypertension, Department of Internal Medicine, The Jikei University School of Medicine, Tokyo, Japan

Yusuke Okabayashi
Division of Nephrology and Hypertension, Department of Internal Medicine, The Jikei University School of Medicine, Tokyo, Japan
Department of Analytic Human Pathology, Nippon Medical School, Tokyo, Japan

Akira Shimizu
Department of Analytic Human Pathology, Nippon Medical School, Tokyo, Japan

Sukesh Manthri, Sindhura Bandaru and Tamer Hudali
Southern Illinois University, Springfield, IL, USA

Anthony Chang
The University of Chicago Medicine, Chicago, IL, USA

Kalyana C. Janga, Sheldon Greenberg, Phone Oo and Umair Ahmed
Department of Nephrology, Maimonides Medical Center, Brooklyn, NY, USA

Kavita Sharma
Department of Infectious Diseases, Maimonides Medical Center, Brooklyn, NY, USA

RafaB Donderski, Magdalena Grajewska, Beata Sulikowska and Jacek Manitius
Department of Nephrology, Hypertension and Internal Medicine, Ludwik Rydygier Collegium Medicum in Bydgoszcz,
Nicolaus Copernicus University in Toruń, Poland

Agnieszka Mikucka and Eugenia Gospodarek-Komkowska
Department of Microbiology, Ludwik Rydygier Collegium Medicum in Bydgoszcz, Nicolaus Copernicus University in Toruń, Poland

List of Contributors

Michelle Lieberman Lubetzky and Stuart Greenstein
Montefiore Einstein Center for Transplantation, Montefiore Medical Center, Albert Einstein College of Medicine, Bronx, NY, USA

Steve Omoruyi Obanor
Montefiore Einstein Center for Transplantation, Montefiore Medical Center, Albert Einstein College of Medicine, Bronx, NY, USA
Department of Internal Medicine, Maimonides Medical Center, Brooklyn, NY, USA

Michelle Gruttadauria and Kayla Applebaum,
Albert Einstein College of Medicine, Bronx, NY, USA

Mohammad Eskandari
Department of Pathology, Montefiore Medical Center, Albert Einstein College of Medicine, Bronx, NY, USA

H. Trimarchi, M. Paulero, T. Rengel, I. González-Hoyos, M. Forrester, F. Lombi, V. Pomeranz and R. Iriarte
Nephrology Service, Hospital Brit'anico de Buenos Aires, Buenos Aires, Argentina

A. Iotti
Pathology Service, Hospital Brit'anico de Buenos Aires, Buenos Aires, Argentina

Ikuyo Narita, Michiko Shimada, Reiichi Murakami, Takeshi Fujita and Hirofumi Tomita
Department of Cardiology and Nephrology, Hirosaki University Graduate School of Medicine, Hirosaki, Japan

Norio Nakamura
Community Medicine, Hirosaki University Graduate School of Medicine, Hirosaki, Japan

Wakako Fukuda,
Murakami Shinmachi Hospital, Aomori, Japan

Joseph Vercellone, Lisa Cohen, Saima Mansuri and Paul S. Kellerman
Department of Internal Medicine, Oakland University William Beaumont School of Medicine, Royal Oak, MI, USA

Ping L. Zhang,
Department of Pathology, Oakland University William Beaumont School of Medicine, Royal Oak, MI, USA

Kalyana C. Janga and Sheldon Greenberg,
Department of Nephrology, Maimonides Medical Center, Brooklyn, NY, USA

Ankur Sinha
Department of Internal Medicine, Maimonides Medical Center, Brooklyn, NY, USA

Kavita Sharma
Department of Infectious Diseases, Maimonides Medical Center, Brooklyn, NY, USA

Arun Sedhain
Nephrology Unit, Department of Medicine, Chitwan Medical College, Bharatpur, Chitwan, Nepal

Kiran Acharya and Amir Khan
Department of Medicine, Chitwan Medical College, Bharatpur, Chitwan, Nepal

Alok Sharma
Department of Renal Pathology and ElectronMicroscopy, National Reference Laboratory, Dr. Lal Pathlabs Ltd, New Delhi, India

Shital Adhikari
Pulmonology and Critical Care Unit, Department of Medicine, Chitwan Medical College, Bharatpur, Chitwan, Nepal

Fernando Perretta
Servicio de Terapia Intensiva del Hospital Dr. Enrique Erill de Escobar, Provincia de Buenos Aires, Argentina
GINEF Argentina (Grupo de Investigaci'on Nefrol'ogica en la Enfermedad de Fabry), Buenos Aires, Argentina

Norberto Antongiovanni
GINEF Argentina (Grupo de Investigaci'on Nefrol'ogica en la Enfermedad de Fabry), Buenos Aires, Argentina
Centro de Infusi'on y Estudio de Enfermedades Lisosomales del Instituto de Nefrolog'ıa Cl'ınica Pergamino, Provincia de Buenos Aires, Argentina

Sebastián Jaurretche
GINEF Argentina (Grupo de Investigacíon Nefrológica en la Enfermedad de Fabry), Buenos Aires, Argentina
Centro de Neurociencias Los Manantiales, Grupo Gamma Rosario, Provincia de Santa Fe, Argentina
Cátedra de Biofísica y Fisiología, Instituto Universitario Italiano de Rosario, Provincia de Santa Fe, Argentina

Salah Termos and Majd AlKabbani
Hepatobiliary and Transplant Unit, Department of Surgery, Al-Amiri Hospital, Kuwait City, Kuwait

Tim Ulinski, Henri Kotobi and Francois Chalard
Pediatric Nephrology, Armand Trousseau Hospital, APHP, Paris, France

Bilal Aoun
Pediatric Nephrology, Armand Trousseau Hospital, APHP, Paris, France
Division of Pediatric Nephrology, Department of Pediatrics, American University of Beirut, Beirut, Lebanon

Index

A

Abmr, 47-51

Achromobacter Xylosoxidans, 159, 162

Acute Myocardial Infarction, 23, 25

Angiomyolipoma, 66-67

Anti-gbm Disease, 54, 58, 115-118

Arteriovenous Fistula, 38, 41-42, 183

Atorvastatin, 23, 34-37, 80

Atypical Haemolytic Uremic Syndrome, 26, 29

B

Bcf, 38-40

Benazepril, 87-89

Bicarbonate Reabsorption, 70

Bilateral Testicular Infarction, 136

Bnp, 138, 156

C

Cerebrospinal Fluid (CSF), 6, 165

Cetuximab, 150-153

Chest X-ray, 53-54, 76, 81, 112, 116, 126, 137, 156

Chronic Kidney Disease, 10, 33-34, 67, 95, 97, 99-101, 106, 111, 141, 157, 159, 169-171, 195

Cisplatin, 87-90, 125-129

Clostridium Difficile, 17, 73, 75

Corticosteroids, 33, 58, 115, 117, 147-148

Creatinine, 1-3, 6-7, 10-11, 16-17, 19-21, 26-27, 30-33, 35, 44, 48, 54, 58, 70, 73, 75, 77, 81, 88, 106, 112, 116, 126, 137-138, 146, 160, 166, 170, 176, 178, 189, 197

Crescentic Glomerulonephritis, 54, 58, 152, 177, 179

D

De Novo Thrombotic Microangiopathy (TMA), 26

Deferoxamine, 107-109

Denosumab, 100-101, 105-106

Doppler Ultrasound, 60-62

E

Eculizumab, 26-29, 43-46, 50, 73-75, 91, 93-94, 152-153

End-stage Renal Disease, 3, 26, 30, 36, 38-39, 43, 107, 109, 148, 186

Escitalopram, 80-82, 85-86

Esrd Patients, 38, 41, 107-108, 111

Ethylene Glycol Intoxication, 173-174

F

Ferric Carboxymaltose, 107-109

Fusidic Acid, 34-37

G

Glomerular Capillary, 1-3, 116-117, 127, 139, 146, 178

Glomerulonephritis, 1-6, 10, 12-16, 30, 33, 48, 53-54, 58-59, 112, 117-118, 125, 136-137, 140, 145-153, 157, 159, 161, 177-180, 190

Goodpasture's Syndrome (GPS), 53

H

Hemodialysis, 2, 17, 38-42, 54, 63-64, 95, 97, 110-111, 114-118, 123, 126, 141-144, 150-152, 157, 160-161, 170, 173-176, 181-183, 185-186

Hepatic Glomerulosclerosis, 145, 148

Hydrocephalus, 6, 10-14

Hyperkalemic, 70, 98-99

Hypocalcemia, 54, 95-98, 106, 130, 132, 152

Hyponatremia, 76-82, 85-86, 88, 130, 132, 134-135

I

Iga Nephropathy, 30-33, 122, 145, 148-149, 152, 161

Iga Vasculitis, 136, 140

Immunosuppression, 20, 28, 32-33, 47-51, 55, 58, 117-119, 163-167

K

Kidney Transplantation, 26-29, 48, 50, 52, 60, 64, 163

M

Metabolic Acidosis, 49, 54, 72, 98, 112, 116, 121, 134, 157, 173-175, 188-189, 191

Metabolic Alkalosis, 95, 97-99, 135

Monoclonal Igg Deposition, 1-2

Mucin-1 Gene, 169-170

N

Nephrogenic Diabetes Insipidus, 87-88

Nephropathy, 15, 18, 20-22, 30-33, 38, 65, 112, 122, 125-129, 145, 148-149, 152, 161-162, 181, 190, 192-195

Nephrotic Syndrome, 13, 15-17, 20-22, 30, 95, 140, 145-148, 157, 169

Nephrotoxicity, 90, 125, 127-129, 142-143, 150

Nontuberculous Mycobacterial Infections, 120

O
Oncocytomas, 66-69
Osteoporosis, 100-101, 105-106

P
Peritoneal Dialysis, 15, 19, 55, 60-61, 111, 114, 159, 162, 183, 185
Peritoneal Fluid, 15, 19-21, 160-161
Plasmapheresis, 47, 50-51, 54-55, 58, 74, 115-119
Podocyturia, 30-33, 194
Porphyria Cutanea Tarda, 107, 109-110
Posttransplant Lymphoproliferative Disorder, 163, 165, 168
Proteinuria, 1-2, 6-7, 10-11, 15-17, 19-21, 24, 30-33, 44, 47-48, 55, 57-58, 88, 112, 116, 121, 126-127, 145, 147, 150-152, 157, 166, 169-171, 188-190, 192-194

R
Renal Artery Thromboembolism (RATE), 23
Renal Cell Carcinoma, 66, 68-69, 164, 166, 168
Renal Replacement Therapy (RRT), 111, 159
Renal Transplant Biopsy, 47, 49
Renal Tubular Acidosis (RTA), 70, 188
Resin Therapy, 95, 98
Rhabdomyolysis, 34-37, 72, 112, 154-158, 162
Rifampicin, 112, 120, 123-124
Rituximab, 15-22, 47-52, 54, 58, 163, 166-168

S
Scleroderma Renal Crisis, 91, 94
Selective Serotonin Reuptake Inhibitors, 80, 85
Shunt Nephritis, 6, 8-14
Siadh, 78, 80-82, 85-88
Slow-infusion Thrombolytic Therapy, 23
Spermatic Cords, 136, 140
Sticky Platelet Syndrome, 60, 62, 64-65
Streptococcus Suis, 159, 162

T
Testicular Lymphoma, 163, 166-167
Thrombocytopaenia, 73, 75
Thrombosis, 23-25, 40, 42, 60-61, 63-65, 137, 139
Thrombotic Microangiopathy (TMA), 26-27, 93, 152
Thrombotic Thrombocytopenic Purpura, 91-92
Tobramycin, 141-144

V
Vancomycin, 6-7, 10-11, 39, 74-75, 137, 141-144, 184-186
Ventriculoperitoneal (Vp) Shunt, 6

CPSIA information can be obtained
at www.ICGtesting.com
Printed in the USA
BVHW012152160619
551142BV00003B/17/P